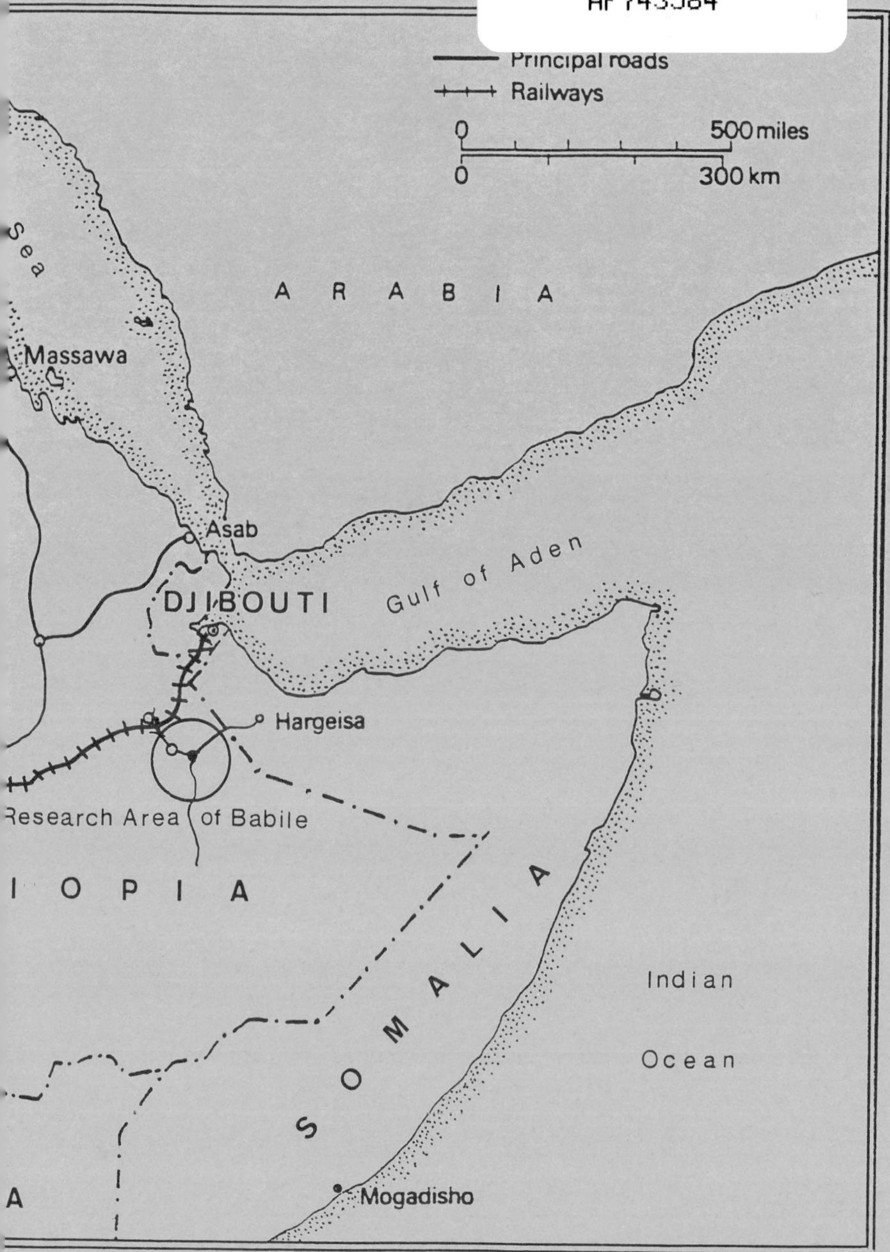
Principal roads
Railways
0
500 miles
0
300 km
Sea
ARABIA
Massawa
Asab
DJIBOUTI
Gulf of Aden
Hargeisa
Research Area of Babile
IOPIA
SOMALIA
Indian Ocean
A
Mogadisho

# Plural Medical Systems in the Horn of Africa

Monographs from the African Studies Centre,
Leiden

# Plural Medical Systems in the Horn of Africa

*The Legacy of 'Sheikh' Hippocrates*

Leendert Jan Slikkerveer

KPI

Kegan Paul International
London and New York

*First published in 1990 by Kegan Paul International Limited*
*PO Box 256, London WC1B 3SW*
*England*

*Distributed by*
*John Wiley and Sons Ltd*
*Southern Cross Trading Estate, 1 Oldlands Way,*
*Bognor Regis, West Sussex PO22 9SA*
*England*

*Routledge, Chapman and Hall Inc*
*29 West 35th Street*
*New York, NY 10001*
*USA*



*The Canterbury Press Pty Ltd*
*Unit 2, 71 Rushdale Street*
*Scoresby, Victoria 3179*
*Australia*

*Produced by Worts-Power Associates*

*Set in Times New Roman by Action Typesetting Limited, Gloucester*
*and printed in Great Britain*
*by Dotesios Printers Ltd., Trowbridge, Wiltshire.*



*British Library Cataloguing in Publication Data*
*Slikkerveer, Leendert Jan,* 1941–
*Plural medical systems in the Horn of Africa: the legacy of "Sheikh" Hippocrates. – (Monographs from the African Studies Centre, Leiden).*
*1. Horn of Africa. Medical services*
*I. Title II. Series*
*362.1'09677*



*ISBN 0-7103-0203-7*

*Library of Congress Cataloging in Publication Data*
*Applied For*

# Contents

# Foreword

The majority of the population in the Third World nations is located in rural areas which have only limited access to national health delivery systems. As populations continue to grow and pressures on national economies increase, the constraints faced by ministries of health in their efforts to expand the cosmopolitan health care system to the rural sectors are expected to become more difficult. Given these serious health planning circumstances, it is critical that we identify, understand, and evaluate the range of indigenous, regional and cosmopolitan therapeutic systems which already exist in most areas and together comprise the national health system. Such an analysis is necessary for national health planners as they seek new strategies for improving the quality of health care available, particularly in the rural areas.

This study is an important landmark in our understanding of the complexities of pluralistic medical systems. It is an unusual study as it provides an overview of the indigenous Oromo and Amhara, the regional Greaco-Arabic, and the cosmopolitan health systems in the Horn of Africa, using a variety of approaches and methodologies.

A socio-historical approach is used to explore the complex development of African, Greaco-Arabic, and European medical traditions in the multi-ethnic community of Babile in the Eastern Highlands of Ethiopia. It is in this historical context that we learn of the link between the Arabic healing tradition in Babile and the medical traditions attributed to 'Sheikh' Hippocrates.

The methodologies of comparative ethnomedicine providc us with insights into each of the alternative medical traditions which co-exist in Babile. Each system is based on its own disease classification structure and each is distinguished by different categories of healers and therapy options.

Using survey methodologies and a multivariate model of trans-cultural health care utilisation, a range of variables such as ethnicity, religion, age, gender, occupation and household size is analysed in terms of the factors which influence choices among the therapeutic options available to the citizens of Babile.

By using this array of approaches and methodologies, it is possible to provide a holistic and comprehensive description, analysis and explanation of the health delivery system characteristic of this part of the Horn of Africa. The author is in a position to recommend ways in which health planners can recognise the variety of medical systems as a national resource base for more culturally appropriate and integrative approaches to health care.

Although this multi-disciplinary approach is limited in this study to the Eastern Highlands of Ethiopia, it is expected to provide an important global model for other studies elsewhere in the developing world. Training and research on this ethnomedical approach to understanding the nature and role of pluralistic health delivery systems are being provided through the Leiden Ethnosystems And Development program (LEAD) in The Netherlands and the Center for Indigenous Knowledge for Agriculture and Rural Development (CIKARD) in the U.S.A.

Prof. Dennis M. Warren
Technology and Social Change Program
Iowa State University, Ames, U.S.A.
April 1988

# Acknowledgements

*Babile*, a multi-ethnic community in the Ethiopian-Somali borderland in the Horn of Africa forms the research area for the study into the health care utilisation process of various medical systems by different ethnic groups in the highlands: Oromo, Somali and Amhara. As a first follow-up study to the preceding 'Rural Health in Ethiopia' project among the *Kottu* Oromo of Hararghe by Buschkens and Slikkerveer (1982), this book is based on an analysis of relevant literature in the medical social sciences and on fieldwork carried out between 1976 and 1982. Several modifications for adaption to the specific pluralist situation in Babile were introduced. These include additional tests for longitudinal health interview and household surveys among different ethnic groups, an expanded conceptual framework for the development of a theoretical model of transcultural health care utilisation, and an extended network of explanatory variables. Improvements in communications and the general logistics of the fieldwork were necessary to permit the team to continue to operate in the highlands under the extremely difficult circumstances of increased guerilla activities, separatist movements and the Ethiopian-Somali warfare in the Ogaden during 1977/1978.

The success and finalisation of this study would not have been possible without the unceasing advice, support and cooperation of a large number of institutions and individuals contributing to the Babile study in a variety of ways. In the first place, I feel most indebted to the former Director and staff of the Institute of Development Research of the University of Addis Ababa and particularly wish to thank Dr. Assefa Mehretu, Dr. Teshome Mulat and Dr. Fasil Gebre Kiros who all strongly supported the study despite the trying situation of the university in Ethiopia immediately after the revolution of 1974.

Also, I owe a great deal to the members of the field team from the study area, Ali Abdi (the team leader), Hamza Adam, Mustafah Abdulahi, Mumi Umer and the late Abdul Hafiz, and to Dr. Ahmed Nagi, Director of the Government Hospital in Dire Dawa and Dr. Zemed of the French Hospital in Dire Dawa and their staff. Mr. Beyenne Haile assisted as driver and logistic assistant in the field. Without their year-long motivation and perseverance, I could not have carried out the research in Babile.

I am much indebted to staff members and colleagues of the Institute of Cultural and Social Studies of the University of Leiden. Especially, the late Professor Emeritus R.A.J. van Lier, who supervised the research projects in Ethiopia and Dr. W.F.L. Buschkens with whom I had the pleasure to share weal and woe during the project. Likewise, Dr. W.H.J.C. Dechering who – in consultation with Dr. R. Niemeyer of the African Studies Centre – so skilfully dedicated much of his time to the design and execution of the rather advanced data analysis. Here, I also thank Professor J.D. Speckmann for his general support, Dr. W.A.R. Shadid for his kind assistance with the translation and interpretation of Arabic manuscripts and medical textbooks and Professor A.J. Drewes of the Faculty of Literature for accompanying me during several fieldtrips to traditional healers and sheikhs of the regional Arabic medical system in the remote areas of the Eastern Highlands of Ethiopia.

Similarly, I wish to thank Drs. W. Teller, Director of the Office for International Cooperation of the University of Leiden, together with staff members Dr. D. Bhalla and Mr. J.H. Jongepier for their continuous provision of advice and administrative support.

Also, I wish to express my gratitude for the financial support of the Netherlands University Foundation for International Co-operation (NUFFIC) in The Hague, where Drs. W.E. Broersma and Drs. H.J. Mastebroek kindly provided the necessary organisational backstopping. I would also like to thank and acknowledge the Netherlands Organization for Scientific Research (NWO) in The Hague for its substantial contribution to the cost of translation and First Edition, the Translation and Editorial Service in Cambridge, U.K., for its correct translation of the original Dutch manuscript into English. Likewise, I feel deeply grateful to Professor H.J. Duller, Chairman of the African Studies Centre in Leiden, for his general support for this study and excellent editing of the English version of the manuscript, and to Dr. G.W. Grootenhuis, General Secretary of the African Studies Centre, for his advice and manifold contributions to the translation and production of the book. Here also, I wish to acknowledge the contribution of Dr. J. Hoorweg of the African Studies Centre. In this context, I would especially like to thank Mrs. Ank Amesz-Uyttenbroek of the Institute of Cultural and Social Studies of the University of Leiden for cheerfully typing the final draft of the manuscript.

I also wish to express my thanks to the Director and staff of the Center for Health Research, Portland, Oregon, U.S.A., respectively Dr. Merwyn R. Greenlick, Dr. Clyde R. Pope and Dr. Donald K. Freeborn, together with Professor Joseph F. Jones, Director of the Center for Sociological Research of Portland State University for their scholarly advice for the preparation of the conceptual framework of the study in Africa, based on their early, pioneering work in health care utilisation research among the population of Oregon, U.S.A. Additionally, I wish to thank Dr. John Hinnant, Dr. Harold Marcus and Dr. David Wiley of the African Studies Center of Michigan State University, East Lansing, Professor Dennis M. Warren of Iowa State University, Ames, Professor Charles Leslie of the University of Delaware, Newark, and Professor Cornelis Ch. Goslinga (Emeritus) of Florida State University, Gainesville, for their academic advice and kind support of this study. I extend my special gratitude to Dr. E.W. Odenwald as well as to Dr. H.J. Stroomer and Drs. F. Gheneti for their meticulous reading of the final draft and Drs. A. de Groot for his mathematical corrections.

Also, I am especially grateful to Professor John Markakis and Professor Dimitri Gutas, both of the Centre for Oriental and African Studies of the University of Crete, Greece, for their kind contributions to the finalisation of the book.

Although it is impossible to mention all those individuals in the Horn of Africa, who contributed to the success of the study, I wish especially to express my gratefulness to the people of Babile, who have so generously cooperated in numerous interviews and surveys, patiently giving so much of their time.

My wife Mady inspired me to this study in many aspects and I wish to thank her and the rest of my family for their generous support of my work.

## Transliteration

Amharic words (abbreviated Am.) are transliterated according to W. Leslau's system in his *Concise Amharic Dictionary*, Wiesbaden 1976. For Arabic words (abbreviated Ar.) the system followed is that of H. Wehr, *A Dictionary of Modern Written Arabic*, edited by J. Milton Cowan, Wiesbaden 1971. The transliteration of Harari (abbreviated Har.) is based on the *Etymological Dictionary of Harari* by W. Leslau, Berkeley 1963, while for Oromifa (abbreviated Or.) the rules followed are those of G.B. Gragg (ed.), *Oromo Dictionary*, East Lansing 1982. For reproduction of terms recorded in the field and not mentioned in the above literature, affiliation is sought as much as possible to the relevant standard notation.

## Illustrations

MAPS



FIGURES

PLATES

*To my wife Mady*

1

# Introduction

*An understanding of the patterns of utilization of medical resources is crucial to the improvement of health care delivery in Africa.*

*P. Stanley Yoder (1982: 16)*

Throughout the African continent, rural health care delivery – more than elsewhere in the world – has come to drift into a situation of crisis. Despite the high technological state of western-styled, cosmopolitan medicine and the allocation of substantial funds to health services, the majority of nations in Sub-Saharan Africa in the course of the eighties are facing an expanding volume of unmet needs, where 70 to 80% of the population have little or no access to primary health care.

In the culture area of Northeast Africa, in particular in Ethiopia and The Horn, the problem of providing essential health services has recently been overshadowed by political transformation and disruption, together with poverty, hunger and starvation as a result of extreme drought conditions during the early seventies and eighties, affecting the whole Sahel region of Africa. Although international agencies, political leaders and planners came to realise that progress in socio-economic development and improvement in health are inseparably linked, and unprecedented aid programmes were launched, different population groups in the periphery, often referred to as 'nationalities', remain almost structurally underserved.

The serious situation in health care in developing countries is beyond a mere assessment in medical or biological terms alone.

With the development of international public health programmes after the Second World War, there was a marked increase in the need for information on the social and cultural factors affecting illness and health, to enable anthropologists and sociologists to contribute to solving health problems in a number of Third World countries. Recently, in addition to ethnomedical studies of traditional medicine and health care coverage there has been growing interest in the health care seeking process in developing countries. Health behaviour, illness behaviour and the utilisation of health care as significant elements in this process have become main issues in the study of medicine, culture and community.

However, the majority of these studies have tended to concentrate on analysing published data and statistics, and on research concerning patients of official health facilities (institution-based research). Although such data occasionally are supplemented by a limited number of socio-epidemiological surveys, only a few have examined the health care seeking process within the context of society as a whole (population-based research – c.f. Newell, 1975; Van Etten 1976; Buschkens and Slikkerveer 1982). Moreover, relatively little attention has been paid to the phenomenon of under-utilisation of 'modern' health care facilities versus other healing systems which has emerged as a specific problem in several developing nations (Buschkens and Slikkerveer 1982; Kroeger 1985). In this respect, the position of ethnic groups in rural areas of Africa and elsewhere, who are at special risk of being underserved, merits specific attention from the social sciences, paving the way for specific future health action. From an interdisciplinary approach to support the WHO global strategy for 'Health for All', there seems today, more than ever, a need to foster the further development of the 'medical social sciences' (Bibeau 1981) for the benefit of the unserved groupings and individuals, not least in this region of Africa.

While in developed countries the study of utilisation of 'mainstream' health care by different groups has dominated in medical sociology research, medical anthropology has focussed on the utilisation of traditional or modern medical systems in developing countries, mostly by one, homogenous population. In the border region of Eastern Ethiopia and Somalia, where an actual situation of a plural medical configuration is complicated by its utilisation of different ethnic groups of Amhara, Oromo and Somali background, a special theoretical framework for the research had to be developed. Combining the promising results of the 'new' ethnomedical approach in medical anthropology with the achievements of transcultural health care science in the West, an attempt is made to develop an appropriate, explanatory model of health care utilisation for this study in the central highlands of the Horn of Africa.

Against the socio-historical background of the acculturation processes at the crossroads of African, Asian and European cultures, where in addition to the existing medical knowledge and practices of local 'Saints', the learnings of 'Sheikh' Hippocrates and Mohammed the 'Prophet', the miracles of Virgin Mary (Maryam) and the 'new science' of travellers, missionaries and colonists from Europe have laid the roots of the present complex situation in medicine, a cross-cultural comparative approach will provide the conceptual orientation of the research. Departing from recent work in Africa of Janzen (1978, 1982), Warren (1979, 1982), Yoder (1982) and Young (1982) regarding illness perception and etiology as part of the health care seeking process, this study links up to the challenging perspective of *medical pluralism* in which patients can resort to perceptions and practices of different co-existing medical systems (Leslie 1977, 1980). Such perspective on the pluralistic character of systems of health care delivery has provided ample scope for the development of a comparative study of the socio-cultural context of biomedical as well as all other medical systems, nowadays referred to as the new or *neo-ethnomedical systems approach* in medical anthropology (Good and Del Vecchio Good, 1980; Eisenberg 1980; Kleinman 1980; Press 1980; Yoder 1982; Slikkerveer 1987). Notwithstanding such widening in the study of ethnomedical systems in the Third World, only limited research efforts have attempted to elucidate the difference in usage of pluralistic medical configurations by various ethnic sub-groups of society. In contrast to a large body of literature, accumulated over the past decades and mostly concerned with explanations of socio-cultural differences in health care utilisation of one 'mainstream' medical system in western countries, few studies in transcultural behaviour sciences have yet related socio-demographic and ethno-cultural factors as sources of variance with cross-cultural patterns of medical knowledge and practices in developing countries (Logan 1977; Harwood 1981).

Hence, the present volume aims to study, from a holistic point of view, all aspects of the pluralistic medical configuration in the Ethiopian-Somali borderland, based on cross-cultural comparisons of existing bio- and ethnomedical systems. This comparison is primarily focussed on behavioural processes of illness perception and management, often referred to as the 'response to illness'. As Fabrega (1974) has indicated, such focus on the health seeking and utilisation behaviour has both theoretical and practical advantages. It no longer regards traditional medicine as 'illegitimate' or 'non-professional', but includes indigenous medical knowledge and practices within the general definition of a medical system. As this study, in contrast with most previous anthropological accounts focussing on either traditional medicine or cosmopolitan medicine in Northeast Africa, approaches the help-seeking process from the participants' point of view, it will enable the development of a theoretical model of transcultural health care utilisation. Through the examination of the relationship and interaction among related variables, certain explanations of differences in usage of existing medical resources by various groups could contribute to finding an answer to the ultimate question: 'Who seeks care, where and why?'

Practically, as Yoder (1982: 16) affirms, the study of utilisation patterns among populations in Africa is important for the improvement of their health care delivery system. In particular, this may have certain implications for the improvement of a future system of primary health care delivery in the area in terms of two recent, most promising WHO guiding principles: the further development of 'ethno- and biomedicine linkage' in primary health care coverage (Bannerman *et al.* 1983) and the 'risk approach in health care' to particular underserved individuals and groups on the periphery (WHO 1984).

After defining the objectives of the study and a short review of relevant theoretical approaches in the medical social sciences in developing countries, particularly in relation to Africa, a description is given of the conceptual framework of the study, and its related model of health care utilisation. Subsequently, an overview is presented of recent planning approaches and policies to the development of rural health care. Following the implications of the present author's involvement in earlier medical anthropological and sociological research in Eastern Ethiopia, the introduction concludes with an account of the structure and arrangement of the book.

## 1.1 Objective of the Study

In the light of the foregoing, the primary objective of the study is to contribute towards increasing knowledge and understanding of the processes whereby members of various groups of the community generally perceive illness and seek health care in a situation of a pluralistic medical configuration, in which different cultures have come into contact with one another. The need for more information derives on the one hand from recent changes in the demand for health care services in developing countries, particularly in rural areas in Africa. On the other hand, during the past decades, applied medical social scientists have become increasingly concerned with the analysis of processes of illness behaviour and utilisation of medical systems. The present study of the health care utilisation process in a plural community in the centre of the Horn of Africa attempts to link up both developments.

To this end, the way in which the social, situational and cultural characteristics of patients as well as the institutional characteristics of health resources determine the pattern of utilisation of existing medical systems are being examined in a multi-ethnic community in the Ethiopian-Somali borderland in the Horn of Africa. *Babile*, the community in question, is situated in the eastern part of the administrative region of Hararghe on the highland slopes near the edge of the Ogaden desert, inhabited by approximately 4000 people from the following ethnic groups: Oromo (40%), Amhara (35%), Somali (15%) and others (10%). The study is based on longitudinal fieldwork from 1976 until 1980 and again in 1982 using a sample of 337 household groups comprising 1351 individuals. The main emphasis is laid on the importance of the historical and socio-cultural context in which the processes of illness behaviour and utilisation are operating in this part of Africa. Ethno-cultural affiliation is specifically included in the analysis as a possible major determinant of health care utilisation by members of different population groups in the research area.

In view of the theoretical, methodological and practical problems and constraints, that lately have hampered further development of both medical social sciences and health care improvement in the Third World, in particular in relation to Africa – which will be indicated in the following sections – a number of secondary objectives are included in this study, which attempt:

1. to describe the various medical systems of the plural medical configuration in the research area. As in the case in almost any society, the medical system in the Horn has a plural character. In addition to the officially recognised, modern medical system, a variety of traditional local, regional, and transitional systems are operational, providing the majority of the rural population with some form of care. With the exception of the limited number of previous studies in Hararghe, few attempts have been made so far to draw the attention of health care planners and policy-makers to the degree of influence exerted by indigenous medical traditions on the formal health system in Ethiopia (Schneider 1975; Buschkens and Slikkerveer 1982). This has produced a distorted and over-simplified picture of the health situation in the area. As a result, the formulation and implementation of effective health care measures and programmes for the local population has lately been severely hampered.
2. to present a disease classification of respondents in the community, differentiated according to the main ethnic sub-groups. As will be discussed in detail in Chapter 2, the general picture emerging from the literature is that perceived morbidity forms one of the most significant determinants of the health care seeking and utilisation process. In developing the analytical model here conceived, further study will be undertaken of the role of perceived morbidity together with ethno-cultural affiliation as independent variables in relation to a number of other independent variables, and subsequently to the dependent variable of utilisation of the plural medical system.
3. to describe the illness and utilisation behaviour of patients in Babile. The successive stages of the course illness is taking and the opportunities for patients to approach the different medical systems in the area by taking one or more 'medical steps' will be established at the level of individual behaviour. The term 'patients' in this context refers to respondents of the sample during a twelve-month period of time and to people who report 'sick' or somehow regard themselves as 'patients'. The analysis of their illness behaviour will provide insight into the overall pattern of health care utilisation of patients in the region. It will then be possible to answer the important question as to what extent the plural character of the community is reflected in the

health care utilisation pattern of available systems of health care delivery. Since the formal health services in the area are badly underutilised by several population groups, the study will particularly attempt to diagnose this rather paradoxical problem, in which socio-cultural and political factors seem to play a dominant role.

4. to provide a basis for the development of a multivariate integration model of health care utilisation for a population group in a transcultural situation. By selecting, testing and adapting a number of earlier theoretical models based on extensive medical anthropological and sociological research into illness behaviour and health care utilisation, the study will attempt to establish an analytical framework capable of serving two objectives: accommodating a number of predisposing and enabling factors together with perceived morbidity and, secondly, taking into account the role of the plural character of available forms of health care in utilisation behaviour. To this end, a general systems approach is introduced to proceed from the individual level of disease management to macrolevel patterns of utilisation of different medical systems of society. As Chapter 2 further explains, the aim here is to incorporate the results of this research into a more generally applicable, explanatory utilisation model for developing countries, largely based on two earlier models of health care utilisation by Greenlick *et al.* (1969) and Kohn and White (1976), which is being developed into a more comprehensive model to account for multiple utilisation of various medical systems.
5. to indicate a number of implications of the study for applied medical-anthropological and sociological research in developing countries. The prime requirement to contribute to the design and implementation of a health programme for the region will be satisfied by presenting specific information concerning the various factors which influence the complex pattern of health care utilisation in rural areas. Decisions concerning the number, type and size of planned medical services are, after all, largely dependent on an assessment of the extent to which the various facilities are actually being used by the population concerned. It is therefore essential to describe and classify the different types of medical systems available in the form of both traditional and transitional as well as cosmopolitan medicine, and to monitor

the ways in which these are being used by local population groups. This is of some importance, since mere registration of under-utilisation and over-utilisation could easily create a misleading impression (Kleczkowski and Pibouleau 1977: 44–48). It will then be possible to contribute to a future regional plan for the area as part of a national plan of action for Ethiopia, which eventually could provide the basis for improving the health of the rural population in this part of Africa.

## 1.2 Medical Social Sciences in Sub-Saharan Africa

In the past, medical and social scientists have concerned themselves increasingly with the study of health care problems in the Third World. Medical doctors and health experts have tended to concentrate on technical and bio-medical matters, while anthropologists focussed their attention on the relationship between culture, community and traditional medicine, studying the socio-cultural context of health and disease in different societies. Later on, development sociologists became concerned with the functioning and organisation of 'modern' health care in Third World countries, often referred to as 'health services research'. Meanwhile, the comparative anthropological – and partly sociological, epidemiological, psychiatric and historical – studies of different medical systems have developed into a new, promising ethnomedical approach providing useful information on different systems of indigenous knowledge, perceptions and practices in the context of health and healing.

Mainly because of the stagnation in the distribution and improvement of medical services, an integrated and interdisciplinary approach to the problem was increasingly sought, and as a result the gap between the social and the biomedical sciences has been closing, although it has not completely disappeared. Concurrently, the recommendations of the final declaration of the WHO/UNICEF International Conference in Alma-Ata (1978: 3, 5) have started to bring about a fundamental change in the relationship between the social and the medical sciences. Paragraph V states:

> *Economic and social development based on a New International Economic Order, is of basic importance to the fullest attainment*

*of health for all and to the reduction of the gap between the health status of developing and developed countries.*

Paragraph VII continues:

*All governments should formulate national policies, strategies and plans of action to launch and sustain primary health care as part of a comprehensive national health system and in coordination with other sectors. To this end, it will be necessary to exercise political will, to mobilize the country's resources and to use available external sources rationally.*

Although this statement still bears the character of a 'declaration of intent', medical social scientists have moved into a new era, in which in addition to non-medical factors of, for example, the political, economic, demographic and institutional backgrounds, tentative models have been designed to analyse the relationship between cultural, social, psycho-social, economic and biological factors involved in current problems of health care delivery (Bibeau 1981).

With reference to earlier reviews of Van Etten (1976), Yoder (1982) and the present author (1982), the following sections deal with an assessment of the 'state of the art' in recent developments in the field of medical anthropology, sociology and ethnomedicine, particularly in relation to Sub-Saharan Africa.

### *1.2.1 Medical anthropological and sociological studies*

Early efforts within anthropology to describe the social and cultural aspects of medicine in Africa have resulted in an over-emphasis on indigenous beliefs and practices, later known in the literature as early studies in 'ethnomedicine' (Fabrega 1972; Lieban 1973, 1977).

During the fifties and sixties, anthropologists directed their attention predominantly to traditional beliefs and practices of tribal groups and populations, mostly in rural areas. Exemplary fieldwork in Africa includes studies in the British tradition of Radcliffe-Brown's structural-functional comparison of basic elements on a microlevel by, for example, Abrahams (1959), Gerlach (1959), Gelfand (1964), Imperato (1966), Hatfield (1968) and Reid (1969). Equally, under the influence of Evans-Pritchard's study of health and healing among the Azande (1937), anthropologists such as

Ackerknecht (1955), Turner (1964) and Horton (1967) focussed their attention on the ritual aspects of health and disease in African society, in which magic and religion were linked with the concept of 'primitive medicine'. This rather deterministic approach focussing on traditional medicine with its neglect of the cosmopolitan, western-oriented medical system in often isolated 'little communities' (Redfield 1956) in the periphery could explain the stereotyped attribution of 'merely traditional', even in cases where 'modern' medicine was available and utilised (Van Etten 1976).

Towards the end of this era, anthropological studies gradually came to pay more attention to the 'dual use' phenomenon involving utilisation of both traditional and modern medicine by the local population. This interest would seem to be linked with the emergence of applied anthropology and its focus on the processes of cultural and social change. Concurrent use of folk healers and physicians has been mostly studied in urban settings lending support to the identification of this concept with urban and sub-urban environments in Africa. The concept of dualism, which, according to Colson and Selby (1974), had been prompted either by differences in traditional interpretation of disease-causation (Foster 1958; Gelfand 1964), or by different socio-demographic characteristics of the population concerned, and in particular of sub-groups (Press 1969; Lieban 1973), generally regards the use of cosmopolitan medicine as an exception. Moreover, this limited view presupposes a rigid dichotomy between biomedical and traditional medicine, disregarding the actual situation in the field, where in addition to the formal health services a wide variety of options for treatment exists.

In the course of the seventies, two major areas of research have predominated in medical anthropological and sociological research. Firstly, expanded ethnomedical studies have focussed on local disease etiology and medical knowledge as components of the help-seeking and utilisation behaviour, thus giving a broader dimension to the study of medical systems in Africa. These include the work of Janzen (1978) in Zaire, Warren (1974) in Ghana and Young (1977) in Ethiopia, in which abundant information is presented on systems of indigenous medical knowledge in relation to healing practices. In these studies, local perceptions on disease etiology are generally classified in terms of 'natural' and 'supernatural' diseases (Warren 1974), 'diseases of God' and 'diseases of men' (Janzen 1978), 'internalising' or 'externalising' in the context of medical systems (Young

1976) and 'natural', 'initial' and 'agent' causes of illness (Bibeau 1979). Although precise definitions of these classifications are difficult to formulate, it has become clear that the study of different types of causal explanations are crucial to the understanding of the health care seeking process. In this way, these studies have not only initiated cross-cultural comparisons of medical systems, thus contributing to the recent development of a wider ethnomedical approach to health and healing in Africa, but they have made a direct link between medical knowledge systems and illness behaviour, which provides a more realistic base for health planning.

Secondly, under the influence of newly developed sociological theories of modernisation on social and cultural change, a number of studies has emphasised the role of cosmopolitan medicine in developing nations. In this respect, Colson and Selby (1974) refer to the important category of studies in *social epidemiology* representing a research focus on socio-cultural factors in relation to disease, particularly among rural populations. In general, this approach is analogous with a tradition in medical sociology, termed *sociology in medicine* centred upon the patient and the sick role (Susser and Watson 1971). Most studies on social epidemiology, or 'social medicine', in Africa have been concerned with general categories of medical problems such as, for instance, mental illness in Tanzania (Aall-Jilek and Jilek 1970), malnutrition in Uganda (Hoorweg and McDowell 1974), childhood diseases and paediatrics in Uganda (Bwibo 1971), Zambia (Voorhoeve 1983) and Kenya (Van Ginneken and Muller 1984; Voorhoeve 1985), infectious diseases in Tanzania (Van Etten and Anten 1972) and family planning in East Africa (Molnos 1973). In addition, several monographs on health and disease have been published describing the general health situation in Chad (Buck *et al.* 1970), East Africa (Gould 1971), Ethiopia (Schaller and Kuls 1972) and Kenya (Vogel *et al.* 1974). In contrast, research in Africa corresponding to the tradition of *sociology of medicine* in terms of the study of the organisation and structure of cosmopolitan health services in the Third World received relatively little attention (Segall 1972; Gish 1973; Schulpen 1975; Van Etten 1976). With a view to the stagnation in rural health development in East Africa, Van Etten (1976: 12) concludes: '. . . *it can be argued that the structure of health services as well as the attitude of the medical profession may be equally important factors impeding a balanced development of the health sector*'.

Only after emergence of recent medical sociology literature on the accessibility and utilisation of health facilities in Western Europe and the United States, the organisational aspects of modern health services in Africa have gained special attention (Benyoussef and Wessen 1975; Van Etten 1976; Kohn and White 1976). Research into this field of formal institutions has frequently stressed the importance of understanding the influence of the structure of services as well as the attitude of the medical staff on the patterns of utilisation by the population. Although it is evident that these studies have provided a major contribution to positive changes in the health care infrastructure in new nations, the interest in the utilisation of the modern health care delivery system prevails, whereas only incidental attention is being paid to the otherwise substantial use of existing traditional and transitional medical systems.

As regards the problem-oriented research efforts of anthropologists and sociologists in the field of health and healing, initially they were mostly engaged in explaining to health personnel: *how traditional beliefs and practices conflicted with western medical assumptions, how social factors influenced health care decisions and how health and disease are simply aspects of total culture patterns, which change only in the company of broader and more comprehensive socio-cultural changes* (Foster and Anderson 1978: 7, 8). In the course of the fifties, anthropologists became increasingly involved with the organisational problems of health care and began making a contribution to setting up and carrying out general public health programmes for the community as a whole. By taking part in epidemiological studies, health information and disease prevention activities and subsequently by becoming members of multi-disciplinary teams, anthropologists, sociologists and social psychologists became involved in the development of international medicine as it entered a new stage of development. McGavran (1979) refers to this classic period as the *public health era*. Bibeau (1981: 358) specifies three levels at which the social sciences made a contribution during this period: a) information concerning local cultures, in order to make direct intervention possible, b) additional information mainly for the benefit of epidemiological research in particular, and c) data concerning factors and principles of local social ecology.

Following this period a new era dawned in the early seventies which Bibeau (1981: 360, 361) describes as the *health political science era*. In the last ten years, the focus of attention in the health sector shifted from regarding the total population as the target group to regional groups, whose health problems are placed in a broader socio-economic and political context. Health care then is primarily linked with the political responsibilities of the society. It is noticeable that in addition to anthropologists, sociologists and social scientists, three additional categories of medical social scientists have become active in health care in developing countries: medical economists, political scientists and health care policy makers. Bibeau (1981: 361–363) also distinguishes between three areas in which social scientists were active in this period: a) community medicine, b) ethnomedicine and c) in clinical settings.

It is worth noting that by the end of the seventies, despite decades of productive fieldwork, medical anthropologists and sociologists in developing countries, together with health planners and administrators, only gradually became aware of the fact that the rather isolationist interest in either traditional or cosmopolitan medicine, as well as the concentration on 'dual use' dichotomy between both systems, had not yet resulted in a better understanding of the complex relationships between medicine, culture and society, let alone in an improvement of health care delivery in Africa, or for that matter, elsewhere in the Third World.

### *1.2.2 The challenge of medical pluralism*

In contrast to the above-mentioned, normative views, a new, more realistic approach has increasingly gained scholarly interest, in which medical systems, according to Leslie's (1977: 9) conceptions, can be regarded as: '. . . *pluralistic structures in different kinds of practitioners and institutional norms*'[1].

Although in Western Europe and the United States – mainly because of unease about technocratic, 'impersonal' treatment, over-medicalisation and the staggering cost of the dominant biomedical system – people have resorted to 'alternative' therapies such as homoeopathy, herbalism, natural healing and holism of the 'new era', the co-existence and utilisation of a wide range of traditional and modern healing systems in many parts of Africa, Asia and Latin America has generally been regarded as a typical phenomenon in the developing world.

Here, in addition to the services of doctors and health workers of mostly urban-oriented, hospital-based, 'modern' health facilities for the elite, different types of indigenous healers of ancient local and regional systems such as Chinese medicine, *Ayurveda, Siddha* and *Unani-Tibbi* have persisted in providing 'alternative' health care to the majority of the population on the periphery[2]. As in cultural pluralism, where two or more cultural systems in prolonged contact have established a mutual accommodation to sustain distinctive ways of life, medical pluralism refers to the historically grounded co-existence of more than one medical system which in a more or less interconnected way seeks to maintain the health status within the community. Although the mere presence of different perceptions and practices does not imply, as Press (1980: 47) indicates: '. . . *that they constitute a functionally integrated system*', a plural medical configuration generally encompasses a society with more than one paradigmatically differentiated medical system. This means that although this concept in the first instance relates to a complex of distinct systems and accompanying categories of health workers and healers, medical pluralism could also include a multiplicity of knowledge and perceptions of ill health, illness behaviour and the use of various forms of health care. In this context Press (1980: 47) concludes: '*Our task must be to determine the extent to which users of the particular medical configuration under study conceptually compartmentalise the various elements, or integrate them into a coherent cognitive system*'. It is clear, that research into the concurrent or multiple utilisation of co-existing medical systems – often referred to as 'healer shopping' – requires a specific methodology, in particular in quantifying such intricate use of services. Chapter 2 deals with some methodological problems in the study of utilisation of plural medical systems. The theoretical implications of the pluralist perspective on medicine have mostly been perceptible in the emergence of new orientations in the medical social sciences. Fundamentally, non-formal medical traditions have no longer been identified as 'irregular' or even 'illegal' variations of a dominant, 'modern' or 'scientific' medical system. Indeed, as Leslie (1980: 191) observes: '*All medical systems can then be conceived of as pluralistic structures in which cosmopolitan medicine is one component in competitive and complementary relationship to numerous "alternative therapies"*.' In addition to reference to such co-existence of multiple systems, medical pluralism also applies to multiple conceptions of disease and illness among patients and their families, multiple categories of healers and health workers and, last but not least, to multiple choices of therapy between and within particular systems. Consequently, an expanding research interest in medical anthropology has recently focussed on medical pluralism in various settings (Leslie 1976, 1978; Janzen 1978; Janzen and Feierman 1979; Rubel 1979; Weidman 1979; Kleinman 1980; Warren *et al.* 1982; Slikkerveer 1982, 1983). As will be demonstrated in the following section, 1.3, these cross-cultural studies of different medical systems have laid the foundation for the further development of a new, comparative study of ethnomedical systems, lately referred to as the *ethnomedical approach to medicine.*

The practical advantages of the pluralistic perspective on medicine in developing countries, particularly in Africa, are manifold. Firstly, the recognition that medical systems may range from relatively 'simple' to 'complex' entities of a multi-systemic continuum enables a more balanced appraisal of the concurrent and serial use of health care that goes beyond the limited 'dual use' dichotomy of either traditional or modern medicine.

Secondly, it provides a more objective base for the interpretation of the sometimes misleadingly termed 'unscientific medicine' as indeed a valuable alternative involving: '*rational use of naturalistic theories to organise and interpret systematic empirical observations*' (Leslie 1977: 7). Such interpretation has paved the way for a functionalistic approach to health care improvement, especially with respect to the development of innovative views on alternative solutions to public health problems in Africa, Asia and Latin America.

Thirdly, as the management of illness episodes is included in this approach, it facilitates the study of the help-seeking and utilisation behaviour of patients. The understanding of overall patterns of utilisation could ascertain dynamic processes of mutual influence among systems, and thus identify areas of interface and friction.

Fourthly, inspired by the example of the People's Republic of China, where traditional medicine has been incorporated successfully within the formal medical system, several ethnomedical studies on medical pluralism have provided a challenge to the utilisation of local and regional medical traditions and functionaries within future health plans for developing countries, particularly in Zaire (Bibeau 1982; Yoder 1982), Ethiopia (Slikkerveer 1982), Ghana (Warren *et al.* 1982) and Nigeria (Brink 1982)[3].

## 1.3 The Development of a Comparative Health Care Science

Within medical anthropology, the relatively recent pluralist perspective on medicine has further widened the research interest to the cross-cultural comparison of different medical systems in developing countries. As the holistic study of medical knowledge and practices within a particular socio-cultural context has led to a new ethnomedical approach in the medical social sciences, promising research has developed into a theoretical framework, distinct from the biomedical paradigm. Parallel to such development of cross-culturally valid concepts and definitions for the analysis of the situation predominant in Third World countries, a field of trans-cultural health care science has been evolving in the course of the seventies in Western Europe and the United States. Primarily focussed on the variety of cultural and sub-cultural groups in industrialised nations, a similar comparative approach to different health care beliefs, values and practices has resulted in a number of well-documented studies of health, illness and healing among various minority groups. In the following sections, implications of both ethnomedical and transcultural health care research for the development of a transcultural view on health and illness problems of specific groups in developing countries, and in particular in the Horn of Africa, will be ascertained, especially in relation to the design of an explanatory model of health care utilisation.

### *1.3.1 The new ethnomedical approach to medicine in Africa*

As the pluralist perspective on medicine became a major issue in medical anthropological and sociological studies in the late seventies, it has given impetus to the further development of the comparative study of ethnomedical systems, ultimately resulting in the new ethnomedical approach to the research of: '*. . . the ideological and cultural bases of any medical system, including the official sector of Western medicine*' (Press 1980: 45)[4]. Before looking at the comparative foundations of this approach, it seems useful to identify appropriate definitions of what constitutes a 'medical system', respectively an 'ethnomedical system'.

In the course of the development of medical anthropology as a sub-discipline a range of definitions of a 'medical system' has appeared in the literature, reflecting different perspectives and orientations. In addition to Glick's (1967: 32) working definition of a medical system as: '. . . *a patterned set of ideas and practices having to do with illness*', Kleinman (1978, 1980: 50) has developed a structural model of a health care system, applicable to research both in developed and developing societies, conceiving it as: '. . . *a local cultural system composed of three overlapping parts: the popular, professional and folk sectors*'. Dunn (1976: 135) places a medical system, or 'system of health care delivery' in its historico-geographical context, describing it as: '. . . *the pattern of social institutions and cultural traditions that evolves from deliberate behaviour to enhance health, whether or not the outcome of particular items of behaviour is ill health*'. Stressing the medical-ecological interaction between behaviour and socio-cultural structure, Dunn offers here a highly useful classification of *local, regional* and *cosmopolitan* medical systems. Moreover, such distinction has major methodological implications for the analysis of complex pluralistic configurations as are, for instance, operating in the area of the Horn of Africa. In addition to Foster and Anderson's (1978) definition of medical systems focussing on the health promoting beliefs and actions together with knowledge and skills, Press (1980: 47) presents a more comprehensive conception of a medical system. He speaks of: '*A patterned, interrelated body of values and deliberate practices, governed by a single paradigm of the meaning, identification, prevention, and treatment of sickness*', offering ample scope for comparison of different forms of health care.

Early medical-anthropological interest in the socio-cultural context of 'alternative' medicine has led to the rather dichotomous definition of ethnomedical systems distinct from biomedical systems as: '. . . *those beliefs and practices relating to disease which are the products of indigenous cultural development and not explicitly derived from the conceptual framework of modern medicine*' (Hughes 1968: 88). Subsequently Fabrega (1977) in his conception of medical institutions follows the classic differentiation between social science research in biomedicine and in ethnomedicine, recognising, however, that the term ethnomedicine has ethnocentric connotations. The need to define the plural character of medical systems encompassing a wider variety of knowledge, perceptions, practices and behaviour related to health and disease has called for a holistic approach to the study of the socio-cultural context of both modern and alternative medical systems, as suggested by Press (1980), Leslie (1980), Kleinman (1980) and Yoder (1982). Consequently, the former distinction between a medical system as 'bio-medical', and 'lay' health practices as 'ethnomedical' can be ignored, since in this new approach both definitions basically refer to the same conceptions: all medical knowledge and practices within a given socio-cultural context, including self-treatment, traditional medicine and biomedical health care. By using such a conception of a medical system, it has become possible to develop a valid comparative study of ethnomedical systems, based on different criteria for labelling, classification and cross-cultural comparison.

Press' (1980) definition offers one basis for comparison, looking at specific functions of all medical systems: a) meaning, b) identification, c) prevention and d) treatment of illness. A second basis for comparison is offered by Yoder (1982), who calls attention to the way in which any medical system is linked with a particular form of social organisation, as for instance social groups in Africa, based on lineage affiliation.

Further to these functional and socio-cultural foundations, a third promising basis for comparison has evolved from a behavioural perspective, focussing on the management of illness episodes, which include all actions from symptom perception, lay and professional consultation, medical care, contact and recovery until rehabilitation. According to such research interest, not only the crucial role of lineage groups in the *quest for therapy* among patients can be highlighted – as Janzen (1978) did for the Bakonge in Zaire – but it widens ethnomedical research to include the dynamic aspects of help-seeking and utilisation processes. As Yoder (1982: 16) observes: '*Following episodes of illness through time also reveals how diagnoses change, efficacy is evaluated, and alternative treatments are sought.*'

In addition to the theoretical advantages of such dynamic forms of study on the management of illness episodes, it practically offers applied-oriented research into the help-seeking and utilisation behaviour of patients in the Third World. With reference to the initial citation at the start of this introduction of Yoder's (1982: 16) conclusion on the importance of the understanding of the utilisation behaviour for health care improvement in Africa, it has become clear that the empirical study of such behaviour provides insight in the actual way, in which people cope with illness, and, at the same time, in the functioning of the health care system, offering a realistic base for health care planning and programming.

The present study attempts to combine such theoretical and practical implications by making the management of illness episodes of the different groups in the Babile area the behavioural focus of the research.

### *1.3.2 Transcultural perspectives on health care*

In medical sociology, a large body of literature has accumulated in the last two decades on the study of differences in health care utilisation in Western Europe and the United States. In spite of an increasing number of alternative resources of health care, most studies have concentrated on the use of 'mainstream' medicine, examining several sets of factors as possible determinants of variation in health services utilisation. McKinlay (1972) in his early review of utilisation literature has defined six sets of such factors: economic, socio-demographic, geographic, social-psychological, socio-cultural and organisational. Although all these six variables seem to be important to the understanding of differential health care utilisation, it has been almost impossible to select specific factors as the sole explanation of difference in the use of health services. The absence of a single theory or approach that has earned general consensus has partly been explained by the general descriptive character of these studies. As Denton (1978) notes: '*What is needed is research examining the relationships among the six variables and determining their relative importance in utilisation.*' This supports the need for additional research in medical sociology into the relative effects of different variables on health care utilisation. Such research could develop *a multivariate model* of health care utilisation, as has been initiated by the early work of Suchman (1965). His systematic study of the extent of the belief in modern medicine among ethnic groups in New York City has at the same time laid the foundation for further research concentrating on ethnicity as an important factor in health care utilisation behaviour.

Parallel to the previously described development of cross-culturally valid concepts and definitions into a comparative science of ethnomedicine in developing countries, a field of transcultural health care science has been evolved towards the eighties in the West as: '*an evolving body of knowledge and practices regarding health-illness care patterns from a comparative perspective of at least two or more designated cultures* . . .' (Leininger 1976: 3). In addition to the theoretical advantage of conceiving the nature, direction and scope of transcultural health care phenomena, an important sub-field of *transcultural nursing* has developed as a new area of understanding and serving different cultural groups in western pluralist societies. Primarily focussed on the variety of cultural and sub-cultural groups in industrialised nations, a comparative approach to different health care beliefs, values, and practices has resulted in well-documented studies of, for example, Iranian, Papago, Jewish, Belgian, Chinese, Haitian, Italian, Mexican, Navaho and Puerto Rican ethnic groups in North America in relation to illness behaviour and health care (Leininger 1976, 1978; Harwood 1981). The contribution of these studies has mostly been apparent in the applied field of teaching and providing transcultural care and nursing for minorities. Later on, several of these studies embarked on the *health culture* concept to develop the transcultural view in medicine as a prerequisite to interethnic communication in health care (Weidman 1977, 1979).

Similarly, anthropological involvement in the clinical setting of psychiatric disorders among European and North American ethnic groups has developed into *transcultural psychiatry*, in which culture-bound disorders, folk healing, family and childhood problems and doctor-patient relationships have been extensively studied (Chrisman and Maretzki 1984). Although the transcultural behavioural sciences in general are interested in ecological and socio-cultural influences on human behaviour in both western and non-western societies, most of these early applied studies remained focussed on the problematic situation of minority groups in the developed world (Branch and Paxton 1976; Brink 1976; Leiniger 1976, 1978; Redlener and Scott 1979; Lefley 1979; Weidman 1979). Their implications, however, in terms of the development of a transcultural view on health and healing problems of specific groups of the population in the Third World should reinforce current cross-cultural research efforts in the anthropological study of ethno-medical systems in Africa, Latin America and Asia.

### 1.3.3 Towards a model of transcultural health care utilisation

In the light of the foregoing it seems fruitful to employ a medical pluralist perspective in order to classify the different co-existing medical systems and sub-systems within the socio-cultural context of the community of Babile, according to Dunn's (1977) earlier mentioned, historico-geographic typology. Taking additionally the management of illness episodes as the behavioural basis for the comparative ethnomedical analysis, it becomes possible to study the situation in the Horn of Africa from a holistic point of view: examining all aspects of local knowledge, practices and behaviour in relation to health and illness. As mentioned above, a complicating factor, however, is the fact that in addition to the existing pluralistic configuration in health care, patients belong to different ethnic groups of the plural society in the region. Indeed, as the population in the Horn of Africa is anything but homogeneous, and 'nationalities' retain their lifestyle and behaviour according to their sub-culture, a specific approach is needed to examine and analyse differential utilisation patterns of co-existing medical systems in relation to patients from various groups of the society. In other words, here a transcultural view of the problem of the help-seeking and utilisation behaviour is an added prerequisite to the understanding of the dynamic process of multiple use of different services by various ethnic groups.

In this study, therefore, a theoretical model is designed for the description and explanation of transcultural health care utilisation, providing the conceptual framework for the analysis of the health-seeking and utilisation process in this part of Africa. Such a model could not only elucidate the complex illness behaviour within a pluralistic medical configuration, but also ascertain causes of differential and under-utilisation of particular medical resources, critical to the understanding of problems of health care delivery in rural areas. Theoretically, the model should not only approach different sets of causative factors in a descriptive way, but additionally should, in an explanatory way, examine the relationships among specific sets of variables and determine their relative importance in differential utilisation patterns. Following Suchman's (1965) model of utilisation mentioned above, a multivariate model of transcultural health care utilisation will be designed for this study, based on previous models of Greenlick *et al.* (1969)

and Kohn and White (1976). Practically, it could identify specific minority groups as 'risk groups' to whom relatively more medical attention could be paid in future health plans. Chapter 2 deals further with the theoretical and methodological considerations of the model.

## 1.4 Rural Health Care Planning and Development in Africa

'Modern' or 'Western' medicine, of which Leslie (1977: 5) remarks: '*At the end of the Middle Ages, scientific research and forms of professional association in Europe began a development which led eventually to the worldwide traditions of cosmopolitan medicine,*' spread with the expansion of Europe and the rise of modern science. During the ages of the great colonial powers, missionaries, travellers and colonists started to provide the local population in the tropics with limited medical assistance, mostly of a curative nature (Van Amelsvoort 1964). In the course of the second half of the nineteenth century, which witnessed rapid technical developments in western medicine and the gradual introduction of more 'ethical' colonial policies, preventive mass campaigns were initiated for the benefit of the local population. At the same time, curative health care started to reach rural areas from urban centres, albeit on a limited scale. However, health care still remained largely organised by central government along western lines. During this period, a start was made in providing health education, equally based on western concepts.

At the beginning of this century, in Western Europe in particular, the first systematic planning of social services was introduced and after the Second World War developments accelerated as a result of changes in perception of the role of the state in relation to the public sector. This marked the beginning of the period in which the liberal state evolved into the welfare state, in which social medicine came to play an important role (Mannheim 1940). The subsequent approach to initial health care planning in Third World countries was largely based on the conviction that existing types of formal health services were inequitably distributed both geographically and socially, thereby denying the majority of the population its basic right to health care. This became dramatically evident during the fifties and sixties, the period of decolonisation, when it became clear that the developing countries did not have the financial resources to sustain expensive western medicine – which retained a therapeutic nature centred around chemotherapy and antibiotics – such as was practiced by the former colonial powers. As a result, modern health care continues to be available largely to rich urban elite groups whereas 70 to 80% of the rural masses remains badly underserved (WHO 1978; Rifkin 1981: 477–386).

Inspired by the new ideas on planning, a number of international public health programmes were designed and implemented. However, for decades they continued to be based on the assumption that improving health care largely depends on developing and implementing programmes on a proper bio-medical basis to which the members of the target groups will then respond enthusiastically. Despite the high technical quality of many of these programmes, several ended in failure. For example, the Rockefeller Foundation was responsible for a programme to control and treat hookworm in Ceylon based on western methods, but after six years was still unable to eradicate the disease (Philips 1955: 265–305). It has since gradually become apparent that bio-medical programmes, introduced in areas where traditional, indigenous and unorthodox systems are still strongly represented, will encounter active opposition and criticism. Foster and Anderson (1978: 22) make the following observation: '*The initial high hopes of international medical specialists time after time have been dashed, as they have found to their astonishment that seemingly technologically sound programmes have failed completely or achieved only partial success.*' When, in 1942, the Institute of Inter-American Affairs developed a number of public health programmes in conjunction with several Latin American governments, the ethnocentric concept of the superiority of western medicine formed a stumbling-block to the introduction of curative and preventive health care via an organised system of health centres. Utilisation of available medical services by the local population was far less than expected (Foster 1952: 5–16). When the World Health Organisation (WHO) was set up after the Second World War, and an international administrative system was created with the aim of extending modern health care on a world-wide scale, similar problems were encountered.

In the sixties, the inequitable geographical and social distribution of medical facilities received the attention of economic development experts and planners, such as Myrdal (1968: 1531–1619), whose main thesis was that an integrated model of socio-economic planning should necessarily recognise the significance of mutual links between health care and other social, economic, institutional and policy factors in the development process. He warned against an isolationist approach to health planning which ignores the importance of increasing agricultural production, improving education and health care and, more generally, tackling the problem of poverty on a massive scale. Health care indeed is not a 'bottomless pit' for national budgets but rather an 'investment in man' (Myrdal 1968: 1541). This kind of development strategy for Third World countries was later amplified and developed in more detail by a number of health care experts such as King (1966), Bryant (1969), Worth and Shah (1969), Gish (1971), Rifkin and Kaplinsky (1973) and Elliott (1979).

A central feature of this latter approach is the integration of health care with the socio-economic and political systems. Despite efforts to shift emphasis from curative to preventive medicine, and to use manpower rather than capital-intensive technology in health care, a situation has developed in which the relatively affluent, educated minority in big cities retained preferential treatment at the expense of the relatively poor, uneducated majority in rural areas. Gradually it became clear, that a wider range of the usually underestimated 'soft factors' is lying at the root of the largely inadequate health care programmes and medical services in developing countries.

### *1.4.1 Recent strategies to improve health services*

Inspired by the rapid development of health care in the West after the Second World War, a similar planning and intervention philosophy was introduced in a number of Third World countries on a modest scale. This mainly came about as a result of the desire to put an end to the inequitable distribution of health care services, and was primarily designed to implement a series of measures to bring modern health care within the reach of a larger section of the population. After the virtual failure of 'investment in capital' which had been inspired by the success of the Marshall Plan in Western Europe after the war, the emphasis was shifted to 'investment in man' (Myrdal 1968). As a result of improved coordination of funds, the decentralisation of planning and organisation, and the implementation and evaluation of health care programmes, attempts were made to achieve the primary objective of providing modern health care facilities for the entire population.

Three strategies have successively been designed to improve the low coverage of medical services and were subsequently implemented as part of health care planning efforts in developing countries, in particular in rural areas: facility based services, the community-oriented approach and primary health care.

## Facility-based services

Roughly twenty-five years ago, efforts to improve health care, particularly on the periphery, tended to concentrate on the organisation of the health services and the spread of modern medical knowledge. Attempts were made by governments to reach a larger section of the population by setting up a network of health facilities in rural districts and by creating a hierarchical medical infrastructure of district hospitals and health centres. As part of the country's administrative system, this network provided indispensable, basic health services to the population, usually starting from the centre and extending out to the periphery. King (1966: 2: 4, 2: 5) has pointed out the great advantage of this *referral system* through which the treatment of patients in outlying rural areas is cheaper than at a central point: '*This system is based on the idea that patients are to be treated as close to their homes as possible in the smallest cheapest most simply equipped and most humbly staffed unit that will still look after them adequately.*' However, because there are insufficient health centres which can treat individuals as outpatients in order to allow hospitals to concentrate on referred patients, the system often breaks down in outlying areas. Only a small proportion of the population is being treated by modern health care. This policy barely affected the problem of low coverage and in 1975, a WHO/UNICEF joint study stated that only 15% of the rural and non-privileged urban population in developing countries did have any access to health care services (Djukanovic and Mach 1975). In this context, the United Nations Development Programme (1975: 53) pointed out the '... *inability of conventional Western-inspired [models of] health services to equitably cover the population in developing countries and the failure in many cases to win the confidence of the people.*'

Navarro (1974: 721–742) traced the emphasis on this western-inspired conventional model of health care to the 'Flexnerian' medical model dated from the beginning of the century: the medical doctor occupies a central position within a type of health care organised around medical services and biological, clinical laboratory work. Another disadvantage of the referral system is the fact that it is geared to providing curative care which is expensive and often only temporarily effective (Van Amelsvoort 1979). As a result, preventive measures which are often necessary and of a more permanent nature are not possible because of the limited funds available to rural health care institutions. Were (1978: 7) who arrives at a figure of one health care organisation per 35,000 sq. km in the northeastern province of Kenya, notes with regard to patients: '*If they utilise the facility at all, it is as a last stage before almost certain death. This makes the service non-existent to the majority of the people.*' She concludes: '*Hospitals then acquired the reputation of killing people.*' Despite the fact that efforts have been made to put modern health care staff on a more active basis outside the confines of official buildings and the introduction of more mobile health services during the seventies, the attempts by the health authorities to provide better care in rural areas have not produced the expected results. A considerable stumbling-block is the fact that health services were not used or called in for what Were (1978: 7) describes as '*. . . a base for mobilising people's interests and efforts in health care.*' Because of the consistently urban location of these services, both the geographical and the socio-cultural distance to the rural population even has increased.

In the course of the seventies, it became increasingly apparent that facility-based health care with its emphasis on curative care and professionally trained staff was not coping adequately with the problem of the stagnating distribution of modern health care in rural areas. With the medical knowledge and financial resources available it remained impossible to achieve a significant improvement in the scope of health care in developing countries. This led to the realisation that alternative approaches were necessary in order to bring more health care within the reach of the total population.

## Community-oriented approach

About a decade ago the limitations of facility-based services became more and more apparent and were widely acknowledged. Health care became increasingly intertwined with socio-economic and political considerations, whereby emphasis came to be placed on an integrated approach to development from within the community itself widely known as the community-oriented approach. Attempts were made to obtain a new kind of ancillary staff at village level in outlying rural areas in order to devote more attention to preventive rural health care. These 'village health services' as they were called, were still provided by the medical services but also covered a number of other provisions such as immunisation, maternal and child health, improved water supply, sanitation and health education.

The involvement of the community in health care, which initially was considered merely desirable, soon came to be seen as a necessity. Although there exists a general consensus about the importance of public involvement in health care, there is no unanimity among experts and authorities about the way in which the population can become involved in such health-promoting activities. Rifkin (1981: 378) attempts to divide the different views, ideas and opinions on public involvement in health care into four categories. She adds two recent approaches to the classic concepts of 'public health' and 'community development': *self-care* and *health planning*. While 'public health' concentrated mainly on controlling and eradicating infectious diseases, with medical doctors and sociologists often working together on the engagement with the community, 'community development' has placed greater emphasis on mobilising local groups (grassroots people) to take part in decisions and activities affecting daily life. Health is regarded as a human condition rather than a state achieved through medical service. Advocates of involving the local population in the provision of self-care are keen to point out the inadequacy of health care provided by professional medical staff and urge the organisation of self-care groups. Based on the idea of mutual service, such groups attempt to harness the combined efforts of those involved with the aim of finding solutions to common problems of illness and disease (Robinson and Henry 1977).

The fourth approach, 'health planning', is based on the idea that the coverage of health care can be improved by exploiting additional resources in terms of manpower, finance and materials within the community itself. Its main objective has been to achieve better utilisation and development of health care by using the hitherto untapped resources of the community (Rifkin 1981: 380). Here it should be noted that planning the involvement of the whole community in health care implies on the one hand that non-professional, human resources can be used and on the other, that better use can be made of existing medical services.

### *1.4.2 Primary health care towards 'Health for All'*

In 1977, the Thirtieth World Assembly declared the main social goal of all governments and WHO for the coming decades to be the attainment of 'Health for All by the Year 2000', encompassing a process that eventually will lead to a progressive improvement in the health of the entire world population. Despite differences in health status, morbidity patterns, type of health system and state of socio-economic development in any country, all people should then have a level of health that: '. . . *will permit them to work productively and to participate actively in the social life of the community in which they live*' (WHO 1979: 9). The key to attaining this goal of 'Health for All' is Primary Health Care (PHC) which was defined at the International Conference in Alma-Ata (WHO/UNICEF 1978: 3) as:

> *Primary health care is essential health care made universally accessible to individuals and families in the community by means acceptable to them through their full participation and at a cost that the community and country can afford. It forms an integral part of both the country's health system of which it is the nucleus and of the overall social and economic development of the community.*

The adoption of the primary health care approach implies the establishment of such a new form of health care system with primary health care as the central function and main focus supported by the rest of the system.

The involvement of the members of the community then becomes an important starting point for a more equitable distribution of health services and improved use of them, together with the mobilisation and deployment of new types of health care workers. Not only ancillary staff such as 'medical assistants' and 'primary health workers' are to be involved in rural health care, but non-professionals such as laymen and traditional and transitional healers are also to be part of an integrated system of national health care. A number of recent studies have shown that traditional medicine is an important and operational element of many cultures and that it also provides the most important form of health care for the majority of the population of the Third World.

With regard to the idea of integrating traditional and modern medicine it should first be stipulated that there is no fundamental conflict between the two systems as far as the population is concerned. It is also important to realise that the 50 to 80% of the population which cannot use modern health care, rely on traditional medicine. Consequently the low coverage of modern health care services has created a need for new approaches in response to traditional ideas, practices and perceptions which are prevalent among the population at the present time. The potential role of traditional healers in the official health system is explicitly referred to in the declaration of the WHO/UNICEF Conference (1978: 63) as part of the concept of primary health care: '. . . *these indigenous practitioners become important allies in organising efforts to improve the health of the community.*'

As to the related use of traditional medicines, WHO has estimated that 80% of the world's population mainly rely on local drugs for their primary health needs (cf. Farnsworth 1985). Despite divided opinions among scientists and policymakers in favour or against the incorporation of traditional medicine in national health care systems, it has become clear that – apart from experience of successful integration in the People's Republic of China, India and a number of nations in Africa – utilisation of local medicines and practitioners has accentuated the significance of the two previously mentioned arguments of self-care and health planning for the improvement of the global health situation. It is only through the main objective of the Primary Health Care approach of community involvement, that essential health care indeed can be made universally available to the entire population.

Recent research into the potential contribution of indigenous healers in developing rural health care in Ethiopia, which is beyond the scope of the present study, shows that under specific conditions, the experimental introduction of certain categories of healers could lead to improved coverage by a new syncretic form of national health care (Slikkerveer 1982).

In the Horn of Africa, the general importance of the role of the community in socio-economic development was first recognised and implemented in rural areas in Ethiopia after 1974 as part of the new idea of *Hebretesabawinet* (Am.) or 'Ethiopian socialism'. After the revolution, new government policies on national development were aimed at involving the entire population in expanding and improving local community services (Andargatchew Tiruneh 1981). The ideas of *Harambee* in Kenya and *Ujamaa* in Tanzania (Mbithi and Rasmusson 1977) expressed similar, politically oriented approaches. Although the new policy also involved improving facility-based services, on the whole, coverage of the rural population has only marginally improved. However, it did become apparent that the problems will not be solved only by mere re-allocation of financial resources but rather by gearing health care to the actual needs of the community.

On the basis of first results and experiences in Primary Health Care, at both national and international levels the need has recently been expressed for further research on the contribution of traditional systems of medicine, especially in developing countries. The high priority of health services research and operational studies in improving health care has also been emphasised by the WHO/UNICEF International Conference on Primary Health Care (1978: 29), in paragraph 16:

> *The Conference ... recommends that every national programme should set aside a percentage of its funds for continuing health services research, organise health service research and development units and field areas that operate in parallel with the general implementation process ....*

Later on, in 1982, a WHO Study Group on Research for the Reorientation of National Health Systems stressed this crucial relationship of a wider interest in health systems – known as *health systems research* – as the goal of member states of WHO to achieve health for all. In particular, the population survey, an important issue in this type of research, not only deepens the understanding of patterns of utilisation of different kinds of health services by a population, but relating health care utilisation to cases of illness reveals the volume of unmet needs, identifying illness or disability for which only self-medication or no specific care has been sought: '*The extent of unmet health needs in a population can provide a foundation for health planning*' (WHO 1983: 19). With such WHO commitment to research on help-seeking and utilisation behaviour in different regions of the world within the context of Primary

Health Care development, part of the present study will provide data on the socio-economic and cultural background of the utilisation process in the Horn of Africa, based on a longitudinal population survey in Babile.

## 1.5 Implications of the 'Rural Health in Ethiopia' Project

Prior to the present study, applied medical social science research was conducted in Ethiopia from 1974–1978 as part of the 'Rural Health in Ethiopia' project (RUL 22). Its main purpose was to support government health policy and it resulted from the cooperation between the Institute of Development Research of the University of Addis Ababa and the Institute of Cultural and Social Studies of the University of Leiden, under the guidance of Dr. Assefa Mehretu and the late Professor R.A.J. van Lier. It was financed by the Netherlands University Foundation for International Cooperation (NUFFIC). It was carried out in the Highlands of Hararghe by the present author in cooperation with Dr. W.F.L. Buschkens from our Leiden Institute of Cultural and Social Studies, assisted by Dr. Nagi from Dire Dawa and a team of Ethiopian fieldworkers. During the research project, the illness behaviour of the Eastern Oromo was analysed from a medical-sociological perspective with a view to providing recommendations for future health planning in Ethiopia (Buschkens and Slikkerveer 1982: 118–127).

The most striking result of this study among the highland population which numbers roughly two million, emerged from the household surveys in five different villages, and was the fact that only a small proportion of cases of illness were treated at a government health institution in the area. Under-utilisation of modern health services by the *Kottu*-Oromo (peasants) became apparent from the fact that health stations, health centres and hospitals in the area were not functioning optimally. On the basis of the available statistical medical data, extremely low utilisation rates were calculated of less than *one visit per year per person* to an available health institution. In this way it was established that in Ethiopia, with its present pattern of morbidity and mortality, there exists an almost unacceptably high degree of under-utilisation. In comparison with observed utilisation rates in urban areas it was established that under-utilisation of modern health care in Ethiopia is greatest in rural areas

(Comprehensive Health Service Directory 1977: 212). The concept of access was used, among others, to analyse in depth the under-utilisation which emerged from the population study among the Highland Oromo. This is a sociological concept which has received a good deal of attention in recent studies of behaviour of population groups in the Third World in relation to the development process as a whole (Schaffer 1975; Buijs 1979; Galjart *et al.* 1982). A number of such studies have shown that certain population categories, particularly the poor, ethnic and cultural minorities and rural communities make no use or insufficient use of services provided by the government such as housing, education, loans, agricultural extension, and health care. Government services are often under-utilised because the distance of barrier between institutions and the population is too great.

During this previous research in Hararghe, the whole process of illness behaviour has been considered in terms of a functional relationship between modern health care services as 'producers' on the one hand and the rural population as 'consumers' of medical care on the other. The relationship was expressed in terms of *distance*, the size of which was determined by the characteristics of the population and also by the quality and nature of the services provided. By analogy with the results of recent research into access and participation in developing countries, three aspects or dimensions of distance can be distinguished: geographical dimensions, economic dimensions and socio-cultural dimensions (Buijs 1979). Working on the assumption that the extent of health care utilisation is an expression of the size of this distance, it has become possible to analyse the concept in more detail in terms of various factors which influence the utilisation behaviour process. The concept of *distance reduction* was subsequently introduced as a planning instrument for policy recommendations to improve health care in an attempt to reduce the geographical, economic and socio-cultural distance between government services and the local population in Ethiopia (Buschkens and Slikkerveer 1982: 118–127).

The implications for the present in-depth study as a first follow-up to the 'Rural Health in Ethiopia' Project can be summarised as follows:

> utilisation by the population of Babile of various forms of health care will likewise be analysed in terms of traditional, transitional and modern medical systems;

the problem of under-utilisation of the modern medical system in the research area will be examined more closely in the context of the overall pattern of health care utilisation of all available systems;
on the basis of the theoretical orientation of geographical, economic and socio-cultural factors affecting utilisation, an attempt will be made to interpret the interaction between these factors and a range of additional factors in order to establish the basis for a more elaborate, multivariate model of transcultural health care utilisation;
in keeping with the recommendations formulated earlier to improve health care among the Oromo, an additional attempt will be made to draw conclusions regarding future health care planning for different ethnic groups in the Ethiopian-Somali borderland.

## 1.6 Structure and Arrangement of the Book

In order to achieve the objectives formulated earlier, a description and analysis will be made of the historical, economic and socio-cultural context of illness and disease in this part of the Horn of Africa, based on research into existing resources and fieldwork carried out in the multi-ethnic community of Babile. The historical processes of internal differentiation and external interaction will serve as the background to the process of seeking and obtaining health care within the specific context of the complex present-day society of Ethiopia as a plural society in this part of Africa.

More specifically, Chapter 2 deals with the theoretical orientation of the study, developing the ideas discussed briefly above concerning the objectives of the research, the development of health care in the Third World, and the role medical social sciences can play here. Concepts such as illness behaviour, health care utilisation, medical pluralism, multiple utilisation and under-utilisation are discussed in more detail. The conceptual framework is based on the assumption that various factors influence the complex process of utilisation of medical systems. A brief review of the literature discusses medical-sociological hypotheses and models based on research in the West. Particular attention then is paid to recent studies of health care utilisation in the Third World. In addition, the methodological shortcomings and the potential for analysing this kind of research in developing countries are indicated. The chapter concludes with an account of the methodological framework within which an adapted, analytical model of transcultural health care utilisation can be developed for the situation in Africa as well as in other parts of the Third World.

Chapter 3 describes the socio-cultural context within which utilisation of health care takes place. It gives a brief account of the process of historical development in Ethiopia and the Horn of Africa as an example of a plural society. In addition to a description of the administrative region of Hararghe as a borderland between cultures, an assessment is given of the process of transculturation which, as a result of successive culture contacts and waves of migrants has established the present complex situation in this part of Africa.

Chapter 4 gives an account of the general situation in the research area of Babile. After describing the research and the sample survey, it presents fieldwork data on the community's demographic structure, its ethnic and religious composition, family system and housing together with its economic life and occupational structure. The chapter also contains a brief description of the regional pattern of illness and health. By comparison the results of a study of indigenous classification of disease among the main ethnic sub-groups of Babile will be presented.

Chapter 5 describes the complex and plural character of the health care situation from a historical, socio-cultural perspective. The phenomenon of medical pluralism, made up of various systems in this part of Africa, is developed on the basis of relevant criteria. In this way, the pluralistic medical configuration in Babile is analysed in terms of 'traditional', local Cushitic medicine, regional Arabic and Amhara medicine, 'modern' cosmopolitan medicine and 'transitional' pharmaceutical medicine. Further to indigenous perceptions and practices, a typology of the various types of healers is presented.

Chapter 6 describes the patterns of illness behaviour and health care utilisation of the plural medical system by local population groups and goes on to deal with various factors closely associated with the utilisation process. Phenomena such as differential health care utilisation of the plural medical system and under-utilisation of the 'modern' health facilities in the area are dealt with in detail in view of increasing public health problems among the population.

Chapter 7 introduces a descriptive bivariate analysis of

determinants of utilisation followed by a multivariate analysis in an attempt to interpret and explain the interaction between the various factors regarding utilisation. This renders possible identification of dominant factors as important determinants of transcultural utilisation. As a result, the model can be refined and, more importantly, it can acquire general explanatory value.

Finally, Chapter 8 contains a summary and the conclusion of the study. The implications for medical anthropological and sociological research in developing countries and for planning and improving health care in the Third World, particularly in the Horn of Africa, are also indicated.

## Notes

1. The impetus to start basic research into the plural structure of health care in developing countries was given by Charles Leslie (ed.) among others with the special editions of *Social Science and Medicine* on 'Theoretical Foundations for the Comparative Study of Medical Systems' (1978) and 'Medical Pluralism' (1980).
2. Important studies of the major traditional medical systems of China and India include *The Health Care Delivery System of the People's Republic of China* (Sidel and Sidel 1975); *Asian Medical Systems: a comparative study* (Leslie (ed.) 1977); *Culture and Healing in Asian Societies* (Kleinman *et al.* (eds.) 1978); *Chinese and Western Medical Care in China's Rural Commune: a case study* (Rance 1981); *The Ayurvedic System of Medicine in India* (Udupa 1975) and *Susto, a Folk Illness* (Rubel, O'Neill and Collado-Ardon 1986).
3. In recent years, there has been a good deal of interest in medical, anthropological and sociological research into the integration of traditional healers into official health care in the Third World. Bannerman (1977) drew up a special programme to study traditional medicine for the World Health Organization, in which he formulated a number of specific objectives. In 1981, the Society for Applied Anthropology (AAA) held a symposium in Scotland entitled Utilisation of Indigenous Healers in the National Health Delivery Systems, as a result of which a special edition of *Social Science and Medicine* was published (McEwan 1982, vol. 16 No. 21) with the same title. It

contains, inter alia, an account by Slikkerveer of the problems of involving various categories of traditional healers in Ethiopia (1982: 1859–1872). Reports on a number of experiments in this field are available: on Indonesia (Peng *et al.* 1974), India (Jeffery 1982), Zaire (Bibeau 1982; Yoder 1982) and Ghana (Warren *et al.* 1982) among others. Bannerman, Burton and Ch'en Wen-Chieh (1983) edited a comprehensive manual for WHO on *Traditional Medicine and Health Care Coverage* for developing countries, providing a clear understanding of the functioning of traditional medical systems and their role in primary health care.

4. Ethnomedicine is now one of the major fields of interest of medical anthropology and a number of publications have recently appeared on the subject. They include *Culture, Disease and Healing; Studies in Medical Anthropology* (Landy, (ed.) 1977); *Health and the Human Condition; Perspectives on Medical Anthropology* (Logan and Hunt 1978); *Medical Anthropology* (Foster and Anderson 1978); *Foundations of Medical Anthropology* (Zimmerman 1980) and *Indigenous Knowledge Systems and Development* (Brokensha, Warren and Werner 1980).

# 2

# Theoretical Orientation and Analytical Model

## 2.1 Research into Utilisation of Health Care in the West

This chapter develops the ideas put forward in the Introduction concerning the interface between the medical-biological sciences, the social sciences and the planning of health care. It begins with a short account of the important research which has been conducted in this connection into the utilisation of health care in the West. After a short review of recent utilisation studies in the Third World, it goes on to deal with the specific nature of research in this field on the basis of processes of socio-economic change, transculturation and multiple utilisation of plural medical systems used in the study.

### *2.1.1 Health, illness, illness behaviour and health care utilisation*

As a result of recent developments within Western health care, a number of questions have been raised and problems have arisen which the social sciences could help to solve. Such developments include the shift from an acute to a chronic morbidity profile of the population, the widening of the definition of illness and the concept of health, the developments in preventive health care, the exponential growth of welfare services and mental health care, and the increasing organisation and planning of health care in order to make it more relevant to society (Nuyens *et al.* 1973).

Whilst these problems have arisen in the field of health care, the social sciences, and in particular medical sociology have become increasingly preoccupied with questions arising from health care delivery. This has happened in two ways: on the one hand by emphasising the socio-cultural context of illness, and on the other by devoting attention to the organisation and administration of health care services. The first of these approaches, sociology in medicine, has produced a number of studies of social and cultural factors which influence illness as well as several studies of the medical treatment and the social consequences of illness (Strauss 1957: 200–204; Susser and Watson 1971). Generally speaking, the approach can be characterised as applied scientific research which was initiated primarily in response to a medical problem situation. The tradition of the sociology of medicine is, however, more concerned with formulating sociological theory on the structure of medical services and the role and training of health manpower within various kinds of medical institutions. Concepts such as organisation, cost, role relationships, norms, standards, values and attitudes in relation to medical practice have been studied as factors of human behaviour (Strauss 1957: 200–204; Van Etten 1976: 11; Mechanic 1978: 516; Rosengren 1980). An important question arising in society at large at the present time in relation to medical sociology concerns the social inequality of health care. Despite developments such as democratisation, social levelling, participation, etc., affecting society as a whole, fundamental inequality apparently still persists in the practice of health care. In addition to the unequal distribution of the risk of illness and death per se among individuals and groups (the differential morbidity and mortality pattern), medical services are used to an unequal extent by the individuals and groups concerned. This indicates different types of illness and health behaviour known as 'differential health care consumption'.

As has been noted in 1.4.2, initially, and in particular within medical circles, it was expected that when illness created a demand for consumption, the patient/consumer would behave in accordance with a simple linear model, which can be expressed as follows:

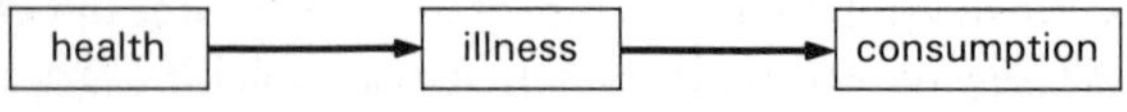


At an early stage, however, it became clear that this process is in fact much more complicated and is being influenced by a number of non-medical factors. This section examines the different ways in which the concept of illness is defined and perceived, how medical demand is influenced by a large number of factors and finally the way in which medical services themselves produce differential consumption. First, the social dimension can be seen in the definition of 'health' by the World Health Organisation as: '*a state of complete physical, mental and social well-being and not merely the absence of disease and infirmity* (Mead 1953: 28). Then, crucial to the study of this process, there is the difference between an objective and a subjective description of ill-health, accurately conveyed in English by the terms disease and illness. While disease literally means 'morbid condition of body' and refers to a condition which can be identified by objective scientific criteria, illness on the other hand refers to an 'unhealthy condition of body' and involves a subjective assessment of the individual feeling unwell (Twaddle 1981). In addition, sickness refers to the social dimension in terms of the ability or failure to meet the obligations of society. Social patterns of interaction between the sick person and the group change when illness appears and the sick person can no longer fulfil his social roles, either wholly or partly. In this sense, illness is not simply an individual condition but a social process accompanied by a specific type of behaviour known as illness behaviour. Existing medical-sociological literature also regards it as a social process in which the sick person goes through a number of stages. Bank *et al.* (1973: 24), for example, emphasise the series of identities which the patient experiences during the course of illness. The authors describe the transition from health to illness as follows:

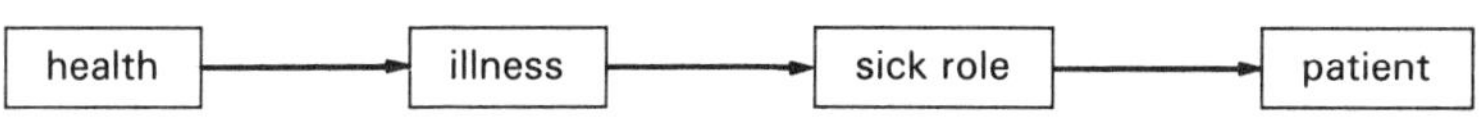


After observing the symptoms of illness, the individual accepts the sick role because his social roles are limited, seeks help from a medical service and finally assumes the role of patient.

Suchman (1964: 114–128) distinguished at an early stage of these discussions between five stages of illness and medical care: 1) *symptom experience*; 2) *assumption of the sick role*; 3) *medical care contact*; 4) *dependent patient role*; 5) *recovery and rehabilitation*. Looking at these five stages, it appears that from the first perception of symptoms, when the individual has not yet taken any action, a succession of events occurs which can ultimately lead to total recovery. Each stage gives rise to specific problems which can result in a choice between various forms of alternative behaviour.

In this context, Nuyens *et al.* (1973: 16) correctly observe that the importance of Suchman's classification primarily consists in rendering illness capable of being described as a dynamic process of successive choices from alternative forms of behaviour. The explanatory aspect of illness behaviour is illustrated by Nuyens *et al.* (1973: 16) in a similar fashion:

> ... *if we take into account the fact that this selection of alternative forms of behaviour or the decision to switch to another form of behaviour is not only dependent on the illness as a biological fact but is partly determined by the various social positions of the individual concerned, in other words, by social, socio-cultural determinants.*

The key influence of socio-cultural determinants on Suchman's first stage of 'symptom experience' has been described in detail in the medical-sociological literature and will be introduced later in the present study as a factor of perceived morbidity in the analytical model. The classic studies by Koos (1954) of health behaviour in Regionsville, a district of New York, showed that perception and interpretation of illness are heavily influenced by social factors, and by the subsequent action taken to seek and obtain treatment. Bice and White (1969) in their comparative study into the use of health care in the United States, Britain and Yugoslavia also came to the conclusion that in the event of symptoms and limited activity by patients, of eight variables examined, perceived morbidity had the greatest influence on the variation in the number of visits to the doctor.

The socio-cultural determination of the process of illness is also expressed by the stage at which use is made of the available medical help. The problem of social inequality among individuals and groups regarding the accessibility of health care presents itself particularly at the symptom stage, the stage of assuming the sick role and the role of patient and that of seeking and obtaining medical help. Therefore, this study will concentrate primarily on these aspects and illness behaviour will constitute a major focus.

Kasl and Cobb (1966: 246) define 'illness behaviour' as '... *an activity undertaken by a person who feels ill to define the state of his health and discover a suitable remedy.*' For the sake of clarity, health behaviour should also be mentioned here: this refers to an action taken by an individual to prevent illness or to discover it at the presymptomatic stage (Kasl and Cobb 1966; Douglass 1971; Behets and Vermost 1972). The latter type of behaviour includes regular health examinations and check-ups, preventive or health-promoting measures and participation in vaccination campaigns. McKinlay (1972) speaks of the 'help-seeking career', defining it as: '*the sequence of stages typically passed through by a person with a real or perceived problem who is on the way to treatment, recovery, rehabilitation, or perhaps even death.*'

More recently, McKinlay (1981) discusses a series of stages in the help-seeking career, divided in two main parts, the *prepatient phase* and the *patienthood phase*. Since it is the transition from one to the next phase that provides the crucial intersection between the 'informal' and 'professional' networks taking care of the patient, the influence of social networks on morbid episodes is indicated in several studies (cf. Cassel 1970, 1974; Cobb 1976; Kaplan *et al.* 1977).

The illness behaviour of individuals or groups generally results in a number of visits to or contacts with a medical practitioner or service. This is usually referred to as 'health care utilisation' and covers a specific type of consumption of medical services often expressed as the number of contacts with doctors and use of hospital beds or prescribed medicines over a certain period of time, for example a year. Health care utilisation can also be expressed as a utilisation ratio based on the number of visits made by patients to doctors or medical services in a year, divided by the size of the total population to which the patients belong. Within the stages of the illness process, there is a certain element of selection of alternative forms of action which, under the influence of certain factors, eventually results in a specific form of health care utilisation. It therefore follows that the volume of utilisation of different medical contacts is a function of the combined behaviour pattern of the patients in question. In other words, the pattern of medical consumption has a differential basis, determined by cultural and social factors.

The complex processes of making decisions to seek and obtain medical help have not been sufficiently identified or explained within current medical-sociological theory. Studies in Western Europe and the United States and, in fewer cases, in a number of Third World countries, have indicated a relationship between certain categories of cultural, social and psychological factors and varying levels of utilisation of medical services (Cockerham 1979). Section 2.1.2 contains a short account of recent social scientific approaches and analytical models of utilisation of medical services in the West.

### *2.1.2 Utilisation studies in the United States and Western Europe*

During the past twenty years, a large number of studies have been conducted in Western Europe and the United States into the differences in utilisation of officially recognised health care facilities. Despite these efforts, it has not proved possible to provide a definitive explanation of why some consumers/patients make use of health care services while others do not. However, there is now sufficient international literature to provide a certain degree of insight into the background to differential utilisation of health care in the West.

After Kasl and Cobb (1966) had taken the first steps towards establishing the determinants of illness and health behaviour, it was McKinlay in particular who managed to classify existing literature on utilisation in the United States and Europe and to group it into six categories. Although he restricts himself to the use of 'official' medical systems, he assumes that some of his findings could apply to utilisation of alternative forms of medicine. After identifying a number of general problems in relation to illness behaviour, McKinlay (1972) has listed a number of approaches, which has provided the base for present theories of health care utilisation, and can be summarised as follows:

#### The economic approach

A good deal of attention has been devoted to the influence of economic factors on differential utilisation. They include the cost of transport to a medical institution, the price of medical care and medicines, and the way of paying for it. The patient's income combined with these factors has produced the concept of 'financial threshold' in relation to utilisation. It used to be assumed that if the price of medical care rose and incomes went down, the level of utilisation would also decline. However, the literature reveals that in the various medical systems investigated, economic and financial factors were not the most important determinants of utilisation. McKinlay (1972) claims the weakness of the economic approach derives from its tendency to relate patients' incomes directly to utilisation. Income should be used not as a determinant but rather as an indicator of socio-economic class. He refers to earlier studies on this aspect by Kadushin (1967), Theodore (1968), McKinlay (1972: 119–120).

### The socio-demographic approach

In studying the effect of socio-demographic factors on health care utilisation, variables such as sex, age, size of household, ethnic origin, marital status, education, religion, etc. are directly linked with utilisation of health care. Various studies have shown that utilisation by women is always less than by men, that it increases with age and is less the lower the patient's socio-economic background (Morris 1967; Antonovsky 1967 and Fink *et al.* 1968). However, this approach still has not been able to provide a satisfactory explanation for differential patterns of utilisation (McKinlay 1972: 121–122).

### The geographical approach

This regards geographical proximity of medical services as an important determinant of utilisation (Lerner 1968; Stoeckle 1969). McKinlay doubts whether, for example, the initiatives in the United States to set up neighbourhood health centres would produce any increase in utilisation. He concludes that further research is needed into the actual effects of geographical proximity on utilisation (McKinlay 1972: 122).

### The socio-psychological approach

This involves relating a number of socio-psychological variables to differential utilisation, using concepts such as 'motivation', 'perception' and 'knowledge', generally favoured by psychologists to explain illness behaviour. Early studies based on this approach include those by Zola (1964), Kegeles (1967) and Rosenstock (1969). The approach also covers fear of diagnosis and treatment, the patient's attitude towards the possibility and recognition of the illness, together with his 'alienation' in relation to medical services. It concentrates primarily on the individual decision-making process in illness behaviour which is often influenced by members of the immediate family or relatives (McKinlay 1972: 122–128).

## The socio-cultural approach

The socio-cultural perspective emphasises the role of socio-cultural determinants on health care utilisation. It assumes, among other things, that life style, value patterns and membership of a social group or class influence the level of utilisation which is explained in terms of the social background of the patient (Suchman 1964, 1966; Coleman *et al.* 1966; McKinlay 1970). McKinlay (1972: 128–132) argues in this context for more sensitive research into the determinants and socio-cultural factors of illness behaviour whereby an attempt must be made to produce a more detailed explanation of concepts.

## The organisational or 'medical services' approach

In the early seventies in particular, some research concentrated on the organisation and administration of health care and the obstacles they created in relation to utilisation of medical facilities. This approach explains differential utilisation mainly in terms of differences in social class, orientation, education and lifestyle between patients and health care personnel. The rigid bureaucratic rules observed in medical institutions are also taken into consideration. McKinlay (1972: 132–138) refers to classical studies by Lefton and Rosengren (1966), Adams and MacDonald (1968), Osofsky (1968) and Walsh and Elling (1968). More recently in the United States discussions revived on the issue of designing a system of health care delivery that meets criteria such as availability, accessibility, acceptability, relevance, affordability and flexibility of services (Twaddle 1981: 126).

In the seventies, a number of studies of health care utilisation in the West showed that it was no longer tenable to assume that, in general, poor groups make relatively less use of health care (Bellin and Geiger 1972; Monteiro 1973; Sparer and Okada 1973; Galvin and Fan 1975; Kosa and Zola 1976). The important role of socio-demographic variables such as sex, age, education and marital status has been further corroborated in studies by Andersen and Barktus (1973), Wan and Soifer (1974) and Garth Taylor *et al.*

(1975). A number of authors have also analysed and developed the role of socio-psychological factors in health care utilisation (Mechanic 1972; Kirscht 1974; Becker 1974; Becker and Maiman 1975). The importance of geographical proximity of a medical institution has also been examined more closely and experimental neighbourhood centres have been set up in the United States with a view to improve utilisation (Ehrenreich and Ehrenreich 1971). Later on, the importance of the socio-political context of health care utilisation, in particular in relation to the organisation of medical services in the West, is pointed out as well (Krause 1977).

From this brief review of the founding literature on utilisation in Western countries it is clear, given the present level of medical-sociological knowledge, that it has been difficult to use one or more of the above factors or groups of factors as a basis for explaining differentiation in utilisation. As has already been mentioned in the Introduction, Denton (1978: 86) observes that more research is necessary to establish the relationship between the different variables and their relative influence on utilisation: '*Only through examining the interactions and interrelationships among the various variables can knowledge reach a level that permits us to offer conclusive answers to the question "Who seek care?"*.' It was Suchman (1965: 2–16) who took a first step towards explaining health care utilisation based on analysis of the interaction between a series of variables. His research dealt with the relationship between health, social structure, attitude to modern medicine and socio-demographic factors as compared with utilisation of health care in the United States, on the basis of which he developed an explanatory scheme of health care utilisation. Several subsequent studies based on his work have been carried out into the role of social factors in relation to medical utilisation in the United States, among others by Berkanovic and Reeder (1973: 134–143) and Geertsen *et al.* (1975: 226–237). On the whole, the promising results suggest that additional research is necessary in this field (Denton 1978: 86).

These standpoints concerning the illness behaviour of individuals and groups are most important in relation to the development of medical-sociological theory. Among those active in the applied field too, especially planners and policy-makers there has been considerable interest in developing social indicators which could be used in conjunction with economic and financial indicators to evaluate the concept of 'quality of life' (Wilcox 1972). As a result of the unequal social and geographical distribution of medical care among the population, the concept of access to medical care has become a prominent feature of many health programmes in recent years and planners have included equality of access in the objectives of their policy. In later publications too, the concept of utilisation has been modified in order to measure the degree of access to health care. A number of authors have used the concept of access to health care in their research (Beck 1973; Aday and Andersen 1975). Penchansky and Thomas (1981: 127–140) refine the concept into a relationship between clients and the medical system consisting of five dimensions.

## Models of health care utilisation

As approaches and concepts have been refined and developed in recent years, and patterns of relations between different variables have been established, theoretical models have been built to describe illness behaviour in a more holistic manner. In essence, these consist of speculative constructs describing a certain area of reality. Since, in general, the studies of health care utilisation attempt to analyse elements from empirical observation together with their inter-relations, they are referred to as formal models and formal relational systems (Lave and March 1975: 3; Dechering 1977: 9–17).

The following types of model have evolved using recent medical-sociological research in the West in an attempt to explain differences in utilisation of health care:

the socio-psychological model;
the access model;
the socio-cultural model.

The first model is based on the approach described earlier in this section of the individual decision-making process in illness behaviour. It emphasises, among other things, concepts such as fear of treatment, attitudes to health care and knowledge concerning the illness (Becker 1974; Kirscht 1974; Mechanic 1978). The second model stresses the geographical and financial accessibility of medical institutions. It regards the ability to pay the cost of health care as a very important determinant of utilisation (Greenlick *et al.* 1972; Bice *et al.* 1972; Monteiro 1973)[1].

By contrast with the access model, the socio-cultural model

stresses the important influence of social and cultural factors on health care utilisation, including the culture of the health care as an institution. As has already been mentioned, Suchman (1965, 1966) found that ethnic origin and socio-economic status were directly related to utilisation of health care. Antonovsky (1972) took this a stage further by pointing out the possibility of antagonism between the culture of the client and that of the agency providing the service. Generally speaking, the socio-cultural model emphasises the complex cultural framework in which health care utilisation takes place and which influences differentiation in utilisation. Berkanovic and Reeder (1974: 93) discuss the operation of the simple access model and conclude as follows: '. . . *there appears to be considerable evidence suggesting that cultural factors are important, independent determinants of volume, category and source of health care*' and they specify a number of areas in which cultural differences may act as barriers between health care staff and their clients. Finally, they wish to see a more complex model of utilisation involving a greater number of variables established and developed.

In the last few years, a number of research workers in this field have attempted to develop complex models by focussing their analysis on the relative influence of a series of variables on patterns of utilisation in the West. Originally the impetus to build explanatory models came from Greenlick *et al.* (1968: 298). They introduced a most promising multi-dimensional approach into this type of research laying the foundation for future development based on the hypothesis that '. . . *different sets of social, economic and situational background characteristics are significant determinants of utilisation in different disease situations.*' Andersen (1968) and Aday and Andersen (1975) developed a behavioural model of utilisation which systematically included various groups of variables. Later on, Kohn and White (1976) developed a model of relationships between systems and individual level variables for the comparison of utilisation of health services in Western Europe, and North and South America. Section 2.3 deals with the significance of these models as part of the discussion of the tentative analytical model for the present study.

Subsequently, attempts for refinement were made by applying a sophisticated methodology, such as multiple regression analysis (Hershey *et al.* 1975: 838–854; Becker *et al.* 1977: 348–366; Dutton

1978: 348–368; Van der Gaag and Van de Ven 1978: 299–312; Hightower 1978: 245–254; Berki and Aschcraft 1979: 1163–1181; Leavitt 1979: 105–112; Brunswick *et al.* 1979: 45–46) and path analysis (Shortell *et al.* 1977: 139–159; Bush and Osterweis 1978: 179–189; Williams *et al.* 313–326) in order to establish the separate and combined effects of a greater number of variables on the utilisation of health care. Studies were also carried out to place differential utilisation within a broader framework of inequity in health and health care (De Jong 1980).

The process of illness behaviour was also approached from the systems theory by Fabrega (1973) using four systems:

the biological system, which includes chemical and biological processes;
the social system, which refers to the relationship between individuals;
the phenomenological system, which concerns the individual's own consciousness;
the individual's memory system, which includes his attitudes towards and experiences of illness (cf. Kane *et al.* 1976: 17–18).

On this basis it has become possible to divide illness behaviour into a larger number of stages and to use an extensive system of factors with a cyclical character. Because of its holistic perspective, this approach, which was later elaborated by Kohn and White (1976), also has the advantage of being capable of wider application. Its significance will be dealt with in this chapter.

In short, various approaches and models of illness behaviour and the utilisation of 'mainstream' health care in the West have been developed in medical-sociological literature, based on the premise that a large number of factors play a role in the process of seeking and obtaining medical help. The approaches, however, are clearly based on one type of health care, namely the official medical system, recognised by the authorities, although increasingly it has been accepted that in most research areas alternative forms of medicine also exist. These include faith healers, herbalists, acupuncturists, yoga healers, etc. For a better understanding of the complete range of medical services it would appear to be necessary to adopt an approach which includes alternative forms of health care. At the same time it must be admitted that most models still have limited explanatory value, since they tend to stress one or two aspects of illness behaviour. In conclusion it can be argued that research into health care utilisation is very important both in terms of the development of medical-sociological theory and in the effective practice of medicine.

The next section contains a more detailed account of the development of theory regarding health care utilisation in a number of Third World countries.

## 2.2 Research into Health Care Utilisation in the Third World

Inspired by the extensive arsenal of socio-cultural epidemiological studies in the West, as described in the previous section, and by the development of applied social science research into health planning, medical anthropologists and sociologists have shown increasing interest in illness behaviour and the utilisation of health care in developing countries. However, the sophisticated research methods of Western medical sociology have not proved entirely suitable for studying and analysing the situation in non-Western societies. Research into the socio-cultural context of illness and health in these areas pre-eminently requires an anthropological approach and a specific research methodology. Moreover, the utilisation of health care has a number of special features which include the plural character of the services, the phenomenon of multiple utilisation ('healer shopping') and the extent of self-care.

The following section describes the development of research into health care utilisation in the Third World and goes on to discuss the specific methodologies involved.

### *2.2.1 Health care utilisation in developing countries*

The introduction briefly discussed the role of the behavioural sciences in medicine and health care in the Third World and referred in particular to important contributions from ethnomedicine and socio-cultural epidemiology to the development of strategies aimed at improving health care. Reference was also made to the literature review by Van Etten (1976) who mapped out for the greater part the contribution of the social sciences to knowledge of illness and health in Africa. He divides the anthropological studies of illness behaviour and utilisation into several categories, the first of which covers a research interest among peasant communities focussed on the *exclusive utilisation of traditional medicine* by the rural population. Empirical studies of this kind chiefly concentrate on local concepts of illness and disease and traditional therapy and cures. Such early studies have been carried out in Latin America and Africa (Abrahams 1959; Gerlach 1959; Press 1969; Lieban 1973).

Van Etten's second category involves research mainly concerned with the *dual use of traditional and modern medicine* in the Third World. The author (1976: 55) attritubes the rise of this type of anthropological research to the alternative use of traditional and modern medical systems within the broader framework of developments of the social sciences: '*The interest in this subject can largely be attributed to the emergence of applied anthropology and its focus on the problems of cultural and social change.*' Colson (1971) divided the various hypotheses in relation to the dual utilisation phenomenon into two categories: a) hypotheses relating to the characteristics of illness, and b) hypotheses relating to the characteristics of the patients.

As regards the first group of hypotheses, Foster (1958: 18) earlier had developed the concept of *folk dichotomy* in his study of illness characteristics, where local groups used different etiological perceptions in order to group illnesses into two categories: those with supernatural origins which were to be treated by traditional medicine and those with natural causes which were to be treated by modern medicine. The result of this division in local etiology is that urban groups were largely associated with modern medicine while the rural population tended to favour traditional medicine (Van Etten 1975: 56). The hypotheses which have been developed from the large numbers of studies into the characteristics of patients are based on the concept of acculturation, which assumes that 'modern' and 'traditional' illness behaviour are directly related to type of housing, level of education, occupation, religion and geographical mobility of the patients (Lieban 1973). The most important determinant affecting utilisation of modern health care according to this approach is the degree of modernity of the patient (cf. Benyoussef and Wessen 1974).

The two approaches from the anthropological literature described above could respectively be referred to as *rural health care utilisation* and *dual health care utilisation*. A third approach has subsequently been developed which mainly involves examining the influence of the medical system on illness behaviour. This has already been noted in the discussion of the development of medical-sociological theory concerning differential utilisation in Europe and the United States during the past twenty years. From this orientation, Foster (1958), Van Amelsvoort (1964), Van Etten (1976) and Buschkens and Slikkerveer (1982), among others, have been regarding the social distance between patients and health personnel as a factor which prevents utilisation of modern services. Van Etten (1976: 90) claims that, as far as the development of modern health care in Tanzania is concerned, changes to the medical system itself, particularly in the structure of accessibility to institutions, resulted in a significant increase in utilisation of modern facilities. In their study of 'social distance' among the rural Oromo of Ethiopia, Buschkens and Slikkerveer (1982) analyse the geographical, economic and socio-cultural distance between the target group and the modern health care facilities. In order to reduce this multi-dimensional distance in rural areas in Ethiopia, the concept of *distance reduction* has been incorporated into their recommendations of health care planning.

Several analytical models of illness behaviour in developing countries have now been developed by analogy with research in medical sociology into illness behaviour and health care utilisation in the West. It should, however, be pointed out that the special nature of these models derives from the complex health care situation in developing countries. Section 2.2.2 deals with this specific situation which is characterised by a wide range of sometimes opposite attitudes, practices and medical resources. As regards research into illness and utilisation behaviour in developing countries, Kroeger (1983: 147–148) makes a distinction between two main types of models which creates some degree of order among the extensive range of variables:

> *phase diagrams* which describe the various steps or phases of decision-making and illness behaviour;
> *determinant models* which concentrate on a series of interpretative variables or determinants of health care utilisation.

*Phase diagrams* describe the various stages of the process of illness behaviour which usually begins with the perception of symptoms and results in the use of a certain form of medical help. As the Introduction showed, Suchman (1965) established the foundations of a process-based approach to illness behaviour and health care utilisation in developing countries with his analysis of five stages. Using this framework, Fabrega (1972) described nine stages of illness behaviour in non-Western countries stressing the importance of different concepts of and attitudes towards illness. Geertsen *et al.* (1975) later introduced a revised version of Suchman's model and came to the conclusion that ethnic origin, social norms and values, attitudes concerning illness and experience of the medical system are particularly important elements of the model. Frankenberg (1976) concentrated on the socio-cultural aspect of illness behaviour and showed that it is not simply an individual action but includes social action inasmuch as it refers to the other members of the group. Finally Chrisman (1977) and Igun (1979) have devised diagrams of a series of steps in illness behaviour which are extensively described as successive stages in the course of an illness.

Generally speaking, the variables in these phase diagrams have been established by qualitative research into a series of cases of illness. Results of such studies continue to be restricted to a limited number of individual experiences of perception of illness, choice of action, use of medical help and finally recovery and rehabilitation.

*Determinant models* of health care utilisation are based on the systems approach to the use of health care and, unlike the predominantly qualitative approach of phase diagrams, classify a number of blocks of variables of constantly increasing numbers of patients. In his study of illness behaviour in Africa, Unschuld (1975: 303–312) points out the significant effect of factors such as economic barriers, communication problems and structural differences on health care utilisation in developing countries. Kohn and White (1976) subsequently developed a comparative model in their WHO/International Collaborative Study of Medical Care Utilisation, the basis for which had been established by the research into utilisation in the West.

As mentioned in Section 2.1.2, Greenlick, Jones and Pope *et al.* (1968, 1969, 1972, 1973) developed in their pioneering work in this field a multi-dimensional model which introduced background characteristics as independent variables, illness situations as intervening variables and utilisation patterns as dependent variables. Andersen (1968) and Aday and Andersen (1975), who were also mentioned in Section 2.1.2, developed a behaviouristic model of utilisation which systematically included a whole range of indicators. The latter research into utilisation of health care in the United States linked health care utilisation to a number of demographic characteristics such as age, sex, race, family income, accommodation and number of days' illness. Together with the World Health Organisation, Kohn and White (1976) developed a 'WHO model' using four blocks of variables: *predisposing factors, enabling factors, perceived morbidity factors* and *health service system factors.*

As part of the latter study, comparative research was carried out into the utilisation of modern health care delivery in twelve areas in seven countries. Predisposing factors included socio-demographic variables such as age, sex, marital status, level of education, etc., while enabling factors included the cost of medical treatment, level of income, etc. Perceived morbidity is the most important determinant of utilisation in this model while health services system factors relate particularly to the organisation of the services provided. The theoretical implications of this type of analytical model for research in the West and in the Third World and the role of a number of such determinants such as perceived illness, financial cost, availability of medical services, etc., produced a number of practical results which, in turn, had important implications for policies to improve health care in the regions studied. In general, research using determinant models, unlike that based on phase diagrams is methodologically quantitative and frequently involves analysing samples from relatively large population groups.

Recent anthropological literature has examined a number of variables or groups of variables which occur in the above models in relation to health care utilisation in developing countries. Before discussing the specific research situation in the Third World and the framework of the analytical model to be used in this study, the following section contains a short account of factors studied to date which affect utilisation of the various forms of health care in developing countries, based, among other sources, on Kroeger (1983) and the author's own research.

First, background characteristics such as *age* and *sex* have been examined and it has been shown that specific age-groups, particularly the elderly, prefer to use traditional forms of medicine. This applies for example to such countries as Ethiopia (Buschkens and

Slikkerveer 1982), Northern India (Kapur 1979), Taiwan (Baker and Perlman 1967) and Nigeria (Uyanga 1979).

*Ethnicity* and *religion* have also emerged as important determinants in various studies. Ethnic and religious affiliation have a significant influence on variations in health care utilisation, not only among emigrants to the United States (Scott 1975) but also in Guatemala (Woods and Graves 1976), Nigeria (Gesler 1979), Honduras (Teller 1973), South Mexico (Fabrega and Manning 1979) and India (Bhardwaj 1975).

On the whole, *level of education* is an important factor and would appear to be related to increasing use of modern health care. This has been shown, for example, in Thailand (Hinderling 1973), Mexico (Fromm and Macobby 1970), Iran (Mohseni 1979) and Tunisia (Benyoussef and Wessen 1974).

*Household size*, in Korea, for example, appears to be directly related to the utilisation of health care; the bigger the household, the greater the preference for traditional medicine (Seo 1976).

Although studies into the relationship between *occupation* and *socio-economic status* on the one hand and health care utilisation on the other are extremely rare, they have established in Ethiopia (Buschkens and Slikkerveer 1982), Nigeria (Gesler 1979) and Mexico (Heller *et al.* 1981) that the preference for modern health care is likely to increase the higher the socio-economic class of the individual concerned. Conversely, members of lower social classes would appear to make more use of traditional medicine, for example in India (Djurfeld and Lindberg 1975) and Colombia (Press 1969).

As regards one of the most important determinants of illness behaviour, *perceived morbidity*, studies in Nigeria (Uyanga 1979) and Zambia (Frankenberg and Leeson 1976) have shown that chronic illnesses are predominantly treated by traditional healers. People prefer to use the modern medical system to treat 'serious' illnesses, for example in Taiwan (Kleinman 1980), Mexico (Young 1981), and India (Gould 1957, 1965). Local etiological and traditional classifications of disease are important factors in this choice. A large number of anthropological studies are available in this field, particularly in relation to Latin America, Asia and Africa (cf. Kroeger 1983). As far as etiological concepts and the type of illness in Africa are concerned, reference has already been made to the concept of *folk dichotomy* introduced by Foster (1958).

*Patient satisfaction*, which relates to the result expected from medical treatment, has also been investigated as a potentially important determinant of utilisation of a specific medical service. Its significance has been confirmed by research in Mexico (De Walt 1977), New Guinea (Feacham 1973) and India (Bhardwaj 1975).

The *geographical accessibility* of modern health care services has already been linked in the classic study by Jolly and King (1966: 2: 6) with utilisation by the local population. The authors regarded geographical distance in developing countries as a '... *critical determinant of medical care* ...'. On the basis of quantitative material they showed that the average number of outpatient visits per person per year declines considerably the greater the distance is between the clinic and the patient's home. The adverse effect of distance on the utilisation of modern health services has been shown in research in India (Ram and Datta 1976), Ethiopia (Buschkens and Slikkerveer 1982), Malaysia (Heller 1982) and Tanzania (Van Etten 1976).

Factors connected with the medical system, also include *acceptance* of the modern system by the local population, particularly of doctors and nursing staff. A series of studies has shown that communication difficulties (Lewis 1955), conflict (Chem 1975; Heggenhougen 1978) or alienation (Banerji 1979) between patients and modern health care personnel can arise.

Finally, the *power of attraction* of the modern system plays a role in utilisation by patients, particularly because of the relatively high quality of treatment. In Ethiopia (Buschkens and Slikkerveer 1982) it was found that patients by-passed the 'referral system' and went straight to hospitals for better treatment; in Tunisia (Benyoussef and Wessen 1974) the population appeared to have a preference for the modern services in the towns. Similar conclusions have been reached in Kenya (Van Luijk 1979) and Mexico (De Walt 1977) while, conversely, the poor quality of treatment in the rural areas of India (Banerji 1979), Indonesia (Young 1981) and Nigeria (Murphy and Baba 1981) discouraged the local population from using modern medical services.

*Financial cost* is not always a major obstacle to utilisation of modern health care. Although traditional medicine was found to be cheaper than modern medicine in Ethiopia (Buschkens and Slikkerveer 1982), India (Bhardwaj 1975) and Bangladesh (Sarder and Chen 1981), the reverse was true in Zaire (Janzen 1978), Kenya

(Good *et al.* 1979) and Taiwan (Cunningham 1970). To summarise, the majority of background factors appear to influence illness behaviour and health care utilisation to a greater or lesser degree. Certain categories of factors might change in the course of the socio-economic development of a particular society without outside intervention, such as education, socio-economic status and geographical accessibility. On the other hand, other important determinants could change as the result of increased confrontation between modern and traditional medicine, health care planning and government policy to such an extent that utilisation of modern health care might increase.

The above review of medical-anthropological and sociological research in this field confirms that no single comprehensive theory or method of approach has so far been developed. Although at first glance there are marked similarities between a number of basic principles of illness behaviour and utilisation in developing countries and in the West, such as the role of several predisposing factors and enabling factors, etiological concepts and traditional classifications of disease, the picture is complicated by socio-psychological factors and alternative treatment strategies. What does clearly emerge from the literature is the fact that two distinct approaches have been used: research into the phases of illness behaviour on the one hand and the studies of the role of various determinants of health care utilisation on the other. The contribution of a number of empirical studies to basic research in this field will consist primarily of developing the conceptual framework within which complete categories of independent variables can be incorporated into an analytical model.

Kroeger (1983: 156) considers that the limitations of a large number of empirical studies of illness behaviour and utilisation which exist at present in developing countries, derive to a great extent from the complicated way of compiling data, the complex decision-making process, a failure to take the influence of social networks sufficiently into account and the various forms in which health care is provided.

It would also be true to say that the majority of existing studies has had modest application to health planning and policy implementation, since most of their research has been limited to qualitative material assembled by means of the cognitive anthropological, ethnographic approach. In addition, many studies have been carried out in specific situations for the benefit of specific groups and have been conducted in the context of a largely static social context which does not take into account ongoing processes of socio-economic and political change.

Mention has already been made of the limitations of a rigid division of health care utilisation into traditional and modern medicine, ignoring the complex reality of a series of co-existing medical systems and sub-systems. In particular, little attention has been paid to the transcultural character of utilisation in developing countries, as a result of which a very one-sided picture has been created. A specific shortcoming lies in the limited attention the majority of studies have paid to separate factors or groups of factors, such as economic, socio-cultural or socio-psychological factors. Analysis of research material has tended to attribute the complexity of the illness process to simple relationships between, for example, a number of independent variables and intervening variables on the one hand and dependent variables in the form of utilisation on the other. By limiting their analysis to *bivariate relationships*, models often have retained a descriptive rather than an explanatory value. So far, the *interactional* characteristics of relevant factors have generally been overlooked. The *multivariate pattern of relationships* between the various variables and their combined effects on health care utilisation are not included in the analysis at the expense of such explanatory value which the model is seeking to achieve. Moreover, bivariate analysis has the disadvantage in this context that it does not identify the dominant factors in utilisation within the interrelation among variables. Kroeger (1983: 153) shares this view stating: '*The need for isolating simple variables from the orchestra as a whole is particularly important for health interventions.*'

The possibility of using and modifying the multi-dimensional models of determinants referred to earlier by Suchman (1965), Greenlick *et al.* (1973) and Kohn and White (1976) which make it possible to analyse the interaction between various variables, will also be examined in relation to the research in eastern Ethiopia. Prior to this, the next section describes the specific character of the fieldwork situation in developing countries, particularly in relation to medical-anthropological research.

## *2.2.2 Medical pluralism, multiple utilisation and under-utilisation*

The interrelations between the different variables which influence the utilisation of medical systems would appear to have a more complex character in developing countries than in industrial countries. Kroeger (1983: 148) points out the enormous diversity within the societies concerned: '*There exists a wider range of health services, both in quality and quantity, as well as in socio-economic conditions, such as family size, income, social networks.*' Again, changes in attitudes and practices in relation to illness and health which are the result of ongoing processes of socio-economic, political and cultural change in the Third World are also important factors.

Another extremely important aspect with regard to the situation in health care delivery in developing countries – as has already been mentioned – is the presence of several co-existing medical systems. The complex situation in a large number of Third World countries inhabited by regional or local population groups with separate medical traditions, requires a specific research methodology in order to analyse concepts of illness and health within the appropriate socio-cultural context. Medical traditions have tended to develop along the same lines as the historical processes of acculturation and transculturation between the various major cultures in the Third World. By analogy with the classic comparative study of cultural systems by Redfield (1956: 70–104) such a complex medical system may be regarded as '. . . *comprised of little and great traditions which have interacted in the past and which are still interacting today.*' Great and little medical traditions function alongside and in conjunction with one another and there is a certain amount of interdependence between them. To obtain a better understanding of the reciprocal nature of traditional and modern medical systems the concept of *transculturation* from Ortiz (1970) will be adopted for the present research.

Generally speaking, if the nature of a society in an area has been determined by different cultures and waves of immigration, the cultures concerned will have influenced one another as a result of a process of continuing contact. This process, which may be unilateral from one culture to another or reciprocal between cultures is known as 'acculturation', and has been defined by Redfield, Linton and Herskovits (1936: 203) as follows: *Acculturation comprehends those phenomena which result when groups of individuals having different cultures come into continuous first-hand contact with subsequent changes in the original cultural patterns of either or both groups.* In a complex process of acculturation between different cultures, particularly in the transitional area, there is a constant exchange of religious, linguistic, political, military, artistic, scientific and legal elements. Since the various cultures in this part of Africa have influenced one another to a great extent, it would be useful to investigate whether transculturation would not be a useful concept to analyse the reciprocal nature of successive cultural contacts. Ortiz (1970: ix) who used this concept for the first time in his analysis of the development of Cuban society, defines transculturation as follows: *It is a process in which both parts of the equation are modified, a process from which a new reality emerges, transformed and complex, a reality that is not a mechanical agglomeration of traits or even a mosaic but a new phenomenon, original and independent.* From the viewpoint of the typical transcultural situation in which health care in Eastern Ethiopia is provided, Chapter 5 will attempt to classify traditional, transitional and modern systems of health care delivery on the basis of relevant historico-geographical criteria, in combination with present phenomena of health, disease and healing.

In general, the medical resources available to the population consist of a wide range of home remedies and practices, folk healers, herbal doctors, masseurs, traditional birth attendants, spiritual healers, charlatans, drug vendors, public and private clinics, hospitals, medical doctors and specialists. In addition, in the majority of developing countries, cosmopolitan medicine has been incorporated as 'modern medicine' into the state system and a blind eye has often been turned to other medical traditions as non-formal or unofficial practices. In some cases, however, they have been declared illegal. As indicated in the introduction, several medical-anthropological studies of the interweaving of traditional and modern medicine in the Third World have recently successfully been coupled with WHO programmes for the integration of different systems of health care delivery.

In view of such diversity in traditions, institutions and patterns of behaviour related to health and illness, it is as Yoder (1982: 8) notes: '*... not surprising, then, that there is no consensus about the definition of "medical system".*' Kleinman (1973:57) has presented a conception of medicine as: '. . . *an organised system of ideas and practices concerning illness, a system which is grounded in, and derives its structure from, a given cultural context*', which later on was worked out in his model for the comparison of medical systems as cultural systems. Dunn (1977: 135) defines a medical system, or system of health care delivery as: '. . . *the pattern of social institutions and cultural traditions that evolves from deliberate behaviour to enhance health, whether or not the customs of particular items of behaviour is ill health*', stressing the medical-ecological interaction between behaviour and socio-cultural structure. In addition to Foster and Anderson's (1978) definition of medical systems focussing on the health promoting beliefs and actions, and scientific knowledge and skills, Press (1980: 47) presents a more comprehensive conception of a medical system. He defines it as a: '. . . *patterned, interrelated body of values and deliberate practices, governed by a single paradigm of the meaning, identification, prevention, and treatment of sickness*.' The operational aspect of his definition, which offers a valid basis for comparison, is that it leaves ample scope for a pluralistic perspective on different forms of health care.

Early medical-anthropological interest in the socio-cultural context of 'alternative' medicine has led to the definition of ethno-medical systems – rather distinct from biomedical systems – as: '. . . *those beliefs and practices relating to disease which are the products of indigenous cultural development and not explicitly derived from the conceptual framework of modern medicine*' (Hughes 1968: 88). Subsequently Fabrega (1977) in his conception of medical institutions follows the classic differentiation between social science research in biomedicine and in ethnomedicine, recognising, however, that the term ethnomedicine has ethnocentric connotations. The need to define the plural character of medical systems encompassing a wider variety of knowledge, perceptions, practices and behaviour related to health and disease has called for a holistic approach to the study of the socio-cultural context of both modern and alternative medical systems. In this respect, Press (1980: 45) indicates ethnomedical studies should focus on: '. . . *the ideological and cultural bases of any medical system, including the official sector of Western biomedicine*', thus essentially levelling the definitions of both medical systems and ethnomedical systems. Kleinman (1978: 85) in his model of a health care system makes a distinction between three 'social arenas' in which illness is experienced and treated: popular, professional and folk arenas. Together they form the internal structure of a national system of health care. The *popular arena* includes the immediate family, relations and the activities of the community with regard to illness and treatment. Previous studies have indicated that in both the West and the Third World, approximately 70 to 90% of all cases of illness are treated in this sector (Hulka *et al.* 1972; Zola 1972). At the same time, decisions concerning action to treat illness are largely taken in this sector. The *folk arena* is a sector in which non-professional healers operate while the *professional arena* covers modern and occasionally officially recognised traditional medicine such as Chinese, Ayurvedic and Unani medicine.

Assuming Dunn's (1977: 135) socio-cultural definition of a medical system allows the classification of complex systems of health care delivery according to their geographical and cultural setting: . . . *thus there are local medical systems, a category which can accommodate most systems of 'primitive' or 'folk' medicine; regional medical systems, such as Ayurvedic, Unani, and Chinese medicine; and the cosmopolitan medical system (often referred to as 'modern', 'scientific', or 'Western' medicine).*

He relates the complex forms of health care, in terms of different opinions, practices and officials, to the development process of the society concerned, on the basis of which he classifies local, regional and cosmopolitan medical systems within a particular society. By applying this socio-cultural approach to the wide range of medical traditions it has become possible, by analogy with the sociological concept of a *plural society* (Furnivall 1939; Van Lier 1949, 1977; Smith 1965; Speckmann 1966) yielding a specific differentiation in complex societies, to define all forms of health care in the Third World accurately, and to analyse them as plural medical systems. The concept of the plural society which was originally introduced by Furnivall (1939) as the plural economy to describe colonial societies, was developed by Van Lier (1949; 1977) in his study of Suriname into a specific description of a particular kind of society composed of different elements. The plural nature of such a society consists of differentiation in terms of ethnic origin, language, religion and economic activity. Unlike a pluralistic society which is characterised by unity of ethnic origin, language and religion within a single culture, but which consists of numerous segments as the result of far-reaching divisions of labour and specialisation, a plural society is made up of groups of people from different cultures (Van Lier 1977: 7, 8). Leslie (1978, 1980), has presented a solid basis for the pluralistic approach to the study and analysis of complex medical traditions in developing countries. Bhardwaj (1980: 209) employs a definition of medical pluralism in which the plural character of various medical principles or philosophies finds expression: '... *the synchronic existence in a society of more than one medicine system grounded in different principles or based on different world views*.' Minochoa (1980: 217–218) points out two meanings which can be attached to this idea. On the one hand it can mean: '... *the co-existence of multiple systems of medicine, including what are called folk systems, popular systems, traditional professionalised systems*...', while it can also refer to '... *pluralism in the types of personnel who contribute to the practice of modern medicine*.' On the basis of the classification of medical systems used in this study, which includes the different attitudes and practices of the population with regard to ill health, the emphasis is mainly on the response of the population to a situation of medical pluralism. Analysis of the illness behaviour which has been studied will confirm the significance of pluralism at the level of utilisation of various medical systems. The plural nature of the medical system in Babile is expressed in the local, regional and cosmopolitan medical systems which have evolved over the years, and are being used by the population in various ways. This makes it possible to abandon the fairly rigid dichotomy between traditional and modern systems of medicine in favour of a more empirical model of health care utilisation (cf. Leslie 1980).

The idea of medical pluralism is an important aspect of the study of one particular form of medicine which contains elements of both traditional and modern systems: an unofficial system of pharmaceutical medicine where, on a large scale, a commercial form of chemotherapy is often practised by illegal drug vendors and needlemen (Unschuld 1977). In their research into the utilisation of health care by the Oromo in the administrative region of Hararghe, Ethiopia, Buschkens and Slikkerveer (1982: 53) introduced the concept of a *transitional medical system* where drug vendors represent the final link in the sales chain: 'a sales organisation of the modern pharmaceutical industry which is finding a good market among the population of developing countries.' Chapter 5 contains a more detailed account of this particular system. As a result of the introduction of a plural perspective to health care, the application of medical anthropological and sociological research has been considerably widened. Information concerning alternative therapies, practices and attitudes can make an important contribution towards planning and improving health care delivery. As mentioned in the introduction a number of international programmes and symposia have recently been organised on the viability of using and integrating traditional medical systems within the official system. Moreover, the use of a pluralistic approach in studying processes of help-seeking and utilisation behaviour of various systems has introduced a new stage in socio-scientific research in developing countries. Slikkerveer (1982: 1860) divides the major hypotheses and research results of anthropological literature into three main categories and notes that, after the classic, normative approaches to the study of traditional versus modern medicine: in contrast to the (above-mentioned) rather normative view, recently a totally new approach to the perspective of medical pluralism has increasingly gained scholarly interest, especially with respect to the development of innovative views on alternative solutions in the complex field of medical care in the Third World.

Recent studies have shown that the illness behaviour of patients in developing countries with co-existing medical systems in some cases results in a characteristic pattern of multiple utilisation. In other words, patients consult several medical institutions concurrently or consecutively. Kroeger (1983: 153) comments as follows: *'The concurrent of serial use of different healing systems seems to be a typical feature of transitional societies of the developing world.'* This phenomenon of different healers treating the same illness without any process of referral between them has also been described in the literature as *healer shopping* (Kroeger 1983: 153 – 155). A similar form of utilisation has been observed as a combination of visits to both traditional and modern healers, where the nature of the illness and local etiological concepts play a particularly important role (Bhardwaj 1975; Djurfeld and Lindberg 1975; Kasteler *et al.* 1976; Greene *et al.* 1979). Buschkens and Slikkerveer (1982: 101, 103) who use the term *flow-through cases* for a number of illness episodes where patients make successive use of different medical systems, have shown that in the general pattern of utilisation, there is a slight tendency away from traditional medicine in favour of transitional and modern systems.

A problem which has a direct bearing on plural and multiple utilisation of alternative medical resources in developing countries is that which is described in the literature as under-utilisation of the modern system. Section 2.1.2 has already mentioned a number of studies of health care utilisation in the West in which differential utilisation of health care has been explained in terms of socio-economic or socio-psychological factors. In the sixties as a result of the *War on Poverty*, a good deal of attention in the United States was devoted to low-income and poverty groups who made relatively little use of health care. Wide-ranging studies such as *The Health Gap* by Kane *et al.* (1976) and *Poverty and Health* by Kosa and Zola (1976) revealed a number of barriers which result in under-utilisation of health services by specific groups. Fink (1969) analysed the under-utilisation of health care by means of comprehensive patient studies, explaining low patient ratios in terms of the inadequate functioning of medical services. In their study of utilisation of maternal and child health, McKinlay and McKinlay (1972: 369 – 381) made a distinction between utilisers and non-utilisers; the latter category referring to people who make insufficient use of existing services.

The crucial problem of population coverage has already been mentioned in relation to health care facilities in developing countries, noting in particular the inequitable distribution of health care. Although there is a great need for a national health service, a large part of the rural population appears to make little or no use of it. In view of the various co-existing medical systems in the Third World, Bryant (1971: 319) described this problem succinctly as follows: '. . . *many who need health care don't come for it and many who don't need it do.*'

Gunawan (1972) considered the problem of under-utilisaton to be the specific feature of modern health care in Indonesia. Chabot (1973: 52) concluded in his comparative study of four health centres in Java and Bali that under-utilisation of government health services in Indonesia is very high in rural areas, mainly because of the quality of the medical services provided. Morley (1976: 56, 57) divides the population of developing countries into three categories in relation to health care utilisation shown as A, B, and C. in Fig. 2.1. His extensive research leads him to the conclusion that 30 – 60% of the

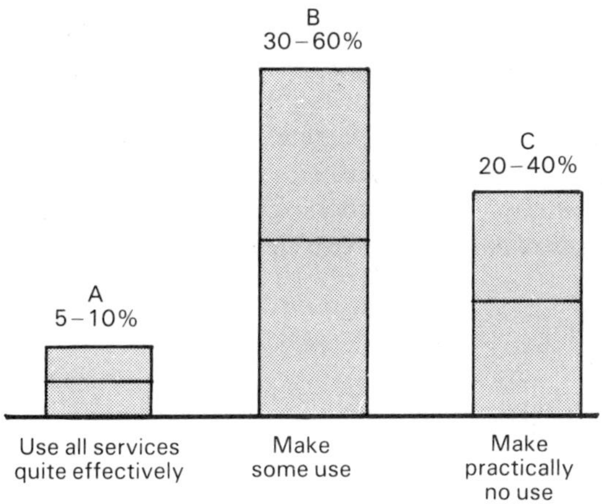


Figure 2.1: *Utilisation of health care in an average developing country (Morley 1976: 57)*

population (category B) make reasonable use of medical services, although the individuals concerned have less knowledge of modern health care than members of category A and are also from a lower economic class. Category C, which can vary in size, consists of individuals who receive very little modern health care or none at all.

Utilisation of health care is indicated by the number of contacts patients have with representatives of health care institutions, expressed in utilisation ratios or attendance rates. Because of the nature and the quality of the services provided, and because of the needs and expectations of the population, it has not been possible to establish a universally valid parameter of a desired utilisation ratio. On the basis of estimates of the need for intra-mural and extramural care, King (1966: 2:5, 2:6) stated in this connection that '... *two adult and three child attendances per person per year constitute a convenient basis for planning'*. In a relatively 'young' population as found in the majority of developing countries, where half the population is less that 15 years old, this amounts to approximately 2.5 visits per person per year. Unfortunately it must be said that such a norm, which is in any case rather arbitrary, refers to an idealised picture of the future which cannot be achieved for the time being in the Third World. WHO, realising that ultimately: '... *the inability of health services to meet the basic needs of the population might be adopted as a criterion for the underdevelopment of these services*', has established its own utilisation norm for planning and design of health care facilities in developing countries (Kleckzkowski and Pibouleau 1976: 13). Using a number of recent utilisation studies, the authors give the following *minimum utilisation threshold* for effective elementary health care:

| | | |
|---|---|---|
| 10 – 20 | preventive contacts | per 100 inhabitants per annum |
| 80 – 120 | curative contacts | |
| 6 – 8 | hospital admissions or | |
| 30 – 50 | hospital days | |

It should be remembered that this elementary health care threshold in developing countries is much lower than the demand for health care in societies with a higher standard of living such as in the West, where utilisation of modern health care is two to four times higher than in the Third World. Buschkens and Slikkerveer (1982: 107) attempt to quantify under-utilisation of the modern medical system by the local Oromo population in Eastern Ethiopia. Instead of the 'ideal' utilisation ratio used by King (1966) of 2.5 visits per person per year, they found a ratio of 0.09 which is among the lowest utilisation ratios in the Third World.

Finally, the phenomenon of self-care in the context of illness behaviour in the Third World should be mentioned. Community-based research needs to be carried out to reach a better understanding of the backgrounds of individuals who try to treat themselves exclusively by means of self-care within the family or the local community. Research of this kind is still limited, and, moreover, hampered by the absence of generally accepted definitions and concepts of lay practices, self-care, etiology, etc. However, it is true to say that self-care and family therapy have been observed in developing countries and other parts of the world on a large scale (Kleinman 1980).

With the help of the approaches and models described above which have been developed to study the complex process of illness behaviour and health care utilisation in developing countries, and in the light of the specific situation in the Third World in relation to illness and health, Section 2.3 attempts to devise a suitable approach for the present investigation based on previous research. At the same time, a tentative model will be developed especially for the research in this part of Africa.

## 2.3 The Analysis of the Health Care Seeking Process

The previous sections have reviewed various approaches and models in relation to the study of help-seeking and utilisation behaviour. A number of problems and limitations have been discussed and the specific situation in developing countries has been described by means of several examples. This section deals first with the conceptual framework which has been chosen to study the complex patterns of utilisation of existing systems of health care delivery. The analytical model of determinants of utilisation and its components will then be described at length. Finally, a tentative analytical model will be presented in schematic terms for the approach to the situation in Northeast Africa.

### *2.3.1. The systems approach to illness – and utilisation behaviour*

The utilisation of medical systems is a complex phenomenon occurring within a framework to which a general system approach applies. In principle this perspective is based on the idea that social systems and sub-systems can be taken as complex, dynamic, self-organising, selective componenents of social reality (Hoefnagel 1978). In this context, a system is taken to be a combination of elements between which a specific patterns of relations exists. Engel (1962) and Sheldon (1970) have conveniently placed the various elements and levels of utilisation of medical system within a general systems theory of disease and medical care. Within this theoretical orientation, it is possible to regard the individual as a psycho-biological sub-system interacting in an environment of external natural and social systems, as indicated schematically in Fig. 2.2. Within this pattern of relations, man's psycho-biological sub-system provides him with information concerning his internal and

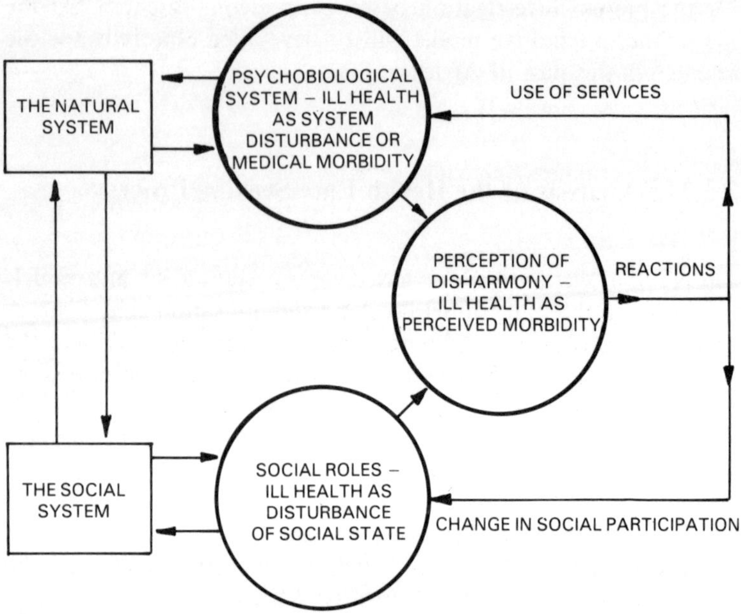


Figure 2.2: *Model of relationships between the individual and social systems (Kohn and White 1976: 11)*

external systems and enables him to use this information in decision-making and implementing behaviour.

The medical concept of illness refers to a disturbance in the individual's psycho-biological system which has been identified and classified by medicine. Perception of the disturbance in the psycho-biological system consists of a comparison of the information of symptoms with the information stored by the external systems, from which an imbalance emerges. Finally, recognition of the disturbance determines perceived morbidity which prompts the individual to act in order to remedy the situation. Kohn and White (1976: 11) include this action or series of actions within the process of illness behaviour: *The major processes of health, illness and care are . . . essentially adaptive and regulatory, and the corresponding behaviour is directed either toward the psycho-biological system through the seeking of treatment or towards altering the system of social connections or toward some combination of these.*

Earlier in this chapter the process of help-seeking and utilisation behaviour in the event of illness was described in terms of an interrelated series of stages at the individual level together with the influence of various factors on the way in which these stages develop. For the purposes of this study, the process-oriented definition of illness behaviour by Kasl and Cobb (1966: 246 – 266) mentioned earlier in section 2.2.1 is most convenient. Such a process, which is curative in character, is different from the process of consulting institutions when symptoms have not been observed and which is mainly geared towards maintaining and promoting health. This latter process is described by Kasl and Cobb (1966: 246 – 266) as health behaviour. In the context of the systems approach referred to here, illness behaviour may be regarded as a process in which the individual using health care takes action to restore the balance both in his internal psycho-biological system and in the external social system. The utilisation of health care can then be regarded as a specific form of consumer behaviour in which interaction between the individual's psycho-biological system and the social system takes place. The pattern of interaction is highly complex and is influenced to varying degrees by biological, psychological, social and cultural factors. In order to gain a better understanding of the interrelation between these processes and the influence of the various factors on utilisation of the medical system, the following section explains the model to be used in the present study.

### *2.3.2 The analytical model and its components*

Because of the specific features of health care in developing countries, such as medical pluralism, multiple utilisation and underutilisation of health care services, a multi-dimensional model is needed in order to describe, analyse and explain the complex processes of illness behaviour and health care utilisation in the specific context of the Horn of Africa.

In order to remedy the shortcomings often arising from the study of a limited series of factors, an attempt will be made to introduce more dimensions into the analysis by examining the role of various determinants in terms of *blocks of variables*. Subsequently not only the direct relationship between independent and dependent variables will be examined, but the interrelation and interaction between variables will also be considered in conjunction with utilisation. Finally, in accordance with the social reality of various co-existing medical systems, a differentiation in the dependent variables will be introduced. Thus, utilisation of the plural medical system will be divided into utilisation of traditional, transitional and modern medical systems, giving scope to the situation of transculturation in the research area.

This model has been developed on the basis of national and comparative, international experience of the application of a general systems approach to ascertain the complex forces in the utilisation of health care services in the West. Inspired on the one hand by the multi-dimensional models of Suchman (1965), Anderson (1968), Greenlick *et al.* (1973) and Kohn and White (1976) and on the other by the previous research carried out in East Africa by Buschkens and Slikkerveer (1982), an adapted model of transcultural health care utilisation has been designed to analyse a number of selected factors which to a certain extent mutually relate and interact in conjunction with utilisation of a plural medical system in Babile.[2]

The model in Figure 2.3 identifies a series of factors which interact with utilisation to varying degrees. They can be divided into a number of 'blocks' which include systems variables and variables at the individual level. In accordance with this model, relevant factors have been divided into five blocks of variables in the analytical scheme:

| | |
|---|---|
| *at the individual level:* | |
| as independent variables: | predisposing factors; |
| | enabling factors; |
| | perceived morbidity factors; |
| *at the system level:* | |
| as independent variables: | factors of the plural medical system; |
| as dependent variables: | factors of health care utilisation. |

The model identifies various blocks of factors which will form part of the analysis of utilisation behaviour. They include the above system variables of the plural medical system and the three types of variables at the individual level: predisposing factors, enabling

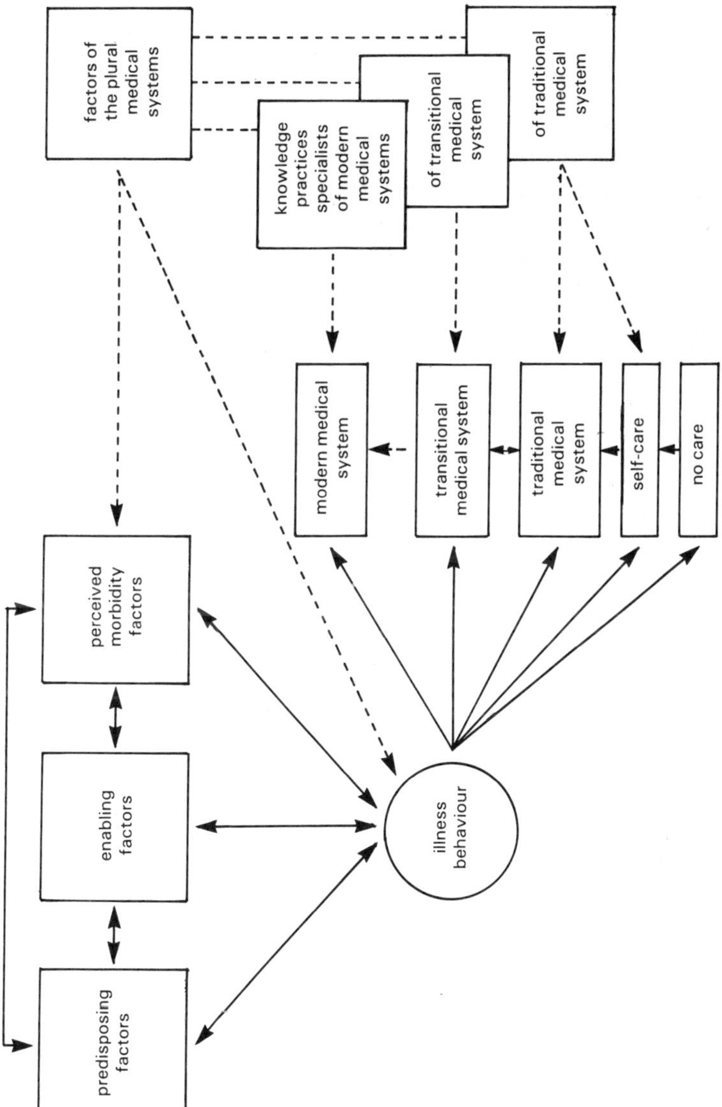


Figure 2.3: *Multivariate model of transcultural health care utilisation*

factors and perceived morbidity factors. These factors, together with the accompanying concepts, variables, indicators and categories will now be defined and described separately within the context of the various blocks of the model.

## Predisposing factors

From the literature survey presented in the previous section it can be inferred that a decision at the individual level to use health care facilities in the event of illness is influenced by a number of socio-demographic and psycho-social factors. These may either encourage or discourage utilisation of systems of health care delivery. In general they determine willingness to make use of health care services at the individual level. In the context of the present research, they comprise personal factors which reflect the socio-cultural background of the patient. Misinterpretations are more likely to arise in relation to 'soft' psycho-social factors such as opinion and attitudes, rather than 'hard' socio-demographic factors such as sex, age and education, which are largely factual. Psycho-social factors are also frequently affected by external influences. The socio-demographic factors selected for this research comprise eight variables: sex, age, ethnic affiliation, education, religion, occupation of the head of the household, size of the household and marital status. It is also clear from the literature that factors such as attitudes, opinions of health care staff and services, together with knowledge concerning the function of the individual's psycho-biological system also have a bearing on utilisation of health care. These psycho-social factors are extremely difficult to assess, but an attempt has been made to include five in the present analysis: opinions of the medical knowledge and skills of the transitional medical system, opinions of the attitude of transitional personnel to patients, opinions of the medical knowledge and skills of the modern medical system, opinions of the attitude of modern personnel to patients and the presence of elementary medical-biological knowledge on the part of patients.

Table 2.1 sets out the predisposing factors of the model and describes them in more detail.

## Enabling factors

Just as decision-making in the context of illness behaviour is influenced by predisposing factors, so enabling factors may be

Table 2.1 *Predisposing factors: concepts, variables, indicators and categories*

| concept | variable | indicator | category |
|---|---|---|---|
| socio-demographic characteristics | sex | sex | man<br>woman |
| | age | age | 0 – 15<br>16 – 25<br>26 – 45<br>46 – 65<br>66 + |
| | education | number of years of schooling | no primary school<br>secondary education |
| | ethnicity | ethnicity | Oromo<br>Amhara<br>Somali<br>other |
| | religion | religion | Muslim<br>Christian<br>other |
| | profession of the household head | profession | farmer<br>merchant<br>civil servant<br>other |
| | household composition | household size | 1 – 3 members<br>4 – 6 members<br>7 + members |
| | marital status | marital status | married<br>not-married<br>widowed/separated |
| psycho-social | attitudes towards health care | opinion on quality of the transitional medical system | no opinion<br>low<br>medium<br>high |
| | attitudes towards health care | opinion on attitude of transitional functionaries towards patients | no opinion<br>low<br>medium<br>high |
| | attitudes towards health care | opinion on quality of the modern medical systems | no opinion<br>low<br>medium<br>high |
| | attitudes towards health care | opinion on attitude of modern staff towards patients | no opinion<br>low<br>medium<br>high |
| | knowledge of own body | medical-biological knowledge | no knowledge<br>some knowledge |

Table 2.2 *Enabling factors: concepts, variables, indicators and categories*

| concept | variable | indicator | category |
|---|---|---|---|
| socio-economic status | SES | income of household, land owned, and state of house | poor<br>average<br>rich |
| financial costs | costs of treatment by traditional medical system | cost paid | none<br>– 1 bir*<br>2 – 5 bir<br>6 + bir |
| | cost of treatment by transitional medical system | cost paid | – 1 bir<br>2 – 5 bir<br>6 + bir |
| | cost of treatment by modern medical system | cost paid | none<br>– 1 bir<br>2 – 5 bir<br>6 + bir |

*1.0 Ethiopian bir = approximately US $0.5

regarded as parameters affecting the cost aspect of this behaviour which can hardly be changed by the individual. As the review of the literature shows, these refer in general to factors which determine the possibility of using health care at the individual level. In this context the patient's ability to pay for treatment, which is expressed by his socio-economic status, is considered. In addition, amounts which have been paid for medical treatment by representatives of the medical system can also be included in this category. Table 2.2 describes enabling factors in more detail.

## Perceived morbidity factors

The majority of studies into the utilisation of health care services have shown that perceived morbidity is a major determinant of utilisation. The studies of Koos (1954) in Regionsville showed already that socio-cultural determinants strongly influence the perception and interpretation of illness to varying degrees and this has subsequently been confirmed by extensive medical anthropological and sociological research. In the context of the present investigation, perceived morbidity is defined as the observation and interpretation of symptoms of illness which initiate the decision-making process of seeking and obtaining medical help. This subjective picture may conform to the objective picture according to medical standards but need not necessarily do so. Although there is a link between the two, the model employed here is based on the individual's perception of morbidity, initiating the decision-making process.

The review of the literature also discussed the socio-cultural influence on the conception of illness, particularly in developing countries. A local, traditional classification of illness may have an influence on the choice of type of health care. In addition to the objective, international classification of the World Health Organisation (WHO 1977 – 1978) a number of indigenous, etiological categories of concepts were encountered in the research area. They include 'naturalistic' etiologies which the local population regard as natural and 'personalistic' illnesses of supernatural origin often resulting from purposeful intervention of sensate agents (cf. Foster 1983). Chapter 4 contains a full account of perceived etiologies as reported during the health interview survey, presenting a disease classification of the two main ethnic groups in Babile, the Amhara and Oromo.

As regards the duration of reported illnesses, a distinction has been made between acute and chronic illnesses which can influence utilisation of health care to varying degrees. Partly using the population's own criterion to distinguish between the above categories, illnesses of up to a month were regarded as acute while those lasting from one to twelve months or more were regarded as chronic. Table 2.3. specifies perceived morbidity factors in greater detail.

Table 2.3 *Perceived morbidity factors: concepts, variables and indicators*

| concept | variable | indicator | category |
|---|---|---|---|
| perceived morbidity | illness | deviation from health and/or social dysfunction | ill<br>not ill |
| | traditional classification of illness | idem | naturalistic<br>personalistic |
| | duration of illness | idem | acute<br>chronic |

## Factors of the plural medical system

The review of the literature has indicated that the influence of the medical system on the choice of type of health care can be expressed, among other aspects, in terms of geographical or financial accessibility of the medical system. In general sociological theory, these concepts are known as *availability* and *accessibility* of services and in recent studies of developing countries they have been extended to include functional and cultural dimensions. In their international explanatory model, Kohn and White (1976) regard accessibility of health care as an important determinant of utilisation when the features of the system are constant for the individuals under investigation.

It is noticeable that the above studies are largely based on officially recognised systems of health care whilst excluding alternative systems to a large extent. In the light of the unequal distribution of health care services referred to earlier and the fact that 50 – 80% of the population of the Third World use some form of traditional medicine, such an approach renders an incomplete picture of the role of system factors in health care utilisation in developing countries. Buschkens and Slikkerveer (1982) differentiate the concept of access according to the type of medical system, i.e. traditional, transitional or modern, which makes it feasible to compare the varying degree of influence system factors have on the utilisation behaviour of the local population.

Two concepts will be used in this study for research into the accessibility of the various medical systems available: geographical accessibility and financial accessibility. Table 2.4 sets out in detail the factors of the plural medical system which will be analysed in the research.

Table 2.4 *Factors of the plural medical system: concepts, variables and indicators*

| concept | variable | indicator | category |
|---|---|---|---|
| geographical accessibility | geographical availability of medical system | geographical distance to medical system | 0 – 8 km<br>8 + km |
| financial accessibility | financial organisation of medical system | financial arrangement for access and treatment | free<br>1 bir<br>1 bir |

## Utilisation factors of the plural medical system

The systems approach shows that utilisation of various medical systems in Eastern Ethiopia essentially can be regarded as a specific form of consumer behaviour resulting from a complex pattern of behaviour and interaction between producers and consumers of medical services. Within this orientation, it is not intended here to give a more detailed analysis of the atypical nature of such behaviour which is, for example, initiated by illness, often allows few options, does not involve a fixed sum of money and to a large extent takes place outside existing market mechanisms. However, it is important to underline that the emphasis is on the determinants of utilisation of the plural medical system where it is assumed that predisposing factors and perceived morbidity factors are independent variables at the individual level, while system factors are independent variables at system level which influence utilisation of medical services as a dependent variable at the same level. Here, utilisation is measured as reported instances of contact with a medical institution or its representation as a result of illness over a period of twelve months. Since complete and accurate interpretation of reported illness behaviour cannot be obtained solely by means of health interviews, a methodology has been developed to adapt to the specific requirements of the situation in Babile: a multi-ethnic community in transition in which several types of medical systems are being used by its population. As Kroeger (1985) notes, consistency in interview answers, validity of illness reporting over recall periods and validity of reporting health care utilisation pose particular methodological problems which require a modification of current models from industrialised countries. In this respect, an attempt has been made to improve the quality of data through a combination of repeated re-interviewing, the use of lists of 'tracer conditions' together with actually following indicated illness episodes of participants in the field during the twelve months of the health care utilisation survey in the research area.

In the light of the special features – referred to earlier – of multiple utilisation of alternative, local and regional medical systems in a number of developing countries, the analysis of data is based on the total number of contacts which respondents have had with various systems in the event of illness. It refers to the total scores of utilisation at system level observed and reported by the patients in the sample. Table 2.5 shows factors of utilisation of the plural medical system specified by concepts, variables and indicators.

On the basis of the approach outlined above and bearing in mind the general limitations of this kind of research, the present study of

Table 2.5 *Factors of utilisation of the plural medical system: concepts, variables and indicators*

| concept | variable | indicator | category |
|---|---|---|---|
| utilisation of the plural medical system | contacts of patients | contacts during the twelve months of the survey | traditional, transitional and modern medical system |

health care utilisation in the multi-ethnic community in Eastern Ethiopia attempts, firstly, to make certain statements concerning the relationship between pre-selected, independent variables on the one hand and dependent variables on the other. Secondly, by applying the techniques of bivariate analysis it will be possible to describe the various factors which influence the help-seeking and utilisation behaviour of the different population groups concerned. Thirdly, with the help of multivariate techniques an attempt will be made to describe the interrelation and interaction between the independent variables in relation to the dependent variables of utilisation of health care and incorporate them in the different blocks of the analytical model. By application of multivariate analysis it will eventually be possible to identify predictors of illness and utilisation behaviour. Because the material is analysed in stages, Chapters 6 and 7 will deal in more detail with the methodological and analytical aspects of the research.

In conclusion, utilisation of the plural medical system in the transcultural situation in the Horn of Africa is a complex process, determined in principle by interaction among psycho-biological, individual systems and the social system. Analysis of the pattern of interactions and interrelations will focus on the various components of the adapted analytical model where the role of the selected factors will be examined as potentially important determinants of utilisation of health care. However, before the fieldwork data are presented and analysed, the next chapter will provide a socio-historical sketch of Ethiopia as a country in the process of development. This serves as background to the research, emphasising the transcultural and plural aspects of the society which is reflected in the complex medical world of the community as a whole.

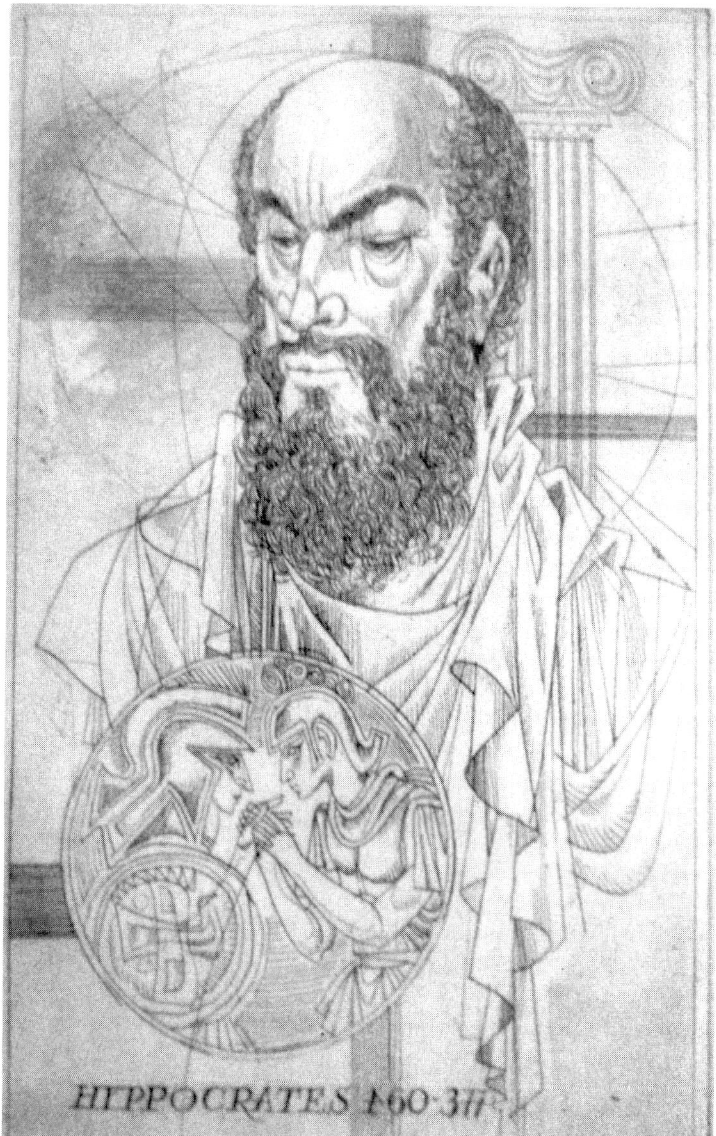


*Hippocrates of Kos (460-370 B.C.). Etching by the Hungarian artist Janos Kass (1984). Private collection of Prof. Dimitri Gutas, Crete, Greece.*

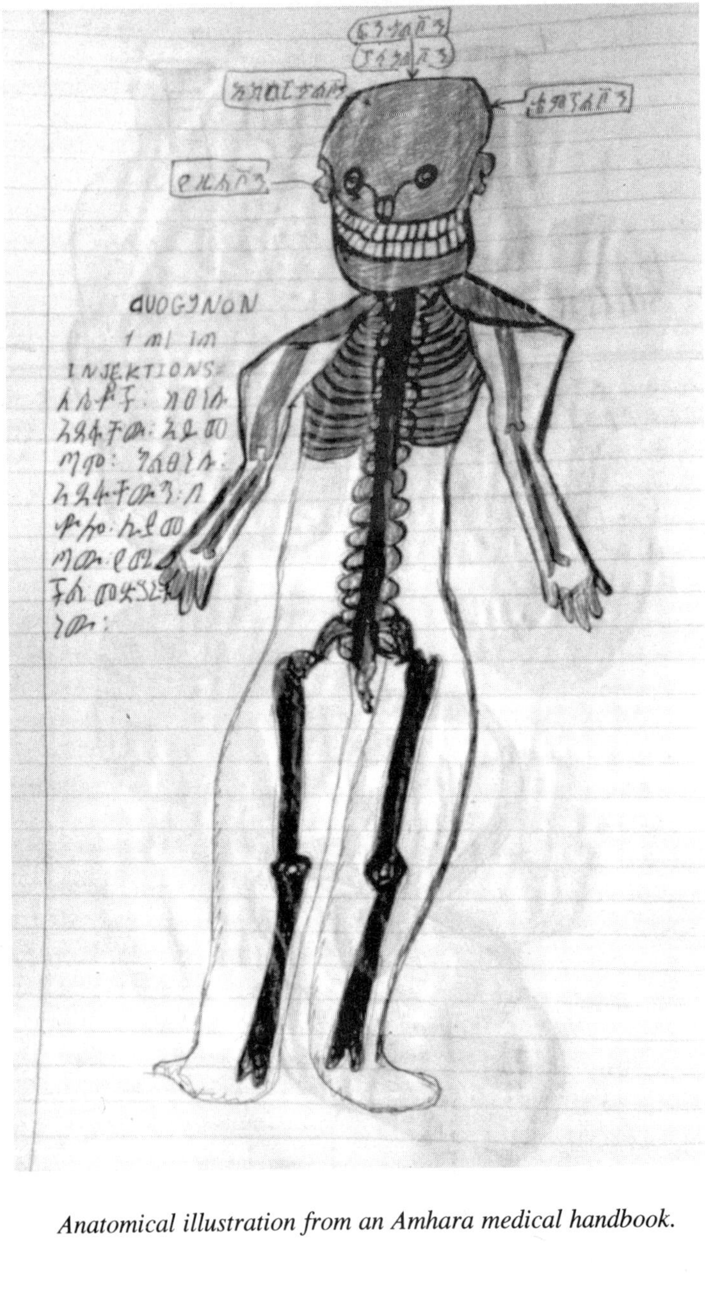


*Anatomical illustration from an Amhara medical handbook.*

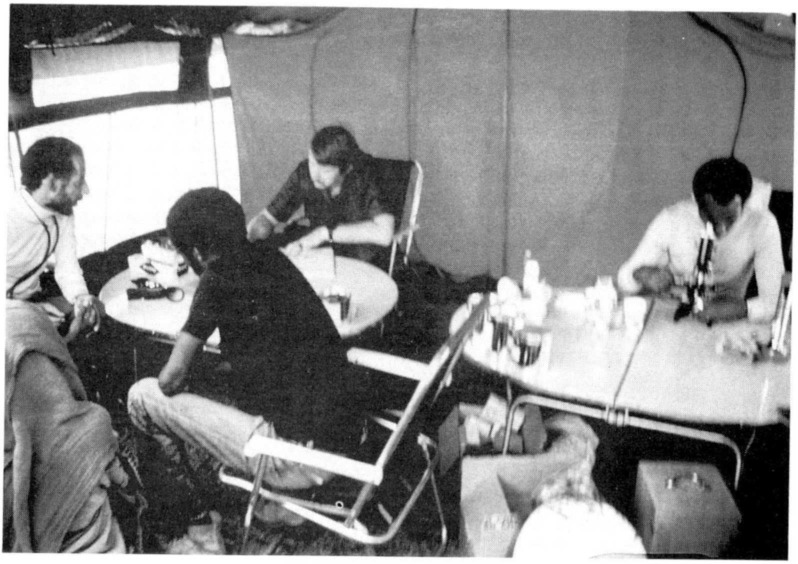

*The field team conducting a health survey in the research tent.*

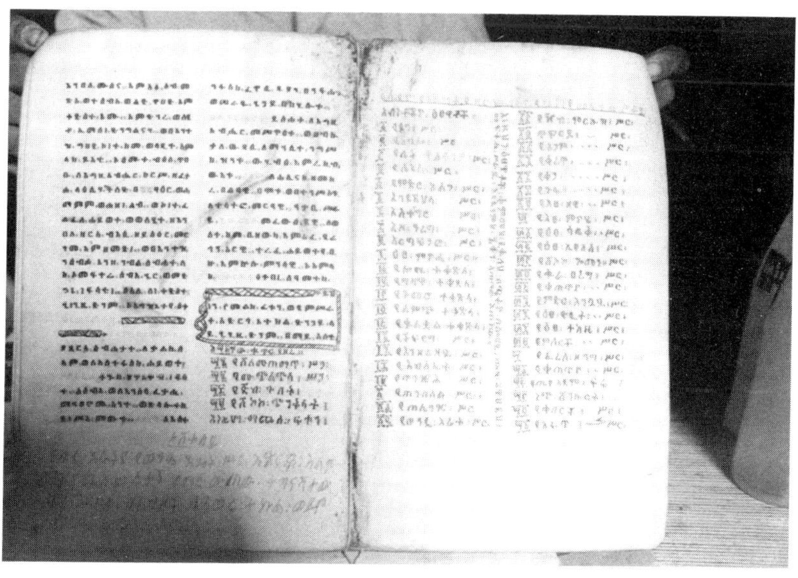

*Two pages of a medical textbook of the 'meshaf-gelach'.*

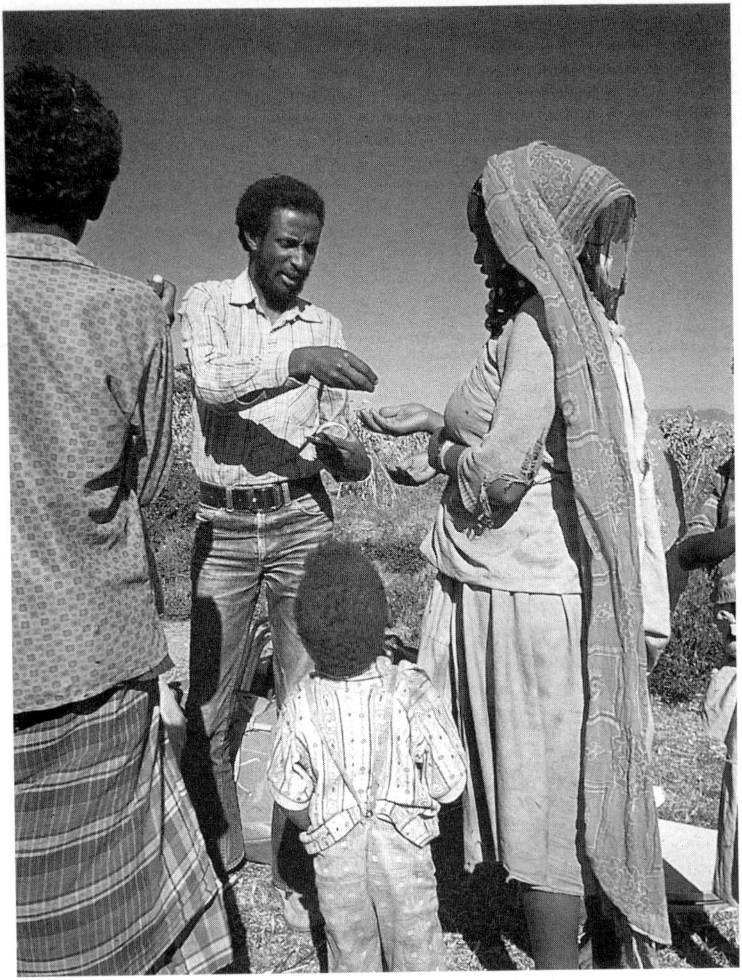

*Handing out medicines during the household surveys.*

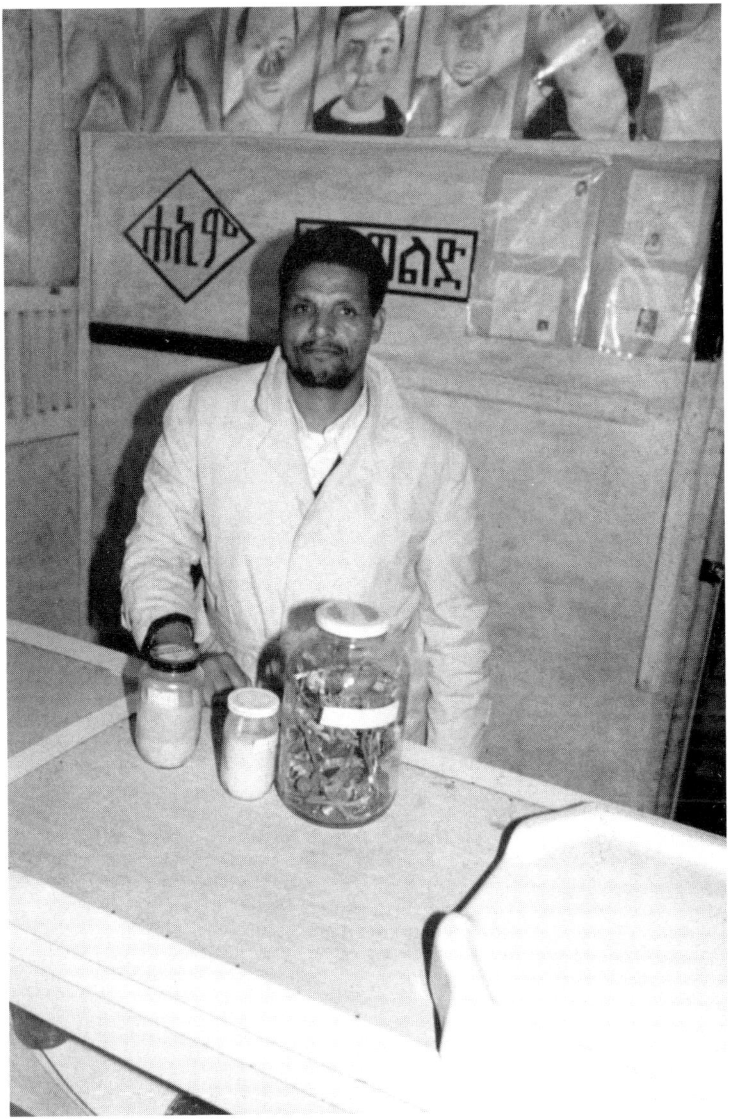


*A medehani tenija showing some of his traditional medicines in his clinic.*

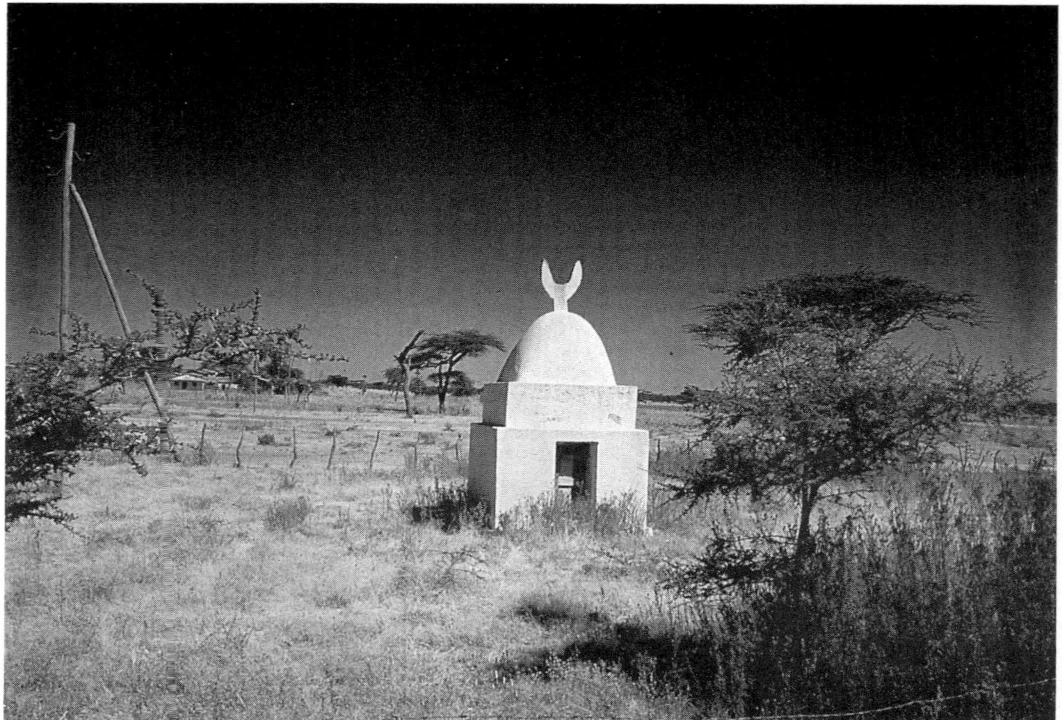

*The tomb of Sheikh Hussein, a local Oromo saint, on the Harar-Jijiga road.*

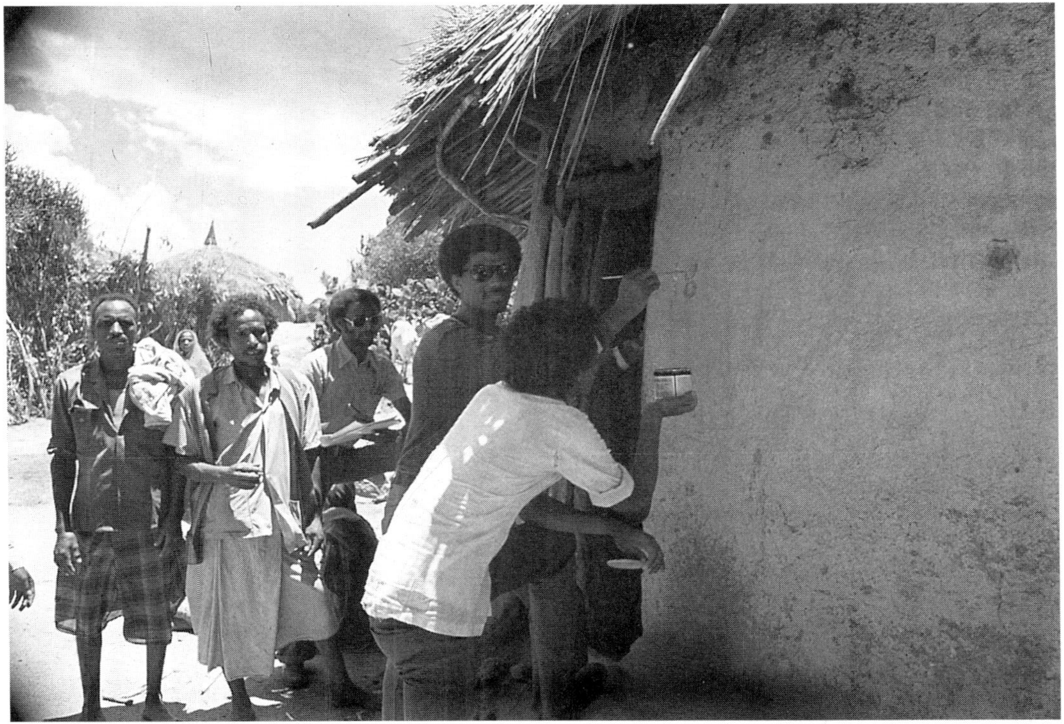

*The team marking the houses in Babile during the health interview surveys.*

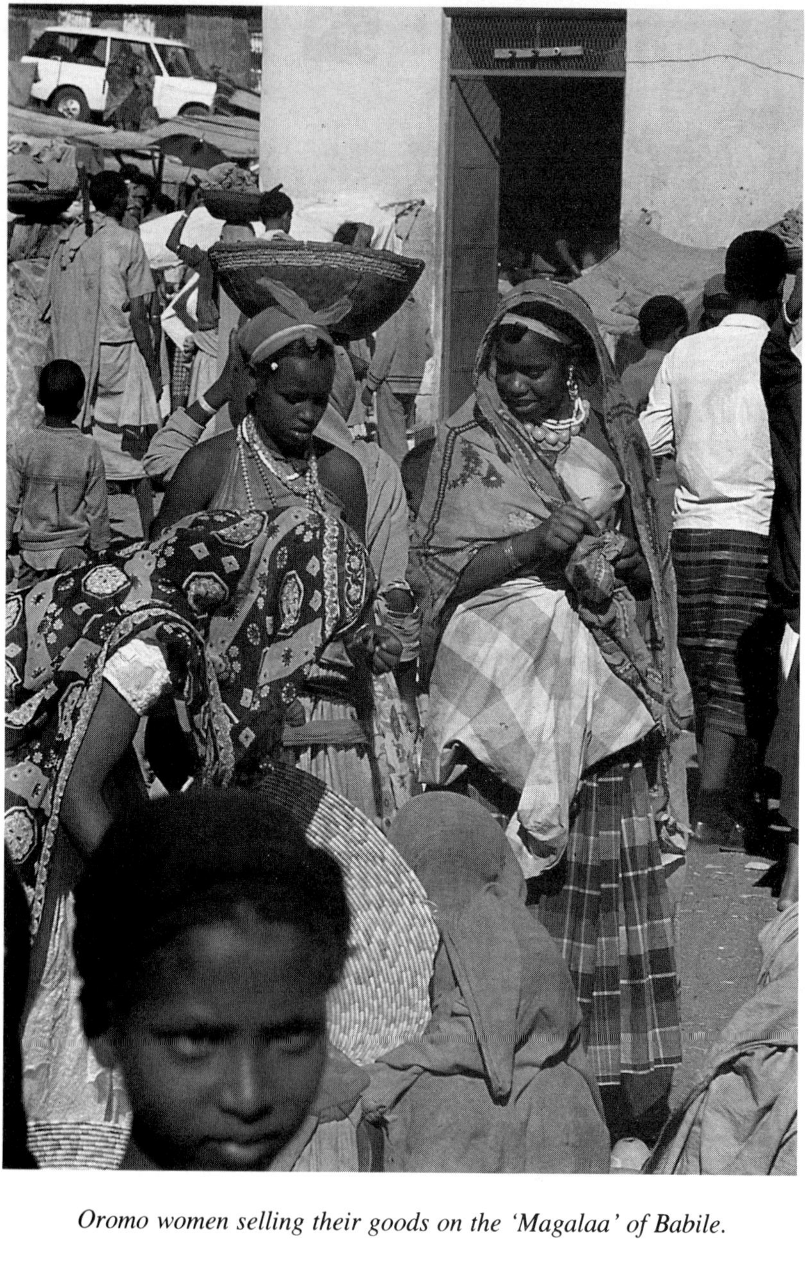

*Oromo women selling their goods on the 'Magalaa' of Babile.*

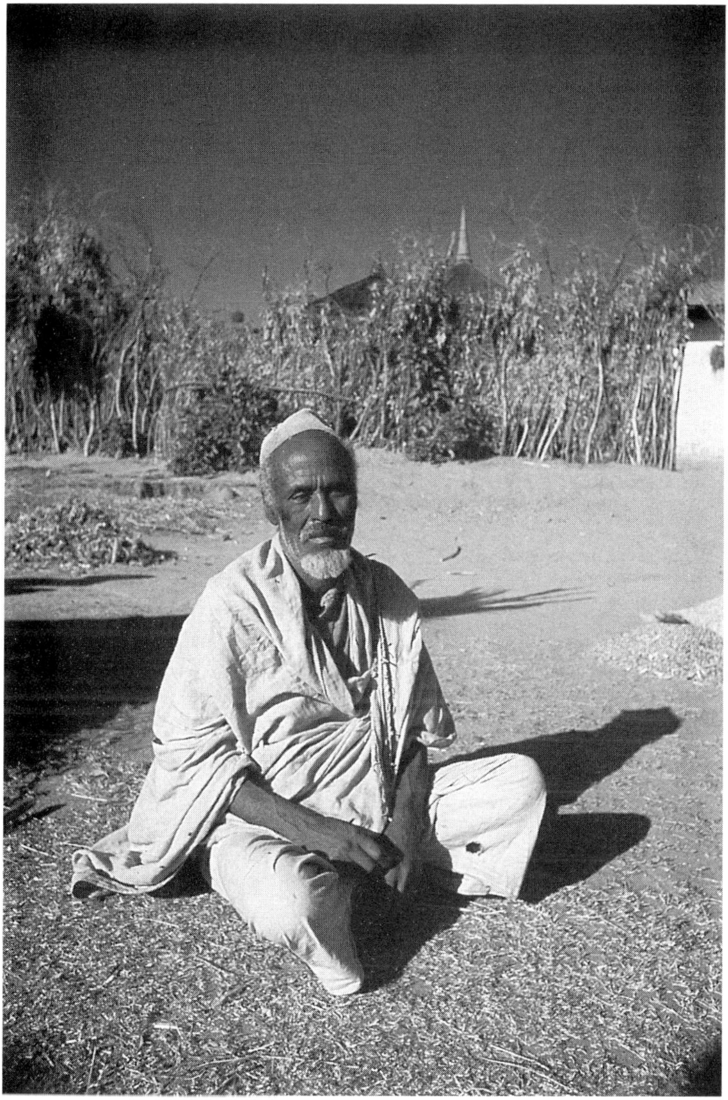

*Sheikh Abdullahi, a local 'ogeessa' from Hararghe.*

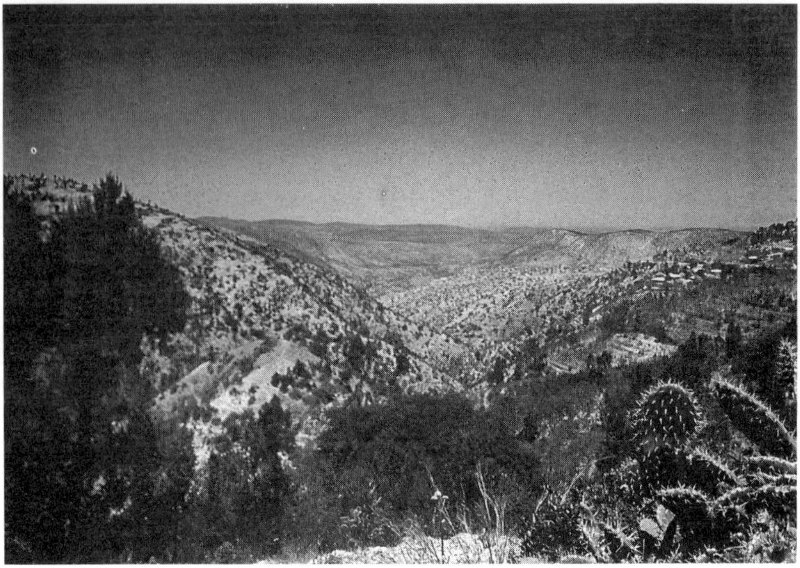

*View on the Eastern Highlands near the Ethiopian-Somali border.*

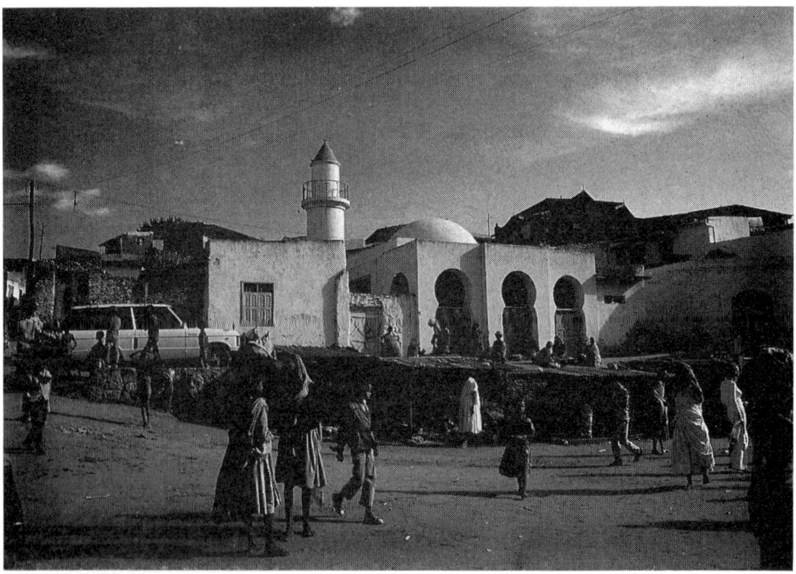

*The marketplace in the centre of the ancient walled city of Harar.*

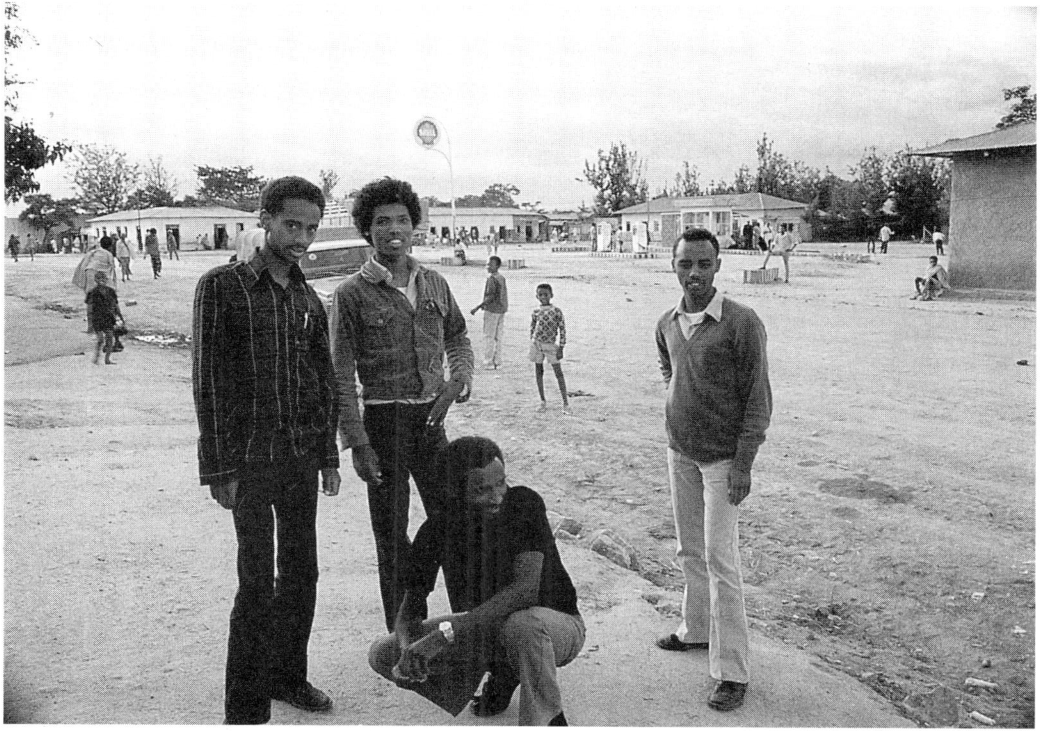

*The members of the field team at the central square of Babile: Hamza Adam, Mumi Umer, Ali Abdi (team leader, sitting on his heels), and Mustafa Abdullahi (from left to right).*

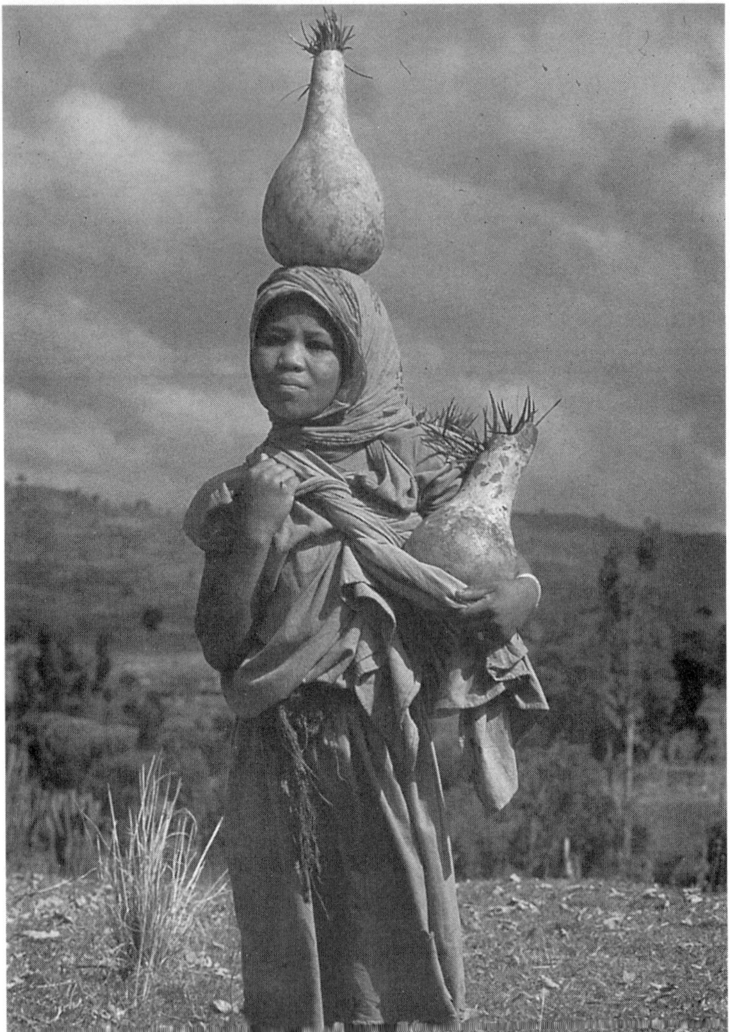

*A young Oromo girl carrying water home in two calabashes.*

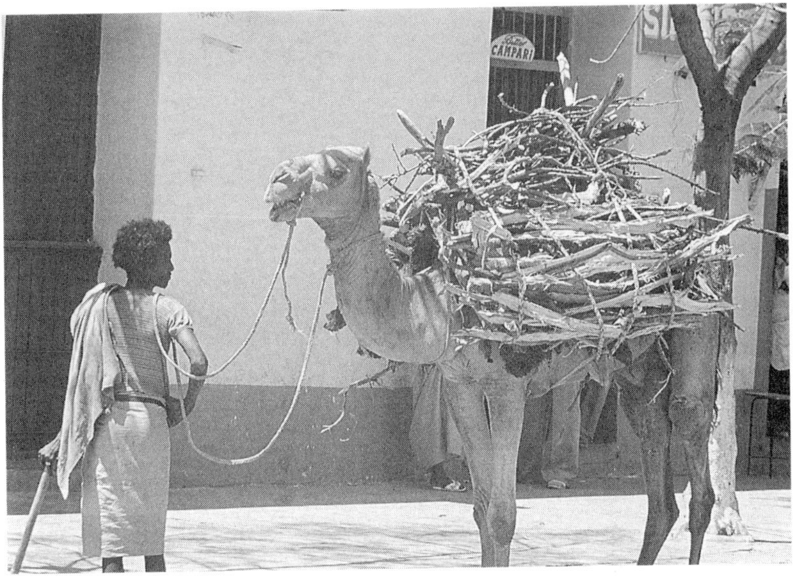


*A Somali offering fire-wood for sale at the market in Babile.*

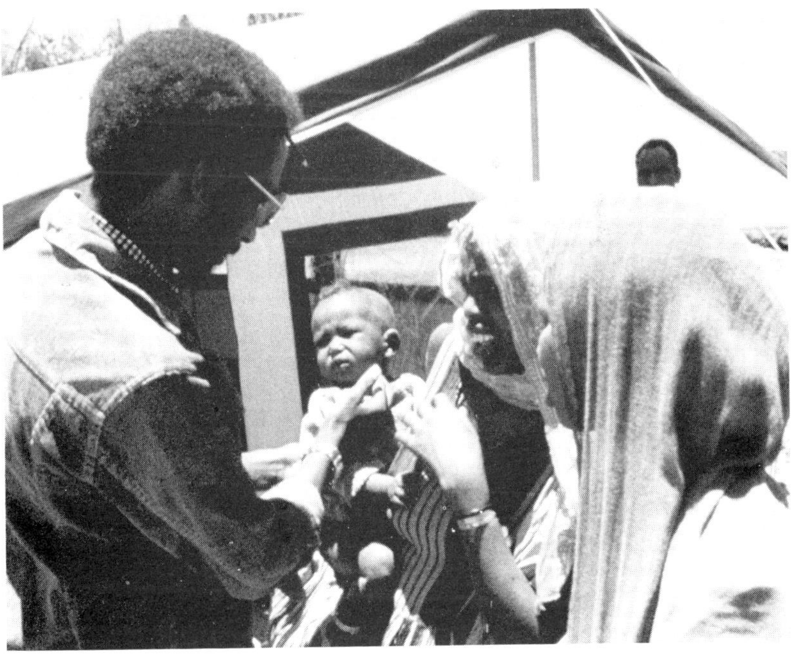

*Treatment of children's trachoma by one of the dressers during the health interview survey in Babile.*

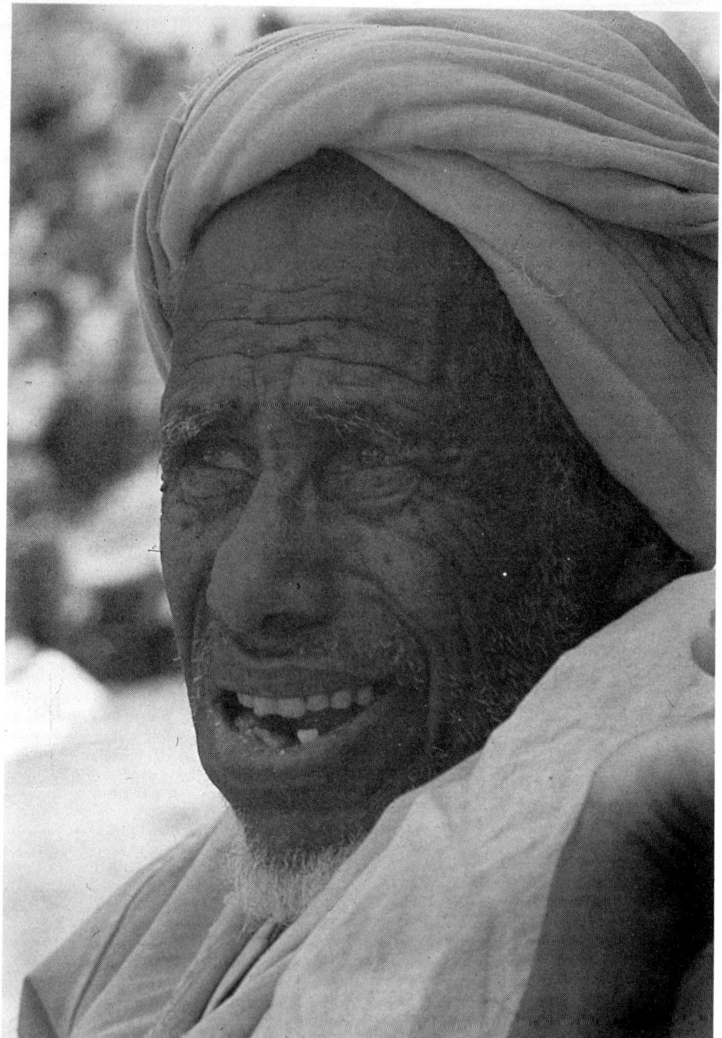

*Yusuf, a local Oromo chief from the nearby village Ganda Helele.*

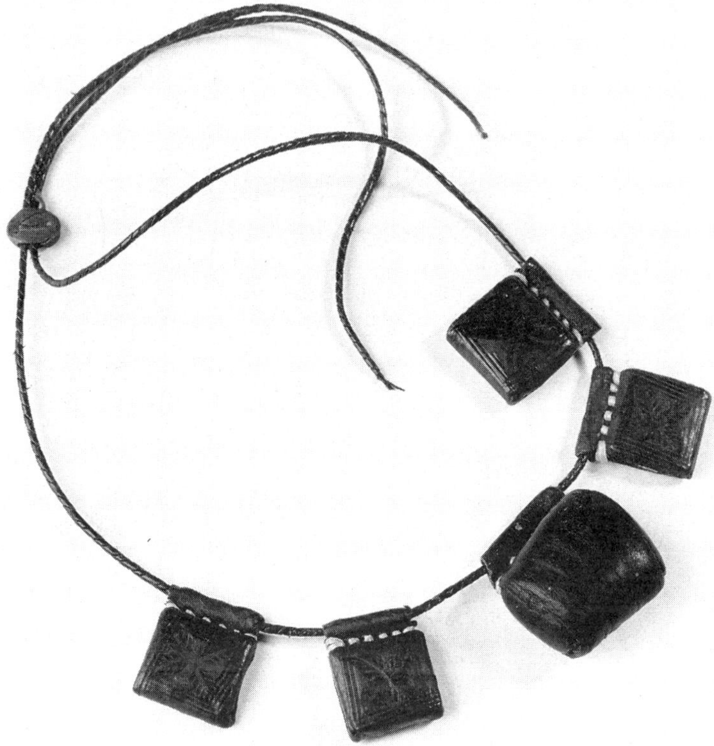

*Arabic amulet or 'kartasa'.*

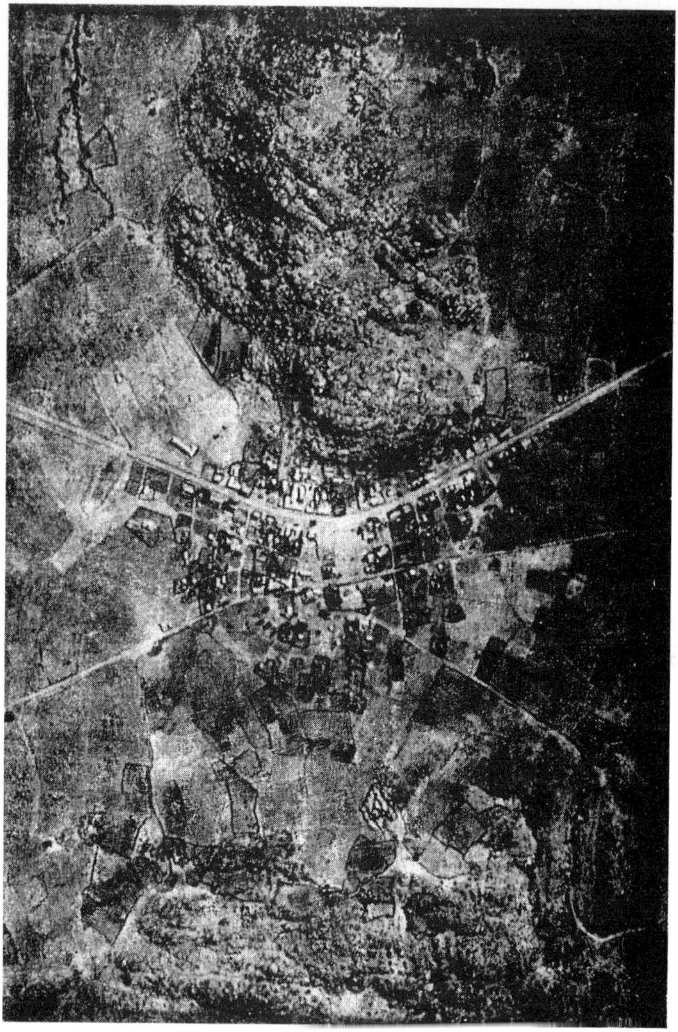

*Aerial view of Babile and its environs (Department of Geography, Addis Ababa University, Ethiopia).*

## Notes

1. Schaffer (1975) and Schaffer and Huang Wen-Hsien (1975) regard access to goods, services and means of production in developing countries as a relationship between the population and the referral agency. In this connection Buijs (1979) and Galjart and Buijs (eds.) (1982), among others, introduced the concept of distance in their analysis of the problems of access and participation in developing countries, noting geographical, financial and cultural dimensions. As regards the acccessibility of health care, Penchansky and Thomas (1981) develop a number of specific dimensions, i.e. accommodation, affordability and acceptability. Accessibility in relation to basic health care has also been extended by the International Conference at Alma-Ata (WHO/UNICEF 1978: 58, 59) as follows: '*Accessibility implies the continuing and organised supply of care that is geographically, financially, culturally and functionally within easy reach of the whole community.*'
2. A highly refined and detailed version of the international model of use devised by Kohn and White (1976) is used by Nuyens *et al.* (1978) in an extensive medical-sociological study of primary health care in Belgium. The research emphasises medical utilisation of the official health care facilities of the state. In the concluding publication of the study entitled *De Eerste Lijn is Krom,* Nuyens (1980) notes that there are two basic patterns of health care consumption in Belgium: the elderly and people with a low level of education are consumers of general practitioners, while younger people and those with a higher level of education are direct consumers of medical specialists. This pattern is described as the 'double circuit' in Belgian health care delivery.

# 3

# Ethiopia and the Horn of Africa

Before proceeding to the central theme of the study – the processes involved in the utilisation of the various medical systems in Northeast Africa – it would be useful first to present a short description of the socio-cultural background in which these processes are taking place. Therefore, an account will be given of the historical processes of socio-cultural differentiation and recent socio-economic development that have taken place in Ethiopia, being an example of a complex multi-ethnic society in the Horn of Africa. The pluralistic nature of the society will provide the basis for the later presentation of the medical-anthropological and sociological material collected in the research area of Babile.

Since this area is situated in the Eastern Highlands of Hararghe, on the verge of the Ogaden desert in the frontier land with Somalia and Djibouti, it seems useful then, to present a short socio-graphic outline focussed on the process of transculturation resulting from the different waves of population groups and cultures.

## 3.1 Synopsis of the Culture Area

Ethiopia and the Horn of Africa form a distinct region in Northeast Africa, which, since the Middle Ages, remained rather isolated from European influences, with the exception of the Portuguese searching for Prester John. Egypt and the later colonial powers did not

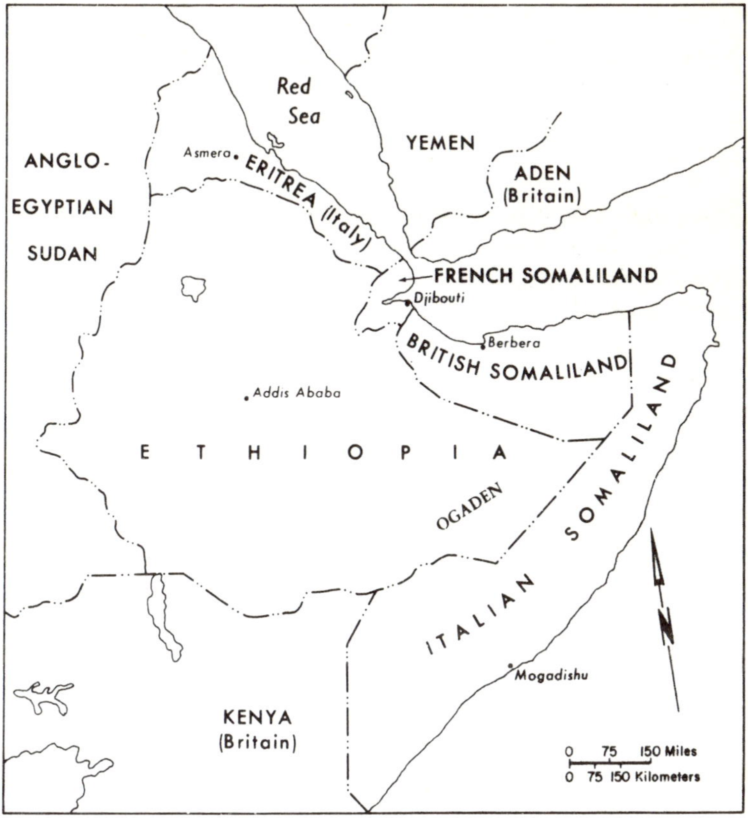


Map 3.1: *Ethiopia and The Horn of Africa around 1935 (Nelson and Kaplan 1980)*

penetrate into this part of Africa until after the opening of the Suez Canal in 1869. Britain, France, Italy and Ethiopia then divided the area into British Somaliland, French Somaliland, Italian Eritrea and Italian Somaliland, but Ethiopia under Emperor Menelik II resisted foreign invasions and maintained its independence (cf. Harrison Church *et. al.* 1977, Nelson and Kapland 1980).

By the end of the nineteenth century Ethiopia's territory had expanded substantially to the South and East under the successive conquests of Menelik. Finally, in 1962, Eritrea was finally incorporated into Ethiopia under Haile Selassie.[1] Map 3.1 shows the geo-political situation in the Horn of Africa around 1935.

In the meantime, Italian Somaliland had become a United Nations Trust Territory in 1950, and after achieving independence in 1960, it was joined with the British Somaliland Protectorate to form the present Somali Republic. French Somaliland, later known as Territoire Français Afar et Isa (TFAI) achieved independence as Djiboubi on 27 June 1977.

Hunter and Whitten (1975: 105) define the concept of culture area as: *a part of the earth's surface on which more or less related groups of people, over many millenia, worked out a variety of adaptive mechanisms for survival, beginning with a common heritage, social and ideological systems, and related languages.*

In the region of Northeast Africa, they rather refer to a transitional area between the great culture areas of the Middle East and Africa comprising the intersection between the agriculture and cattle cultures of the East Horn and the pastoralists of the Eastern Highlands. In this context, it is interesting to ascertain to what extent the situation under study can be described as a *culture area* or whether an alternative concept is needed.

## 3.2 Ethiopia: a Nation in Transition

In order to place the complex medical system in Eastern Highlands within the socio-cultural context of the present differentiated society, it becomes important to approach the Ethiopian situation in the light of the sociological typology of heterogeneous societies which distinguishes between plural and pluralistic societies. Contrary to conventional classification of Ethiopian society as an 'advanced Semitic civilisation area' (Ullendorff 1973; Trimingham 1976), an 'ethnographic museum' (Conti Rossini 1928; Haberland 1936; Lewis 1965) or as a 'developing country' (Ginzberg and Smith 1967; Clapham 1969; Hoben 1972), for the purpose of this study, the distribution of the ethnic groups, languages and major cultures in the Horn of Africa will be regarded as the result of two socio-cultural processes of internal differentiation and external interaction (cf. Levine 1974: 17 – 23).

### *3.2.1 The geographical and historical background*

Ethiopia, formerly also known as Abyssinia, has been a socialist republic since 1974. It covers an area of roughly 1,222,00 square kilometres. The country is triangular in shape with the apex to the north and lies between latitude 3° and 18° north and longitude 33° and 48° east. It borders the Red Sea in the North, Somalia in the south-east, Kenya in the south and Sudan in the west, forming an important point of intersection between Africa, Asia and Europe. Approximately two-thirds of the country consists of mountains ranging in height from 300 to 6000 metres, which rise from the extensive coastal plains as part of the volcanic East African Rift Valley. The mountains are divided from south-east to north-west by the Great Rift Valley into two major ranges, the Western or Central Highlands and the Eastern Highlands.

The most important river is the Blue Nile (Am: *Abbaya*) which fascinated such explorers as Alexander the Great, Julius Caesar and, much later, James Bruce and Richard Burton. Via Lake Tana and the Tis Isat Falls (Am.), the Blue Nile joins the White Nile some thousand kilometres west at Khartoum in the Sudan, from where it flows into the Mediterranean. In the southeast, the Juba and the Wabi Shebeli and in the north the Barka all flow in an eastern direction. The Awash River in the Rift Valley runs northeast and finally silts up in the salt marshes of the Afar Lowlands.

Traditionally, Ethiopians have classified the country's natural regions as four separate climatic zones, characterised by a combination of height, climate and type of vegetation. The term *quolla* (Am.) refers to the low-lying hot dry plains, such as the Danakil Lowlands, the Awash Valley, the savannas of the Somali Plateau, and the Ogaden desert, thinly populated by pastoral nomads,

*Woina dega* (Am.) is the zone which lies between 1830 and 2240 metres and includes a large part of the Ethiopian Plateau and most of the Hararghe Highlands. This is where most of the inhabitants of Ethiopia live. The predominantly agricultural population combine arable farming with livestock farming and exhibit a typical settlement pattern of thousands of scattered peasant villages (Am. and Or.: *ganda*) each consisting of 5 to 50 households. The main crops grown here are millet *teff* (Am.), coffee, *chat* (Am.) and cotton. Oranges, bananas and olives are also grown in certain places. *Dega* (Am.) consists of the sparsely populated area which lies between 2440 metres and 3600 metres. This area is extremely humid and mountainous, the vegetation consisting of grasses, shrubs and scattered pine forests. The fourth and final zone known as *wureg* (Am.) lies at more than 3600 metres and includes the higher mountains of the Semien Highlands, east of Lake Tana, the Choke Highlands of Gojam, the Gughe Highlands and the southwestern part of the Hararghe Highlands. It is a relatively cool area which does not contain any permanent settlements or agriculture (Harrison and Church *et al.* 1977: 209–211; Slikkerveer 1986).

Little is known about the earliest prehistoric times of Ethiopia, but contemporary archaeology in East Africa stresses the importance of the recent discoveries of hominid fossils (approximately 4 million years BC) in the Omo Valley and at Hadar, among other places, for the development of theories about the origins of man (Johanson and Edey 1981). At the beginning of the Late Stone Age (± 9000 BC) two different Afro-Mediterranean cultures inhabited the region, the *Wilton* and the *Hargeisa*, whose descendants changed from being hunters and food gatherers into simple arabie and livestock farmers, at the end of the third millenium. Historical research suggests that the Proto-Ethiopians of the third millenium spoke six related languages which derive from Hamito-Semitic or Afro-Asian, namely classical Egyptian, Berber, Chad, Semitic, Cushitic and Omotic. Levine (1974: 28) who explains the differentiation of peoples and cultures in the multi-ethnic society of 'Greater Ethiopia' from a neo-social evolutionary perspective, concludes: *By 2000 BC the proto-Ethiopians were beginning to separate in groups with different languages and cultures, a process that went on more or less continuously until very recent times and was accelerated by the differential impact of external forces on indigenous cultures.*

On the assumption that the main population groups in the area during this early period were farmers of the Afro-Mediterranean type, speaking three main Afro-Asiatic languages (Semitic, Cushitic and Omotic), Levine (1974: 29) reconstucts the historical processes of internal differentiation and external interaction of this original society by dividing the population into five main groups: the Northern, Central and Eastern Cushitic, the Northern and Central Semitic speaking groups and the Southern Omotic speaking peoples. The introduction of an Ethio-Sabai culture complex with a Semitic language, handwriting and architecture and Sabai religion and political symbolism had a strong influence on the development of Ethiopia. Later, Semitic colonists from Southern Arabia and Central Cushites founded a new Kingdom of Aksum on the Central Plateau. From the fourth to the sixth centuries, the advent of Syrian missionaries produced another major change in the ethno-cultural composition of northern Ethiopia: they brought Christianity to the *Ge'ez* speaking population. Ethiopian Christianity, which in terms of liturgy, sacred music, terminology and church architecture is Syrian in origin, quickly became the core of the ethnic identity of the Aksumites and their descendants, the Tigray and the Amhara. Subsequently, Amhara started to be baptised as Christians. Aksum developed into an important Christian empire in East Africa with contacts with the Byzantine Empire, and influence extending to Yemen and the whole of the Red Sea.

Under the influence of the Muslim Arabs who had founded Zeila, Berbera and other trading centres along the Somali coast, islamisation continued during the tenth, eleventh and twelfth centuries from the Dahlak Archipelago, the Danakil Lowlands and Somali coastal plain to Sidamo in the south, East Shoa and Hararghe in the east and around Lake Zway in the west. A number of Muslim states were established on the fringes of the Ethiopian kingdom, the most important of which was the Sultanate of Ifat in Shoa. In about 1200, the Argobba and Harari were also converted to Islam. In the following century, the Harari developed the town of Harar into the most important Islamic centre in the Horn of Africa.

Once the ethnic groups had split up into separate cultures, they continued to interact by way of trade, wars, religion, migration, marriage and the provision of services. As well as interacting internally with one another, the ethnic groups also responded to the periodic incursions of foreign peoples and cultures. Levine (1974: 64–68) speaks in this connection of a process of 'creative incorporation'.

During the sixteenth century, the Ethiopian kingdom was completely devastated by the ravages of the Islamic armies of the Sultanate of Adal on the Red Sea. In order to prevent its complete demise, the Ethiopians finally turned to the Portuguese for help. After various changes of fortune, the Muslim troops were finally defeated at the battle of Lake Tana and the legendary Muslim leader

Ahmed 'Gran' was killed. Harar then became the last outpost of Islam in Ethiopia, from where attacks were launched on Christians from time to time. Although the Muslim threat to the state of Ethiopia had receded, frequent wars had left the country devastated and extremely weak. This situation directly gave rise to a new threat to both Christians and Muslims: the major Oromo migrations which were to dominate events in Ethiopia for the next three centuries. In the early sixteenth century, the Oromo moved from the south in a circular movement into the highlands in the south and east in a desperate search for land to meet the needs of their growing numbers. They settled in the principalities of Shoa, Amhara and Lasta and left only Tigray, the former Aksum, untouched. The Muslim area around Harar was also invaded by the Oromo who settled everywhere except in the city itself. The Imam of Harar was forced to move to Aussa, from where he managed to retain control of Harar until the mid-seventeenth century. Harar remained an independent emirate until it was taken by Emperor Menelik II towards the end of the nineteenth century.

As a result of foreign contacts, the first moves were made during the reign of the Emperor Theodore II (1855 – 1869) to introduce reforms in government and finances, innovations in agriculture and the use of modern technology. It was during this period that the basis was laid for the establishment of the modern Ethiopian state. During the reign of Menelik II (1889 – 1913) the prestige of the kingdom increased and the development of Ethiopia into a modern state was further stimulated. His policies included the gradual conquest of the adjoining Muslim areas and the establishment of Ethiopian authority there. The conquests of Emperor Menelik are important because, as a result, the Muslim and traditional African areas in the east, south and west which had been lost since the Oromo invasion, were re-absorbed into the kingdom. Moreover, the security of the major caravan routes in the area was substantially increased.

The composition of Ethiopian society also changed considerably. The homogeneity, which had been reached on the Northern Plateau during a century-long process of integration between Amhara and Tigray was interrupted by the influx of a large number of population groups of various origins and cultures. The Christian groups from the north gradually came to be a dominant minority within the new state, which had important consequences for the development of Ethiopia in the twentieth century and for policies pursued by central government in relation to peripheral areas.

In 1923 Ethiopia was admitted to the League of Nations and treaties were signed with Italy, Belgium, England and France. Foreign advisors were recruited, ministers were appointed and a modern government machinery was set up to undertake executive tasks, the organisation of the army and financial matters. In 1936 this process was interrupted when Italian fascist forces under Mussolini occupied the country and annexed it as an Italian colony. When East Africa was liberated in 1941 by the allied forces, Emperor Haile Selassie, aided by Britain, returned to Addis Ababa after five years of exile and soon regained control of the whole country. The temporary Italian occupation disrupted many traditional and political processes and institutions; on the other hand, a number of innovations were introduced relating to infrastructure, communications and social services, such as hospitals and clinics. This situation provided the Emperor with an opportunity to accelerate the process of reconstructing and revitalising the country in the period immediately after the Second World War.

This short geo-historical overview on Ethiopia shows how ecological circumstances and historical events have formed two major elements in the history of Ethiopia. The complex, physical geography of Ethiopia has made a large contribution to the preservation of an independent state in a part of Northeast Africa which, since the beginning of the seventh century and later during the colonial and neo-colonial periods, has come under increasing external pressure. As a result, a society developed which managed to preserve its own identity. Linking up with these developments, the historical processes of internal differentiation and external interaction has had a significant impact on the creation of the present heterogeneous society. The next section deals with the complex contemporary, socio-cultural differentiation on the basis of the historical processes described above, emphasising the plural character of Ethiopian society.

### *3.2.2 Socio-cultural differentiation*

Although an official census has not been conducted in Ethiopia, recent estimates (1984) suggest that the population of Ethiopia consists of approximately 42 million inhabitants or an average of 34 inhabitants per square kilometre.[2] This number varies widely from one area to another: the *woina dega* (Am.) in the highlands, for example, has the highest population density of rural areas where the majority of the population live (approximately 90%). Population growth is estimated at approximately 2.9% per year. Estimates concerning the composition of the population suggest that 45% are under the age of 15, 50% are 15 – 60 and 5% older than 60 years. If present trends continue, the total number of inhabitants will be 52 million by the year 2000.

The heterogeneous nature of Ethiopian society is clearly reflected in the complexity of its population structure. If an attempt is made to make a distinction on the basis of differences in origin, ethnicity, language, religion, etc., then it becomes clear that there are various religions, dozens of main ethnic groups, upwards of seventy languages, and more than two hundred dialects. A large number of authors, including Noel-Buxton (1932), Broekhuizen (1935), Brummelkamp (1956), Haberland (1963), Pankhurst (1968), Ullendorff (1973), Trimingham (1976) and Harrison Church *et al.* (1977) have used historical, regional, linguistic, religious, ecological or socio-cultural classification principles in an attempt to chart the differentiation of peoples and cultures within the political borders of Ethiopia using various classification systems. Abraham Demoz (1968: 36) remarked somewhat cynically in the light of all these different classifications: 'Ethiopia is the despair of the compulsive classifier.'

In order to illustrate the plural nature of Ethiopian society on the basis of the specific heterogeneity of its ethno-cultural composition, it is necessary here to use a type of classification which not only makes allowance for the absence of unity of ethnicity, language, religion, etc., but which is also based, in a historical sense, on the origins of various groups of peoples with different cultures, and on the socio-cultural affinity between such groups. Levine (1974: 33 – 39) has designed such a classification by applying a non-stringent combination of the above criteria to his analysis of the historical processes of internal differentiation of the proto-Ethiopians in a large number of various languages and cultures and of external interaction with surrounding cultures in the west, east and north. He divides the population into nine major ethnic groups and some hundred and fifty smaller groups. The nine major groups consist of the North Eritreans, the Agew, the Amhara-Tigray, the Core Islamic, the Oromo (or Galla), the Lacustrine, the Omotic, the Sudan, and the Caste groups found in smaller entities all over the country. This classification system helps to explain the complex differentiation of ethnic groups throughout the area as a whole, while at the same time a deeper understanding is achieved of the present configuration of the main population groups in the research area (see Map 3.2).

For the present study it suffices to locate the Amhara-Tigray groups as the founders of Ethiopian Christianity and of the Solomonid Dynasty in East Africa. They practise mixed farming consisting of the cultivation of cereals and raising livestock such as sheep, goats and cattle. The Tigray inhabit the western province of Tigray and southern central Eritrea and speak Tigrinya, while the Amhara are scattered in West Wollo, North Shoa, Goyam, Begemdir and Hararghe, but are also found elsewhere. A third group consists of Amhara and Tigray Muslim converts who are found throughout the country.

The Core Islamic group is found in the eastern part of the country. These people have lived for centuries in constant conflict with the Amhara-Tigray peoples of the Central Highlands. They include the Eastern Cushites speaking Afar or Danakil, the Saho and Somali all of whom are nomadic herdsmen in the desert Lowlands of Eastern Eritrea, Tigray, Wollo and Hararghe. The Somali, who constitute a major ethnic group, speak an Eastern Cushitic language related to Oromifa, the language of the Oromo. As far as religion is concerned, the Somali in the coastal areas are strict Muslims while in the interior, various forms of a traditional African religion have survived. This category also includes the southern Ethio-Semitic speaking Argobba and Harari who, as smaller groups of arable farmers and traders, inhabit the Eastern Highlands of Hararghe and its provincial capital Harar. The Oromo, the largest ethnic group who make up one third of the population of Ethiopia, consist of twelve regional sub-groups. They take their name from *Ilma Orma*, the 'sons of Orma' and also used to be known as *Galla*, a term the majority of them regard as derogatory. They speak Oromifa, which is the main language in Ethiopia after the official language Amharinya. Although some earlier authors pinpointed their origins as Southern Arabia and the Horn of Africa (Huntingford 1955; Carulli 1957; Lewis 1960), recent research supports the theory that their origins are more likely to have been in Southern Ethiopia near the lakes in the Great Rift Valley and the Bale Plateau (Herbert S. Lewis 1962, 1965, 1966; Haberland 1963; Levine 1974).

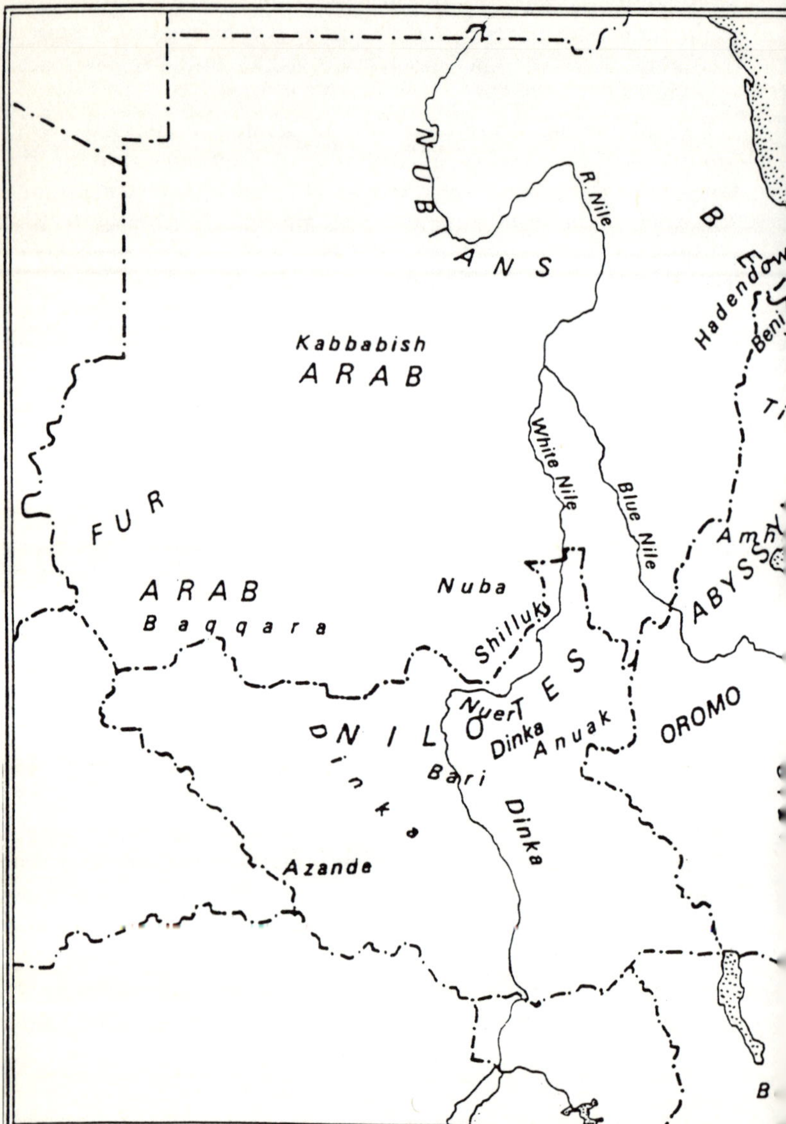


Map 3.2: *Ethnographic map of the Horn of Africa (after Markakis*

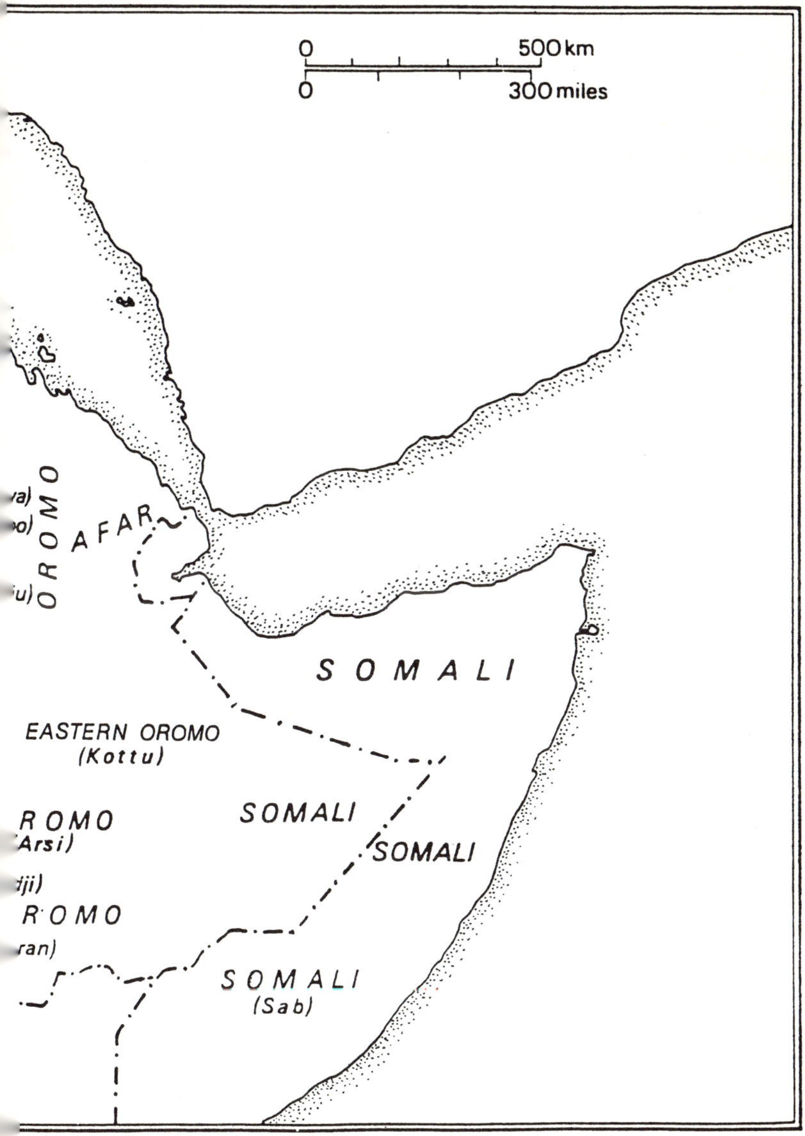
0
500 km
0
300 miles
OROMO
AFAR
SOMALI
EASTERN OROMO
(Kottu)
SOMALI
SOMALI
SOMALI
(Sab)

The great migrations took place at the start of the sixteenth century when the Oromo moved as nomadic herdsmen from Southern Ethiopia and Northern Kenya into the Central and Eastern Highlands. At the beginning of the seventeenth century, the Oromo were to be found in Wollo, Arussi, Hararghe and Wolega where they later settled permanently as farmers. The Borana in the south of Sidamo, who also belong to the Oromo, have retained their nomadic lifestyle which dates from before the great Oromo expansion.

Of the more than seventy languages in Ethiopia, approximately eight are spoken by the larger population groups. Amharic or Amharinya, the official language, is the most widely spoken but Tigrinya and Arabic dominate in Eritrea. The Southern Semitic languages of Amharinya and Tigrinya are associated with *Ge'ez*, the liturgical language of the Ethiopian Church. Although Amharic is spoken by approximately half the population of Ethiopia, Oromifa is spoken by an even greater percentage of the population. Many Ethiopians are bilingual and speak both their own language and passable Amharic (cf. Drewes 1970: 57 – 60). With the exception of Nilotic and non-classified languages in the southwest, the languages and dialects belong to the Afro-Asian family. The pattern of distribution shows that there is a Semitic 'language island' in Ethiopia running from Northern Eritrea to Addis Ababa in the south, surrounded by an extensive area of Cushitic languages and several Nilotic enclaves in the south.

Just as the Horn of Africa shows marked differences in ethnocultural and linguistic terms, so the religious system found in the area is very complex. The original Cushitic groups who practised traditional African religion have come under the influence of the three great monotheistic religions from the Middle East to such an extent that the majority of the present population practise either Christianity, Judaism or Islam. It should, however, be noted that a number of traditional African rites and practices survive within these three main religious systems.

The traditional religions usually have a heavenly deity, surrounded by a variey of supernatural spirits often connected with natural elements such as mountain tops, rivers and trees. Several Cushitic groups, for example, worship *Waaqa* (Or.), the god of the Oromo, *Ateetee* (Or.), the goddess from the Omo district. Belief in a diabolical spirit *Zar* (Am.) is also common. The latter has also been incorporated by the Muslim Oromo into their religious system, as have the *jiinii* (Or.), which are local, often impersonal, spirits (cf. Trimingham 1976: 15 – 33).

In addition to the establishment of Semitic languages, the major socio-cultural changes produced by the historical immigration of Semitic groups from the north and east resulted in the introduction of Judaism, Christianity and Islam into Ethiopia. Judaism was originally introduced among the Agau by early Jewish immigrants who probably moved south as a result of the diaspora in about the sixth century BC[3]. The descendants of these groups include for example the Falasha in the northwest, who worship, among others, the goddess *Sanbat*.

The Ethiopian version of Christianity belongs to the Coptic Monophysitic Church of Egypt from which the Ethiopian Church split in 1948. It does, however, contain a number of local Jewish rites and practices. In particular, the conversion of Cushitic groups resulted in the incorporation of traditional elements in Ethiopian Christianity, which probably established the basis for the unique nature of the Ethiopian Church in this period. Ullendorff (1973: 59) describes this development as follows: '. . . *it brought about a further instalment in the "indigenisation" of monophysitism which, charged more and more with the residue of Judaic and pagan practices and beliefs, assumed a truly national and peculiarly Abyssinian form.*'

Ethiopia is virtually completely surrounded by a belt of Islam which runs from North Sudan, Egypt and Arabia to the coastal areas of Somalia and Kenya. The process of Islamisation – which has been taking place in Northeast Africa from the Arabian Peninsula since the seventh century – has resulted more substantially in almost half of the population being Muslim. The people affected are the northern groups in Eritrea, the groups living in the area along the coast of the Red Sea and the western border area with Sudan, the eastern nomadic Afar and Somali, the Eastern Oromo groups round Harar, Awash, and the larger number of groups round Jima. Unlike Ethiopian Christianity, Islam has made less of a contribution towards cultural and political unity among Muslims. There used to be a number of Muslim states in the east of the country, from which Islamisation began, but the ethno-cultural diversity of the Somali, Afar and Oromo has never been completely harmonised by Islam. There has never really been a Muslim 'bloc' in the east to counterbalance the Christian Amhara and Tigray in the centre.

As far as religious beliefs are concerned, recent estimates suggest that 40 to 50% of the population are Christian, approximately 30 to 40% Muslim and 15% adherents of traditional African religion (Buschkens and Slikkerveer 1982:15).

The social stratification of Ethiopian society is based on a complex series of factors such as ethnicity, degree of incorporation within the state, religion, occupation, etc., of the various groups. Until the 1974 revolution, the society was divided into three social classes: the upper class consisting of the aristocracy nobility, officials and high ranking officers, the clergy, and the working class which included cattle farmers, craftsmen and traders. Given the dominant position of the Amhara and the Tigray, ethnic groups such as the Beni, Barea, Kunama and Sidamo were members of the lowest social class. The Agew, Falasha, Gurage and other caste groups occupied a lowly position in the social order. As will be described later, the drastic socio-economic and political reforms introduced after the revolution have not fundamentally changed this situation.

Generally speaking, the Oromo in Ethiopia belong to the lowest social class, but a distinction should be made between Christian and non-Christian Oromo. The Oromo who have become members of the Ethiopian Church and who have also adopted other elements of the Amhara-Tigray culture often occupy a higher social position than, for example, the Islamic Oromo in the south and east. Among the latter, traces can still be found of the *gadaa* system which involves a certain element of social stratification. It is a class system based on age, which Asmarom Legesse describes as follows (1973: 8): *'The Gada system is a system of classes (luba) that succeed each other every eight years in assuming military, economic and ritual responsibilities. Each gada class remains in power during a specific term (gada) which begins and ends with a formal power transfer ceremony.'* The social position of the other ethnic groups is difficult to determine. The Islamic Somali and Afar groups have consistently been despised by the ruling classes and since they are largely wandering nomads in the peripheral areas, they play a limited role within the political hierarchy of Ethiopian society. Linking up with the differentiation in economic activity between the caste groups in Ethiopia – hunters, fishermen, smiths, potters, weavers and leather workers – reference should finally be made to several slave groups which also have a very low social status (cf. Herbert Lewis 1970).

The above description of Ethiopian society depicts a country inhabited by a large number of groups with significant differences in ethnicity, language, religion, and economic activity. By means of an analysis of the two historical processes mentioned earlier, it becomes possible to attribute this differentiation to a large extent to the advent of people from different cultures, namely the Negroid Sudanese in the west, the Semites in the east and the Mediterranean groups in the north. The differentiation has persisted in the course of history, despite attempts by the central Amhara-Tigray ruling class to establish and maintain national unity by means of 'amharisation'. In some cases, these differences are so great that they amount to serious conflict, for example, the independence struggles in Eritrea and Tigray and the movements supporting Oromo, Somali and Afar separation. The traditional social, political and religious contrasts which are often based on ethno-cultural and economic factors emphasise in a special way the heterogeneous nature of Ethiopian society. Its origins and present form are therefore an outstanding example of a plural society in this part of Africa. This plural nature of Ethiopian society has been an important element in the process of socio-economic change which occurred particularly during and immediately after the era of the Emperor Haile Selassie.

As the following section makes clear, attention in this period focussed chiefly on extending the authority of central government and introducing Amhara cultural values with a view to strengthening national unity. This policy was, however, unable to prevent the recent modernisation process from being delayed and inequitably implemented, with the result that some differences and contrasts have been heightened and have led to renewed tensions. This has had major implications for health care, particularly among the inhabitants of rural areas.

### *3.2.3 Socio-economic development since the Second World War*

Ethiopia is one of the poorest countries in the world. In 1984, gross national per capita income was estimated at 120 US dollars. The economy is largely based on an unproductive agricultural sector, which consists mainly of small, mixed farms with an average size of

3 hectares, the majority of which are still operating at the subsistence level. Approximately 80% of the population is dependent on agriculture but only 15% of the land suitable for cultivation is actually being farmed. Although experts have described Ethiopia's agricultural potential as high, farmers have in the past been confronted with numerous problems. Pankhurst (1968: 216) refers to '... *their situation being one of actual poverty in the midst of potential plenty.*' As a result of drought, bad harvests, insect plagues, looting and war the inhabitants of some areas have been on the brink of starvation on occasions. After the severe drought in 1973, which played an important role in the downfall of Haile Selassie, the famine in Wollo and Tigray became world news in 1984, striking approximately 7 million people and claiming hundreds of thousands of victims.

Industry is still very modest: in 1983 it made a contribution to gross national income of only 16%. In the same year, only 7% of the working popu000luation were employed in the sector. The tertiary sector accounted for 33% of GNP in 1983 and employed 12% of the working population. It has, therefore, undoubtedly experienced greater growth than industry. Nevertheless, it is still underdeveloped. Factors which go hand in hand with a very low GNP, such as a low standard of living, reflected in bad housing, insufficient food, poor health standards, low life-expectancy, high population growth and extensive illiteracy, indicate the relatively early stage of development in which the country still finds itself today (cf. Kleinpenning 1980: 219, 220).

The rise of Ethiopia as a modern state since 1935, which was preceded by the announcement of a constitution in 1931, gave a new impetus to socio-economic development which has continued to progress, particularly since the Second World War. The period since 1941, after the brief Italian occupation, can be divided into two phases: the immediate post-war period until the early 1970s and the recent post-revolutionary period since the military coup of 1974.

After the restoration of the Ethiopian state, and the end of the Second World War, despite war damage and disrupted political relations, a situation developed in which there was a clear need for capital, Western capital goods, modern technology, skills and know-how. International relations with Western countries and Eastern bloc countries were expanded and foreign investment, loans and grants increased. Attempts were made to stimulate economic growth by improving the infrastructure, introducing modern agricultural methods, stepping up agricultural production, and developing modern industry. Major food crops such as cereals, pulses and oilseed were supplemented on a modest scale by a number of cash crops, including coffee, cotton, tobacco, *chat* and sugar cane. In 1962 development of the Awash Valley was begun and in the early seventies approximately one third of the land had been irrigated with a view to large-scale cultivation of cotton and sugar cane (Kleinpenning 1980: 218). The social consequences of irrigation for the local population are described in detail by Van Lier (1968).

At the time, the government paid considerable attention to expanding the education system, which, until the turn of the century, had been in the hands of Christian priests and Islamic teachers. Attempts were made to improve the quality and distribution of education with the help of missionaries, foreign experts and literacy programmes.

As far as modern health care is concerned, during the Italian occupation (1935 – 1941) some two thousand Italian medical doctors formed part of the occupying forces and they carried out a number of extensive preventive health programmes and mass campaigns among the local population. The first steps were also taken to organise systematic health services in rural areas which led to a modest network of clinics and pharmacies (cf. Pankhurst 1973). After the liberation , the government concentrated mainly on training medical staff, implementing public health programmes and extending existing medical services. With the help of a number of international organisations, attempts were made to improve health care even further. The Ministry of Health was set up, followed by the Health Training Institute in Gondar to train medical staff (cf. Gabre Emanual Teka 1975). In the fifties, the network of clinics was expanded with the establishment of five health centres and hospitals in the various provinces and in 1964 the Medical Faculty was opened in Addis Ababa to train doctors and pharmacists (Buschkens and Slikkerveer 1982: 48).

The introduction of Ethiopia's first constitution and parliament have been important constitutional developments. They marked the beginning of a process of democratisation which was strengthened in 1957 by general elections. After the constitution was revised in 1955 the Ethiopian parliament gradually became more and more important. The reform of army and police forces largely consisted of centralising the defence apparatus and improving training and equipment, most of which took place after 1953. In the social field, powerful measure to abolish slavery had started in 1923 when Ethiopia joined the League of Nations, marking an attempt to reduce the traditional divisions between social classes. A number of legal measures were adopted, aimed at replacing the traditional landowner-tenant relationship with an elementary form of labour law. In this period the judicial system was also modernised. The basis of social development in this period was the '1957 – 1982 Plan' sub-divided into a number of Five Year Plans, devised by Yugoslavian experts and implemented by the Ethiopian government.

In the sixties the bulk of bilateral aid was provided by the United States and most of the multilateral aid came from the World Bank (IBRD) and its subsidiaries, the International Development Agency (IDA) and the International Finance Corporation. Technical cooperation between Ethiopia and the Netherlands during this period consisted of a number of projects in the field of health care, agricultural extension and research into food crops (cf. Kurian 1979).

The virtually unchanged power structure and the prolonged absence of democracy in social and political relations, together with widespread dissatisfaction among the majority of the population heralded a period of social and political unrest. In 1974, an emergency developed when living standards deteriorated as a result of inadequate food production and increasing poverty. Finally, the army intervened on 12 September 1974, deposing the Emperor and suspending parliament. The new military junta which consisted of a Provisional Military Administrative Council (PMAC) announced it would be pursuing policies of *Hebretesabawinet* or 'Ethiopian Socialism' based on Marxist-Leninist principles of equality, self-confidence, the value of labour, the importance of common goal and the indivisibility of Ethiopian unity (Alula Abate and Tesfaye Teklu 1980).

Shortly afterwards, reforms were announced by which all land was nationalised and declared the collective property of the population. Banks, factories and trading concerns were also nationalised. Attempts were made to develop the country further by improving the infrastructure and transport and by new investment in the collective industrial sector. Support for these developments was provided mainly by a number of Eastern bloc countries, Cuba and the Soviet Union. To publicise the new socialist policies throughout the country, more than 60,000 secondary school and university students conducted the *Zemecha* or 'Development Through Cooperation Campaign'. Everywhere they went they explained the principles of *Hebretesabawinet* and helped to build up a network of peasant associations and *kebele's*. The campaign, which in subsequent years developed into a major organisation with a total of 28,583 peasant associations, was made up of 7.3 million households (Alula Abate and Tesfaye Teklu 1980).

In the military field, the central authorities were faced with a large number of problems. The army desperately needed to replace old equipment which, since the termination of American aid, had become obsolete and unfit for use. Aid was eventually provided by Ethiopia's new allies, Cuba and the Soviet Union. However, the unity of the new state was threatened by several separatists movements and again there was a major upheaval and political unrest as social and cultural differences reared their heads (cf. Nelson and Kaplan 1980).

Although a number of changes in the internal socio-economic situation have ensued as a result of the international political re-orientation of the Military Council, it is debatable whether fundamental changes as envisaged by the 1974 revolution have in fact taken place. Dissatisfaction among the population has not diminished, there are no signs of democratisation and internal tensions and conflicts in some areas have again risen to serious levels. Despite the desire to replace the old power structure, the social circumstances of the lower social classes and the different ethno-cultural groups in the town and in rural areas do not show any fundamental improvements (cf. Kleinpenning 1980: 219, 236).

If a balance sheet were to be drawn up of Ethiopia's socio-economic development since the Second World War, then it would inevitably lead to the conclusion that the development process has stagnated largely because of internal relations and tensions within the society itself.

## 3.3 Hararghe: Borderland between Cultures

The eastern Administrative Region (Am.: *kifle hager*) of Hararghe covers approximately 259,700 square kilometres and forms the

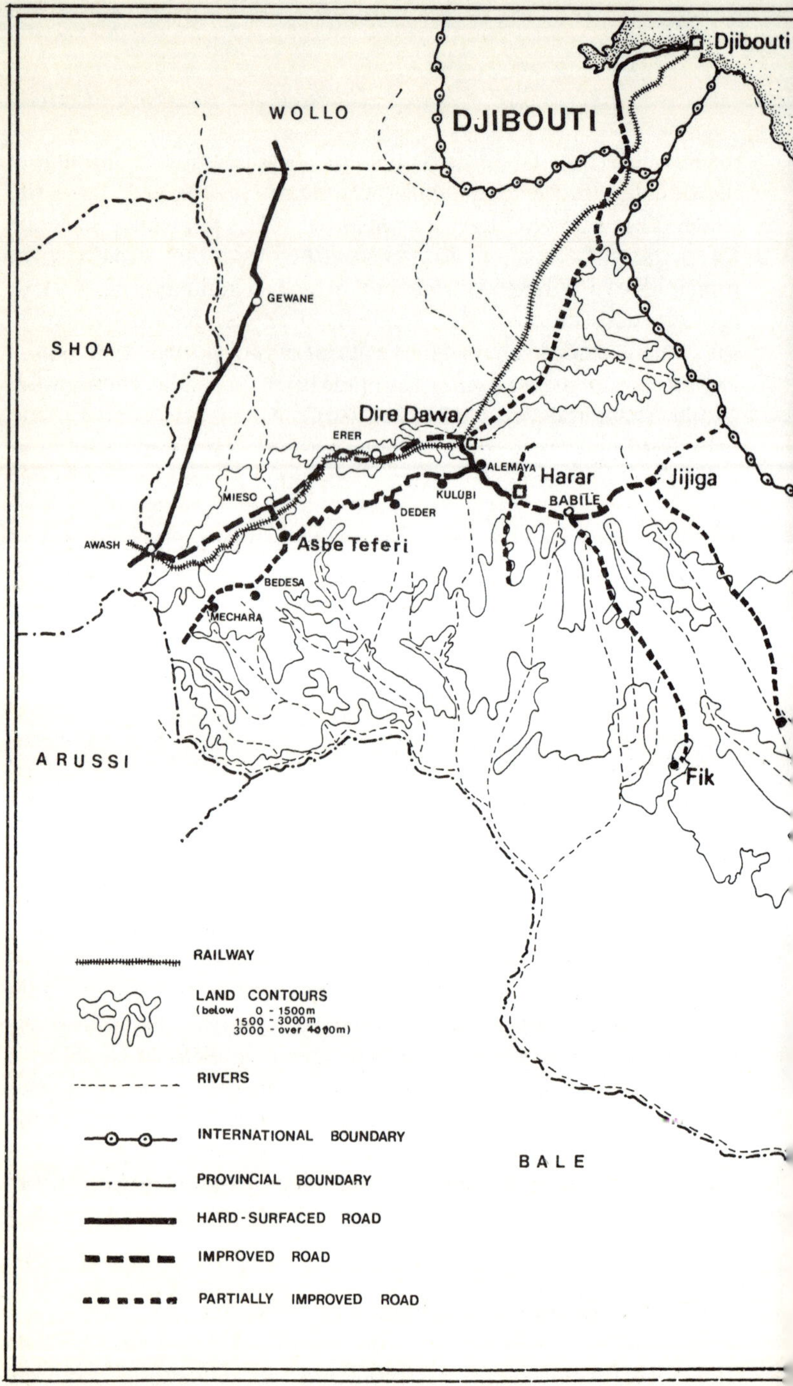


Map 3.3: *The Administrative Region of Hararghe*

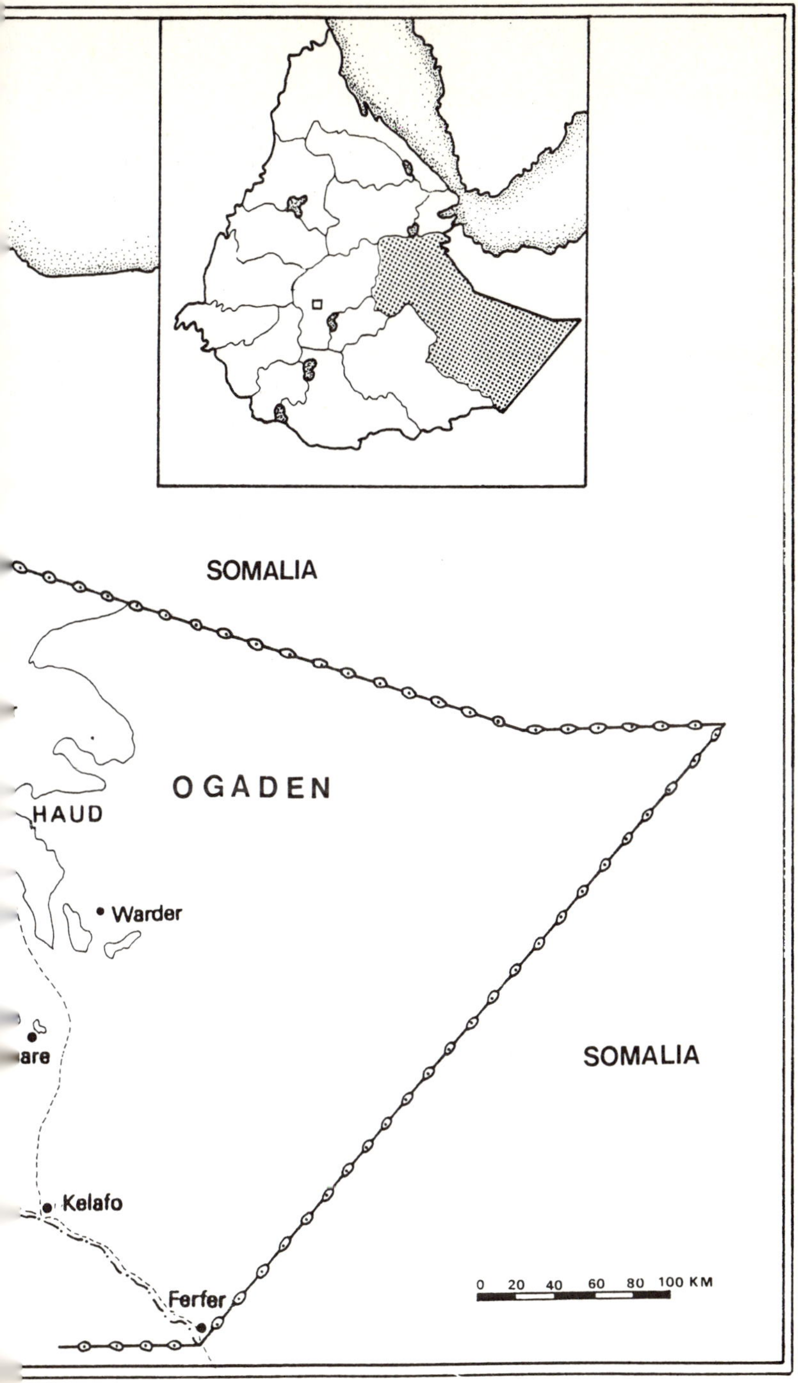
SOMALIA
OGADEN
HAUD
Warder
are
Kelafo
Ferfer
SOMALIA
0 20 40 60 80 100 KM

largest region in the country. It borders Somalia and Djibouti and is divided into thirteen districts (Am. *awraja*), the largest of which is the disputed Ogaden desert between Wabi Shabelli in the west and Somalia in the east. The physical environment in the northwest of the region is determined to a large extent by the mountains of the Hararghe Plateau which are part of the Eastern Highlands of Ethiopia, starting in the west in the district of Bale and running via the Chercher or Ahmar Highlands, the Gara Mulatta massif and the Kondudo Mountains of Jijiga. Hararghe therefore forms the natural transition between the eastern mountains of Ethiopia and the western desert of Somali. Because of its sheer escarpments and deep ravines, the area has made a substantial contribution to the previously mentioned inaccessibility of the eastern flank of the Ethiopian kingdom (cf. Map 3.3).

The majority of inhabitants of the *woina dega* (Am.) live in the high plains where a moderate climate and regular rainfall support a combination of arable farming (plough cultivation) and livestock farming. This area consists of about 20% of the total area of Hararghe and contrasts with the drier surrounding lowlands of the arid Depression in the north, the Ogaden desert in the east and the semi-arid Somali Plateau in the south. The latter areas are sparsely populated by nomads who follow their flocks of goats, sheep, camels and longhorn cattle from one oasis to another within certain tribal boundaries. Two ethnic groups dominate the region: the Cushites and the Semites. The first group consists of the Oromo, Somali and Afar, the second of the Amhara, Tigray, Harari and Argoba. The total population of Hararghe was estimated at more than 4.25 million in 1981, 2.5 million of whom were in the Highlands (Statistical Abstract of Ethiopia 1981). No distinctions as regards ethnic groups are made in these figures. Recent estimates of the distribution of ethnic groups in the area suggest there were 2 million Oromo and 0.9 million Amhara while the remainder of the population consisted of Somali, Argoba, Afar and Arabs.

The Oromo, who ethnically speaking belong to the main Oromo group in Ethiopia, the Barentu, speak Oromifa which is part of the Eastern Cushitic family of languages. They are predominantly Muslims and grow arable crops such as cereals (Am. *teff*), millet, sorghum, coffee and several types of vegetables and fruits, combined with livestock farming on a smaller scale. These inhabitants of Hararghe, like those of other regions, derive considerable prestige from owning cattle, quantity rather than quality being the important factor. In recent years, commercial considerations have seen a decline in coffee production in favour of *chat (Catha edulis)*, which is grown more and more on the irrigated terraces of the highlands around Harar. The leaves of the chat bush contain an addictive drug, and small bundles of leafy twigs are sold as far afield as Southern Arabia.

In Hararghe, the Eastern Oromo, also known as *Kottu* (farmers) or *qottuu* in Oromifa, are found in large numbers of scattered villages (Or: *ganda*) in the districts of Harar Zurya, Habro, Gara Mulatta, Woberra, Gursum and to a less extent in Chercher-Adal-Garaguracha and Dire Dawa-Issa-Gurgura. A small number of Oromo have settled in the towns of Dire Dawa and Harar or live in large rural communities such as Asbe Tafari, Gursum, Alemaya, Hirna, Deder, Gelemso, Bedessa, Gota, Melka Rufa, Dodola, Bedenno, Grawa and Babile.

On the eastern flank of the Hararghe Plateau, where the research community of Babile is located, there are several groups of Islamic Somali who have also settled as farmers. Estimates suggest there are as many as 70,000 of them. Since the conquest of Hararghe at the end of the nineteenth century by Menelik II, several hundred thousand Christian Amhara and Tigray migrated to Hararghe from the Western Highlands where they settled in towns and villages throughout the region.

### *3.3.1 Alternating cultures and migrations*

As the northeastern gateway to Africa and the crossroads of the major caravan routes between the Ethiopian kingdom in the Western Highlands and the Somali trading centres in the eastern coastal plains, Hararghe is not simply a border region in geographic terms; in religious, political and socio-cultural respects it forms the interface between the major Christian, Muslim and traditional African culture streams in the region.

In addition to the previously mentioned, far-reaching differentiation in Ethiopian society, a number of Pan-Ethiopian cultural phenomena have evolved, on the basis of which Levine (1974) uses the term '*Greater Ethiopia*' to refer to a separate cultural area in this region of Northeast Africa.[4] In the research area, however, a number of these general cultural phenomena are less widely found.

The ecological conditions in the highlands and lowlands of Hararghe differ considerably while the various ethnic groups have different economic, social and ideological systems and speak distinct languages. Baxter and Blackhurst (1978: 164) point to a number of problems which arise when Levine (1974) includes the Oromo in his assessment of Greater Ethiopia as one cultural area based on a number of general cultural characteristics. They state: *To attempt to support the type of argument Levine is proposing by appeal to those similarities is to underestimate the consequences of Ethiopia's startlingly varied ecologies (Ethiopia is a miniature version of the continent), political, and economic systems and modes of production and the variable access to fire arms, education and other attributes of power which its different populations have had . . .*

Generally speaking the cultures of the population groups on the periphery, unlike those in the centre, are less homogeneous, so that the concepts of *a marginal area* used by Winick (1958: 38) and *frontier area* by Van Lier (1977: 6) seem to apply better to the complex situation in Hararghe. The first of these concepts stresses an area between two different cultures: *'The culture of communities which are at the periphery of a culture area and whose culture springs from the adjoining new culture areas.'* Van Lier (1977: 6) uses the second to illustrate that the population constantly find themselves in border situation: '. . . with the meaning that modern psychiatry gives to this conception . . .'. For present purposes, it is important to examine both concepts in relation to the situation of the population groups in Hararghe based on socio-historical and cultural developments in the region. At a later stage the consequences for the health situation in this particular area will be indicated.

Leaving aside geographical aspects, the socio-cultural and political significance of the 'border' character of Hararghe is reflected in the historical development of society. For centuries the capital Harar has dominated the region as *Kulturträger* from where Islam spread in waves throughout the whole of Southern Ethiopia. Later, however, towards the end of the nineteenth century, this Islamic centre and the surrounding area came under strong Christian influence as the result of a powerful counter-movement from the west. The large number of subsequent political-military and religious events show how the extensive mountain areas of present-day

Hararghe have for six centuries been the scene of changes of power and influence, wars and battles between the Semitic Amhara-Tigray from the central north, the Core Islamic groups from the east and the Oromo from the south, only interrupted by temporary occupation by the Egyptians and Italians in the nineteenth and twentieth centuries. After the 1974 revolution, Hararghe was again subjected to an attempted annexation, this time from the east. In 1977/1978 this led to the armed frontier dispute with Somalia in the Ogaden desert which Ethiopia eventually won with the help of Russian and Cuban troops (Ogaden Campaign).

Although no clear picture can be obtained of the earliest historical developments in the Eastern Highlands it has become evident that until Islam established itself as an important religious and political force, migrants from the Arabian Peninsula found their way west into Ethiopia via its northeastern coast. In about the sixth century, however, a counter-movement was launched from Aksum, the bastion of Christianity in central Ethiopia, as a result of which Islam could only penetrate further via the Eastern Highlands where central government had virtually no control (Stiehler 1943: 271). The tenth to twelfth centuries marked the first period of systematic expansion by Islam in the Horn of Africa. First, important ports in the Gulf of Aden and the Red Sea were annexed, cutting off the Central Kingdom in the east. There then followed the gradual conversion to Islam of the nomadic groups in the Somali coastal region. Afterwards, Islam spread peacefully via merchants and religious teachers from the east to the Cushitic kingdoms in western Ethiopia and Eastern Shoa. Reports dating from the thirteenth and fourteenth centuries suggest that numerous Muslim states and dynasties came into being in Hararghe at this time. However, at the beginning of the fifteenth century, a monarch of the Solomonid Dynasty, Negus Yeshaqs (1412 – 1429) conquered the states of Ifat and Shoa and later Fatagar and Hadya. This pushed the eastern border of the Central Kingdom back to the north eastern edge of the Somali Plateau. With the death of Zara Yakob (1468), however, the first expansive period of the Christian Solomonid Dynasty came to an end.

During the seventeenth century, the city of Harar was elevated to the status of Sultanate by Abu Bakr and developed into an important Emirate by annexing the surrounding states. During the first half of the sixteenth century Imam Ahmed Ibrahim al-Ghazi, known as Gran, 'the left-handed', conquered key areas of the Central Kingdom such as Bale, Dawaro, Gurage, Hadya and Shoa from his base in Harar. The religious antagonism between fanatical Christians and Muslims who had united to wage a holy war (Ar. *jihād*), formed an important factor in this lengthy struggle. After the death of 'Gran', the Emirate of Harar was weakened by attacks from the Oromo groups who had migrated into the area so that eventually, only the city of Harar remained as an important Islamic centre in the Horn of Africa (Cerulli 1936: 39; Drewes 1976: 71).

It was during this period that the great Oromo expansion took place. In 1567, a large group of fairly nomadic Oromo entered the Harar area from Southern Ethiopia. They settled as farmers on the mountain slopes of the Eastern Highlands and soon formed a new threat to both Muslims and Christians. During the Emirate of Emir Nur, the city flourished again and was protected by a fortified wall against Oromo and Somali attacks. Later, the Oromo became part of the Emirate of Harar and converted to Islam (cf. Muhammad Hassan 1973; Buschkens and Slikkerveer 1982: 21–26). This enabled the Emir to consolidate Harar and gradually expand it into a city-state made up of different groups speaking several languages: Oromifa, Harari and Somali. While the Oromo were in the majority in rural areas, Harari was the main language spoken within the walls of Harar. In the middle of the nineteenth century, during the last phase of independence, the Emirate of Harar was approximately 200 × 150 kilometres in area and within it the community of Babile began to play an important role as the marketplace on the caravan route to the Gulf of Aden (see Map 3.4). Burton (1856), who undertook his famous journey from Zeila to Harar in 1856, described the large number of Galla (Oromo) farmers in the area around Erer returning to their mountain villages from the market at Babile. The route of his journey can be seen on Map 4.4 (see page 150).

During the second half of the nineteenth century, the Suez Canal opened up the hinterland and drew the attention of Europe to East Africa. In order to be one step ahead of the European powers, Egypt launched several attacks on Ethiopia and on 10 October 1875, Rauf Pasha entered Harar and Emir Muhamad Abd-el-Shakur placed himself under the protection of the Khedive. During the period of Egyptian rule, which only lasted for a short time, a modern administrative system was introduced and the outlying Oromo areas in

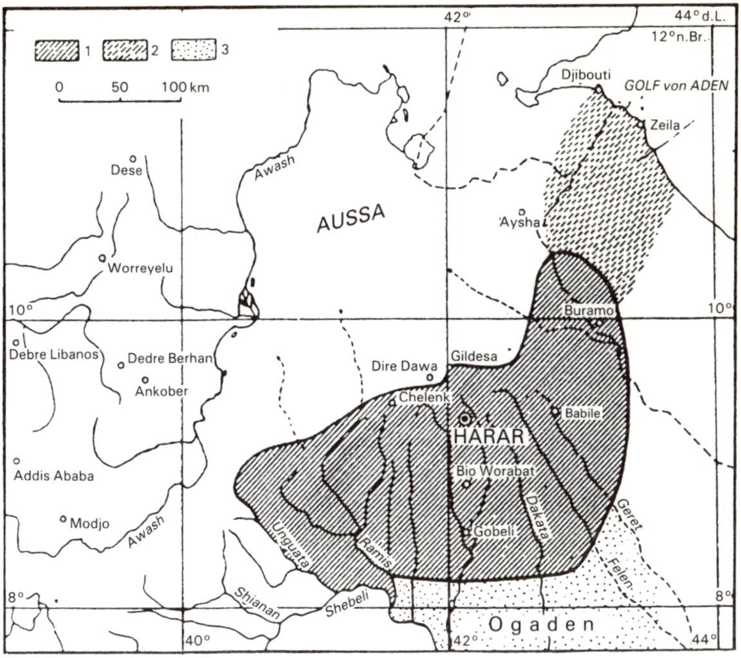


Map 3.4: *The Emirate of Harar at the end of the nineteenth century (Alula Abate 1969)*

which Babile is situated were divided into four regions or *mudiria* (Ar.). It thus became possible to protect the caravan routes with a series of guard posts with the result that the trade (Or. *karaa*) with Zeila and Berbera on the coast increased, so contributing to renewed economic prosperity in Harar.

As indicated earlier, the Amhara had penetrated further and further into Eastern Ethiopia since 1870. At the end of the nineteenth century, under Emperor Menelik II, their expansionist policies eventually focussed on conquering the Emirate of Harar. When Abdulla ibn-Muhammad had all the members of an Italian geographical expedition under Court Porro killed in 1886, the Emperor attacked the Emirate, ostensibly to avenge the deaths as Italy's ally. After a short battle at Chelenko, Harar was annexed as part of the Ethiopian Empire on 6 January 1887 (Perham 1948: 310). Together with all the other conquered territories it was declared part of the Crown Lands of Ethiopia and a feudal system was introduced. Political, administrative, social and military reforms were introduced and at the same time large groups of Amhara began to migrate from the centre of the Empire establishing the basis of the *Pax Amharica* under Menelik. During the short period of Italian occupation (1936 – 1941) the Ogaden desert was absorbed into Italian Somaliland and the remaining parts of Hararghe were divided up into four commissariats. To reduce the influence of the Amhara, the city of Harar was again declared by the Italians to be an independent Islamic centre. On his return from exile in 1941, Emperor Haile Selassie succeeded in using the administrative and financial changes introduced by the Italians and in reducing the power of the local feudal rulers. Powerful expansion of the authority of central government and military strengthening of the area made Hararghe an important Ethiopian province where the process of 'Amharisation' of the indigenous population continued. During the recent war with Somalia in the Ogaden, a military campaign was undertaken from the east which succeeded in penetrating as far as the Awash Valley. In 1978, as noted earlier, after a massive counter-offensive, the Ethiopian government succeeded in recapturing large parts of Hararghe with the help of a large people's army and foreign support from Russia and Cuba.

Constant looting, being driven off their land, high taxes, poor harvests, drought and epidemics have almost permanently caused a sense of insecurity, uncertainty and anxiety among many of the inhabitants. At times of war, great poverty or famine, a crisis developed which seriously threatened the survival of certain groups in this marginal area of The Horn.

From this overview it is clear that the various population groups who presently live on the Hararghe Plateau come from different adjoining culture areas. The wars between the Ethiopian Kingdom and the Afar and Somali under Ahmed 'Gran' involved a struggle between antagonistic, semitised population groups with different religious systems. By contrast, the great Oromo expansion led to the introduction of traditional African authority in an area which only converted to Islam much later. More than half of the present-day Oromo of Hararghe are descended from these migrants from the African cultural areas. The smaller Somali group established themselves as arable farmers in the area having migrated from the Somali coastal region. The culture of the Amhara-Tigray, who migrated to the area *en masse* around the turn of the century, derives from the

Christian Ethiopian Kingdom in the west. The inhabitants of Harar, the Harari who speak a separate South Ethio-Semitic language, are unique in being the only Ethiopian population group to have developed a culture within a single major urban centre. The varying ecological conditions of the highlands and the lowlands forced the various groups to adapt in order to guarantee their survival. For example, the Oromo and the Somali developed a simple form of arable farming based on cereals and oil seeds, while the nomadic Somali practised a system of livestock farming in the low-lying areas.

The difference between the traditional Oromo and Amhara socio-cultural systems are as clear in the plural society of Hararghe as they are in other parts of Ethiopia. The largely individual-orientated authority, which can be seen for example in the hierarchical Amhara administrative system, differs sharply from the collective principles of the Oromo who have retained a number of traditional, economic, political and ritual activities in the village communities based on the 'gada' system. The most striking division, however, is between the two major religions in the area, Christianity and Islam. These phenomena will be discussed in more detail in the description of the socio-graphic survey in Babile.

To summarise, the concepts of *marginal area* and *frontier area* can conveniently be applied to Hararghe with some justification. In linguistic terms, it is a *transitional area* between the culture areas of the Middle East and Africa, and in particular, the cultures of the East Horn and the Eastern Highlands. In these peripheral areas, a society has developed with a complex cultural system, which has its origins to a large extent in the adjoining culture areas. The specific significance of the situation in relation to the crisis which has constantly affected the rural population of Hararghe as a result of conflicts, wars, poor harvests, famine and disease will be dealt with more fully in the account of the health care situation among the different groups in question.

### *3.3.2 Harar and the process of transculturation*

From the preceding socio-historical overview of Hararghe it is clear that the area has been subjected to a highly complex process of alternating cultural influences over the centuries. These include successive contacts with the historical Ethiopian kingdom in the

Western Highlands, the Muslim states in the Somali coastal region, the traditional Oromo groups in the south, the Islamic armies of Egypt, the Christian Amhara of the expansive empire of Menelik II, the Italian occupying forces of Mussolini from Europe and finally, the Amhara bureaucratic system of the modern Ethiopian state, briefly disrupted by the Somali invasion in the late seventies. As a consequence, a number of changes have been experienced by the Oromo, and to a small extent, by the sedentary Somali population and the Amhara-Tigray migrants who settled in the area much later.

As noted in section 1.2.2, generally speaking, when the nature of a society in a given area is largely determined by alternating cultures and migrations, there is a process of assimilation by one society of part of the culture of another, resulting from constant contacts. In this context is it necessary to examine whether the historical contacts between the various cultures in this area have resulted in such reciprocal influences. This will determine whether the concept of *transculturation* put forward by Ortiz (1970) and referred to in section 1.2.2, can provide a better understanding of the reciprocal nature of successive cultural contacts and in particular of the composition of the complex system of health care in this area. The following sections explain and illustrate the transcultural aspect of the society in this border land in more detail in the light of several important consequences of the socio-historical processes in Hararghe which have already been described.

From the tenth to the twelfth centuries, Islamisation of the Ethiopian kingdom and the military organisation of nomads took place under pressure from migrant groups from the Arabian Peninsula, resulting in the fourteenth century in an extensive network of Muslim states and dynasties. As a result, Arabian culture spread throughout the region. Numerous thirteenth-century Arabian manuscripts, most of them religious, found in Harar, Chercher and Arussi, reflect this major cultural force which had established an Islamic frontline in the Eastern Highlands before the existence of the Christian kingdom. However, it did not have any real cohesion. Alula Abate (1969: 40) notes: *'Jedoch bestand, bedingt durch die Oszillation den Machtstellung zwischen Christen und Mohammedanern einerseits sowie andererseits unter den Mohammedanische Staaten selbst zwischen diesen muselmannischen Staaten ein nur lockerer Zusammenhang'.* With the restoration of the

Christian kingdom under the Solomonid Dynasty, a new era dawned in the thirteenth century in the relations between Christians and Muslims. The centuries of conflict which ensued, were not so much caused by political policies but rather by the religious and cultural domination of the islamised population groups in the area. At the root of it, too, was an expansionist movement on the part of Afar and Somali which soon assumed a fanatical religious character. The movement was led to begin with by the local Emir, but when the Afar and Somali combined, the leadership was taken over by the Imam as the 'Defender of the True Faith'. This shift of emphasis changed the character of Islamisation to such an extent that a mass religious war against Ethiopia ensued. Trimingham (1976: 80) comments as follows as regards this war: *'It was transfigured by an ardent fanaticism and turned into "jihad", a religious war.'* As a result, two parties came into being in the Emirate of Harar: the fanatical people's party led by the Emir which sought military victory and the establishment of an Islamic state and the aristocratic party which centred on the Sultan's court which was in favour of trade and peaceful co-existence with the Christian kingdom. This duality eventually led to the disintegration of Islamic authority in Harar.

During the regime of the war-like Ahmed 'Gran', the Muslim area was extended by means of successive military campaigns against the Christians who were forced to convert to Islam or, in some cases, they were executed. After the defeat of 'Gran' by Christian forces assisted by the Portuguese, the Emirate became cut off from coastal trade with the Red Sea and thus with Arabic culture, and the city underwent rapid economic decline as did government and Arabic education and sciences. Subsequently, a defensive process of Islamisation was conducted from Harar along more peaceful lines by means of trade and religious teachers.

Numerous wars had devastated the country which internally had become extremely weak. However, this situation directly contributed to a new threat to both Christians and Muslims: the large-scale Oromo migrations which dominated the next three centuries. Unlike the expansion of the Amhara and the Tigray, which had been largely aimed at political domination, the great Oromo expansion was based on a need for more land for a rapidly growing population and the ritual duty of *gada* to wage war and to launch military expeditions every eight years. Once they had dispersed throughout

Ethiopia, the Oromo groups became isolated from one another, however, and lost much of their original unity. Various types of contact with the peoples they fought or subjugated meant that virtually every Oromo group developed in its own specific way as a result of different religious, cultural, political and social influences. This gave rise to a varied cultural pattern among the Oromo which has spread throughout the highlands (cf. Buschkens and Slikkerveer 1982: 18).

Harar developed into a flourishing centre of trade at the crossroads of the important caravan routes between the Somali coastal towns of Zeila and Berbera and the Ethiopian hinterland. Moreover, the Emirate developed into an Islamic city state with its own special culture. During the great migrations, the Oromo entered the area around Harar where they settled as farmers. Although the political power of the Emirate was broken, the walled city was still able to withstand their attacks. In the early nineteenth century a system of mutual economic dependence developed from the trading relations between Harar and surrounding population groups, as a result of which cultural contacts intensified. During the rule of Emir Muhammad (1856 – 1875), the influence of the Oromo in Harar grew. They were futher absorbed into Islam through close dealings with the Harari. At the same time, as this process of Islamisation was taking place, Arabic music, literature, arts and sciences were spreading more widely among the surrounding groups. The Arabic calendar replaced the traditional method of calculating the time. Consequently, the Oromo like the Somali in the region, underwent major social and cultural changes. The pattern of life which was governed by strict Islamic rules took place to a large extent within village communities, some of which developed into important local markets as a result of contact with Harari and Arab traders. The significance for the ethnic groups in the surrounding area of the spread from Harar of Arabic sciences and the 'great tradition of medicine' will be dealt with in the account of the medical systems in the area (cf. Muhammad Hassan 1973).

When Harar came under the control of the Egyptian khedives in 1875, an expansionist policy in relation to Ethiopia was implemented. The Harari saw the arrival of the Egyptians as an opportunity to resist the growing dominance of the Oromo and handed over their city to Rauf Pasha and his armies without a struggle. Egypt quickly succeeded in turning Harar into a powerful military base and completely subjugating the Oromo living round the city. By the time the Egyptians were forced to withdraw from Harar because of the Mahdi rebellion in the Sudan, a large number of important administrative reforms had been introduced, which were adopted by the new Emir Abdullahi. Demissie Gebre Michael (1974: 22) comments on this period: *'Though their time was rather short and oppressive, they succeeded in registering the land of the neighbouring Galloa tribes and imposed a new land taxation system and established among the Gallas the new administrative positions of Demina, Gerada and Melak.'* The political vacuum in Hararghe after the departure of the Egyptians was exploited by Emperor Menelik II who annexed the province at the end of the last century as part of the Ethiopian Empire. In socio-cultural and political terms this resulted in groups living in the Eastern Highlands again being subjected to a new cultural influence, namely that of the Christian Amhara. In the following period, many Amhara were transferred by the central government to Hararghe in their capacity as government officials, soldiers, teachers or religious leaders. Amhara farmers also moved to the new Crown Land to farm the fertile lands which had once belonged to the Oromo. A large number of new Amhara settlements came into being throughout the province (Am. *katama*) and in 1938 the number of Amhara in Hararghe had increased to approximately 300,000 (Brooke 1956).

Like many other ethnic groups in Ethiopia, the Oromo and Somali were forced to modify their social and cultural systems to that of the Christian Amhara. The Amhara also set in motion the process of 'Amharisation' or *Pax Amharica* which the central government attempted to carry through by making Amarhinya the official language and by introducing a system of health care, education, a banking system, communications, mass media and a legal system.

Major reforms in the field of administration, legislation and the ownership of land were implemented. A feudal rent system (Am. *gebar*) was introduced whereby tenants paid taxes by yielding part of their harvest of crops or by making their labour available to government officials, army officers and, in some cases, representatives of the church. This was temporarily suspended when, for a brief period, Ethiopia together with Eritrea and Somalia became part of the colony of Italian East Africa. The Italians stayed until 1941 and conducted a major programme to develop Ethiopia. This resulted in a number of new developments in Hararghe and elsewhere as regards agriculture, house building, road construction and industry. The attention paid to the province consisted chiefly of extending the network of roads and improving communications. The Italians also tried to create political divisions between the Amhara, the Harari, the Oromo and the Somali, which was in their own interests, by pursuing a pro-Muslim policy. The feudal tenant-system was abolished, with the exception of the land tax system. Part of the tenant-land was reserved for Italian colonists and experimental farms, while the remainder was allocated to the Oromo, Harari and Somali. After the withdrawal of the Italians in 1941, the Amhara quickly restored their authority and a new period of reform and modernisation began. The old tenant-farmer system was re-introduced and the feudal landlords even demanded 'their' rent from the period of the Italian occupation, to which they encountered considerable resistance. Central political and administrative positions and local provincial, district and sub-district positions were mainly occupied by non-indigenous Amhara-Tigray inhabitants of the region. Partly because the Oromo, Somali and Afar no longer played an active role in the dominant political system, their political organisation was substantially weakened and gradually reduced to the level of a ritual institution. Despite the revision of the consititution in 1955 there are still problems regarding equal treatment before the law for the different ethnic and religious groups (Buschkens and Slikkerveer 1982: 31, 32). After the 1974 revolution, the implementation of the 1975 Rural Land Reform Proclamation meant, as far as Hararghe was concerned, that land became collective property and that each household was allowed a holding no bigger than 10 hectares. The students who took part in the Development Through Cooperation Campaign (*Zemecha*) in 1975 were sent throughout the region to organise the new peasant associations on the basis of the traditional rural village communities of approximately 60 to 80 households or administrative regions of approximately 800 hectares. Although the programme of reform was still being implemented while this research was being carried out, and was later seriously delayed by the social and political uncertainty resulting from the 1977 – 1978 border conflict with Somalia, it did represent an attempt to bring about radical change in landownership and existing power structures in rural areas. The unhappy relations between the original inhabitants of the region and national and local government agencies also had an adverse effect on the planned socio-economic development. Despite the fact that farmers in the Highlands managed to increase population in the first instance as a result of the new reforms, fresh armed clashes in Hararghe have created a new crisis for the inhabitants of this area.

To summarise, the one-sided approach to Ethiopian society used in earlier studies which emphasise the Semitic aspect of Ethiopian culture is not only incapable of describing the country as a whole, but is certainly inadequate to describe the situation in Hararghe. This idea of Ethiopia as a 'Semitic outpost in Africa' used by Ullendorff (1973) and to a lesser extent Trimingham (1976), only applies in the border region of Hararghe to the Amhara-Tigray upper stratum of the society. In particular the non-Semitic elements of the complex cultural pattern of the Oromo, Somali and Afar in this area, together with the adjustments which Amhara-Tigray culture has had to make in the Eastern Highlands, argue in favour of a more historical approach to the cultural interaction which has taken place over the centuries. The use of the transcultural perspective in this analysis of the society in this transitional area not only increases understanding of the entire complex social structure, but also creates the possibility of approaching the whole problem of development in the Horn of Africa from a more dynamic point of view by bringing out the various ethno-cultural and religious backgrounds of the population groups concerned. The specific importance of such a transcultural approach to health care problems in the region will be established at a later stage on the basis of an analysis of the existing medical systems and the associated processes of illness behaviour and health care utilisation.

In conclusion it is evident that the current composition of Ethiopian society is largely dependent on the results of two important historical processes: internal differentiation on the part of the various population groups and external interaction by these groups with bordering cultures in this part of Africa. On the basis of the origin of various groups and differentiation in ethnic affiliation, language, religion and economic activity, this heterogeneous society, even in the absence of long-standing colonial rule, can be regarded as a plural society in itself, bearing important implications for the analysis of its socio-economic development. This process, which has been stimulated in all kinds of ways by government, particularly since the Second World War, has suffered from stagnation and disruption, primarily because of internal social and political relations and contrasts. The research area is part of the eastern administrative region of Hararghe which in geographical and socio-cultural terms clearly has the character of a marginal province. It is situated in the transitional area between the Mediterranean and the African cultural areas, on the borders of the Eastern Highlands and the Lowlands of the East Horn. Constant socio-economic, ethno-cultural and political tensions, low production and the symptoms of poverty in food, housing, education and health care, etc., together with frequent armed conflicts, mean that large sections of the rural population additionally find themselves more or less permanently in a psychological 'marginal' position where anxiety and uncertainty are almost permanent factors of daily life.

The process of acculturation which has taken place here between the different cultures and waves of migrants has not been in one direction; reciprocal influences and the incorporation of certain cultural elements (for example relating to social and political organisation, religion and faith in supernatural beings, ritual practices and customs) strongly argue in favour of the adoption of a transcultural perspective to study the divergent social phenomena. Without such knowledge of the extremly complex cultural contacts which have taken place over centuries, it is almost impossible to obtain a proper understanding of the socio-economic development of the society in all its aspects and facets.

Against the background of this approach, the next chapter will attempt to depict the community of Babile where the field study has been carried out, providing the socio-cultural context of medical ideas and practices of the population.

## Notes

1. After the Second World War, Eritrea temporarily became a British Mandate Territory until the United Nations decided to federate it with Ethiopia in 1952. Although Eritrea was autonomous as regards

domestic affairs, its foreign affairs, trade, defence and communications were in the hands of the Ethiopian government. In 1962, Eritrea became part of Ethiopia, a move opposed by some of the local population. Since that time, a number of movements have been fighting a war of independence in an attempt to break away from Ethiopia (cf. Ullendorff 1973; Kleinpenning 1980).

2. Ullendorff (1973: 30, 31) reports on the contribution of aerial photography to demographic research in Ethiopia. By combining detailed aerial shots which record every single dwelling (*tukul*) in the country with samples of the number of inhabitants per household, it is possible to obtain an estimate of the total population.
3. Trimingham (1976: 24 – 25) points out that although Ethiopia is a diocese of the Egyptian Church and the Bishop of the Ethiopian Church (Am. *Abuna*) is always a Copt appointed by the Patriarch of Alexandria, the Ethiopian Church is certainly not a 'satellite' of the Church of Alexandria. '*It is*', he says '*a mistake to call the Abyssinians from the religious point of view, Copts, as many people do* . . .'.
4. The concept of 'field of ethnological study' is closely related to the concept of 'culture area', which, as an anthropological approach to the entire Indonesian Archipelago, can view Indonesia as one ethnological field of study on the basis of a number of pan-Indonesian cultural characteristics among the population groups in the field of social organisation (J. P. B. de Josselin de Jong 1935; P. E. de Josselin de Jong 1977, 1980).

4

# Babile, Community Life in the Highlands

## 4.1 The Structure of a Rural Community

This chapter describes the structure of the research area as a rural community in the Ethiopian-Somali borderland, which forms the focus of the help-seeking and utilisation patterns of different groups of the mountain population.

The nature of the *katama* (Am.) as recent settlements of the central authority in Hararghe are explained in geographical and historical terms and their socio-political implications are briefly indicated. After describing the research and the sample, this section goes on to describe the different methods of the survey. In addition, it presents material based on fieldwork, concerning the demographic structure of Babile, its ethno-religious composition, the family system and housing conditions, and the economic life and occupational structure of the community. Special attention is paid to the social, economic and cultural factors which have been selected for this study as potentially important determinants of illness behaviour and health care utilisation in Babile. In addition, a short account of the regional pattern of illness and health will be presented. By comparison, the results of a study of local disease classification among the two major ethnic groups of Babile will conclude this chapter.

### *4.1.1 Settlement pattern of the katama*

Babile, which is part of the administrative district (Am. *awraja*) of Gursum in the Hararghe Region, is a multi-ethnic, rural community consisting of some 4,000 inhabitants (1982) and lies on the mountain slopes of the Eastern Highlands at an altitude of approximately 2,000 metres, about 30 kilometres southeast of the provincial capital, Harar (see Map 4.1). Situated on the important road connecting Jijiga in the eastern border area with Somalia, which, historically speaking, formed an important caravan route to the port of Berbera on the Gulf of Aden, Babile is a central market place for the surrounding mountain villages. According to local tradition, it is called after the founding Oromo group under Babile[1], one of the four sons of Kallo who settled in the area at the time of the great Oromo migrations during the sixteenth century. The descendants of the four brothers are united in Hararghe in the Confederation of Afran Kallo. The settlement lies on a plateau of the Gondudo mountains, one of the eastern spurs of the Hararghe Plateau between the valleys of the Errer and the Dagata. Towards the south, Babile also forms the gateway to the Ogaden desert and the Somali Plateau via the road junction leading to Fik and Humaro Hadad. As the aerial photograph shows, the original dwellings and buildings are grouped round the central market place (Or. *magalaa*) where the police station, administrative office, road service and primary school were built at the beginning of this century (Plate 16). Vegetation in this part of the highlands consists of grasses, acacias, thorn-bushes and occasional euphorbias. The group of large, shady trees south of the building of the Coptic Church was planted by the parishioners at an earlier date.

Climatically speaking, Babile lies in the transitional tropical zone between the more humid Eastern Highlands in the west and the lower, drier Somali Plateau in the Southeast. In summer, the monsoon blows over the area towards Southeast Asia, while during the winter, a very dry northeast trade wind penetrates the Rift Valley from the Danakil plains. The rains last from April or May to the end of September with maximum precipitation in August. Records are rare and show considerable variation in levels of annual rainfall from one year to another. However, average annual rainfall in the

A Abate HARAR Beilage I

# HOCHLAND VON HARAR

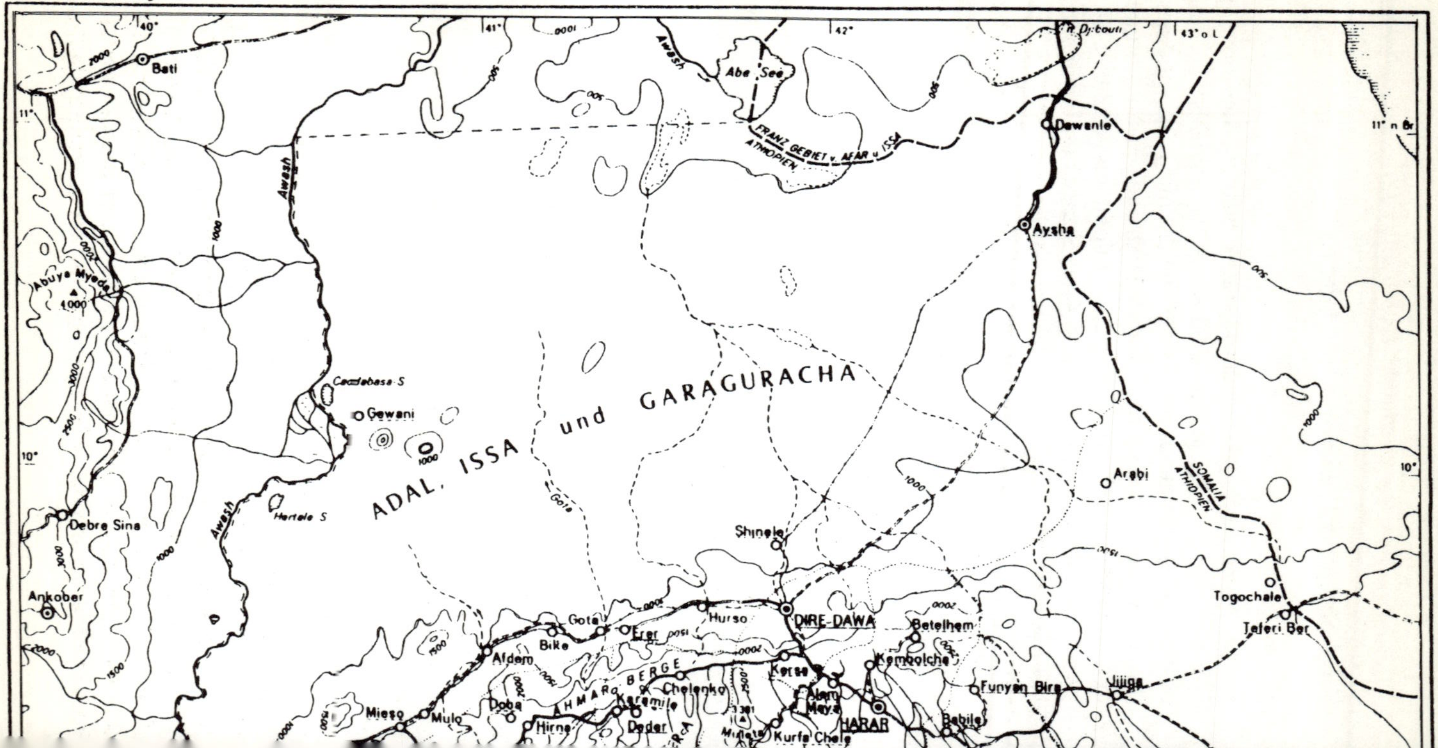

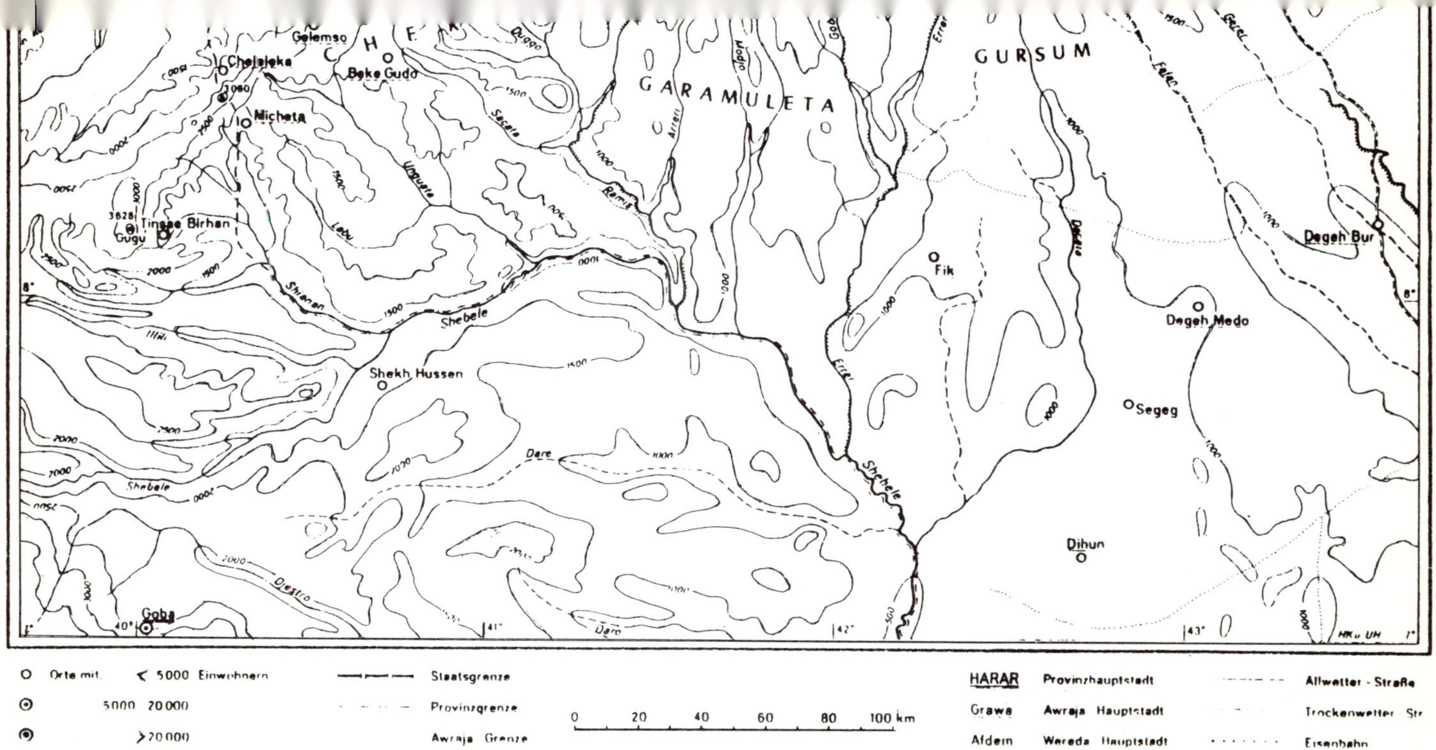


**Map 4.1:** *The Highlands of Hararghe in Eastern Ethiopia (Alula Abate 1969)*

research area is estimated at 900 mm per annum. Average daily maximum temperatures range from 72° to 87°F per year and daily minimum temperatures from 57° to 65°F per year. The community lies at a height of 1,650 metres in the *woina dega* (Am.), the moderate zone roughly between 1,600 and 2,200 metres. The main crops are millet, maize, peanuts, coffee and *chat* (Am.). The zone has a vegetation typical of savannah which, as the ground rises, turns into mountain savannah. Numerous types of shrubs form the ground cover, among which trees such as acacia, ficus and *Euphorbia candelabra* are occasionally to be found. Large mammals such as lion, leopard and elephant inhabit the area, particularly the virtually impenetrable Dagata Valley. Several species of gazelle and deer, including mouse deer, can be seen regularly in these highlands. Seed-eating birds represent a serious threat to the livelihood of local farmers and during the maize and millet harvest they try to keep the large flocks away by throwing stones at them from towers especially built for the purpose.

Little is known about the early history of Babile. At the foot of the steep northern escarpment there are six caves containing beautiful rock paintings, probably dating from the Neolithic period. West of the Erer is the *Erer Kemeyatt* (Am.) where a number of red and black drawings of hunting scenes with bison and gazelles are to be found. There are several old manuscripts in Harar containing descriptions of these scenes (Abdul Hafiz 1976: 3).

Between 1530 and 1540, the Barentu group from Southern Ethiopia entered the area of Bale, Dawaro, Fatagar and Adal as part of the major Oromo migrations of the sixteenth century. They settled on the mountain slopes of the Eastern Highlands as livestock and arable farmers. As mentioned before, Islam spread from the Emirate of Harar across Southern and Eastern Ethiopia and this was how the Oromo in Hararghe, including those living in Babile, first experienced its influences. The Islamisation of the Oromo was so effective during the short period of Egyptian occupation of Harar towards the end of the last century, that virtually all groups were converted to Islam at this time. Two exceptions were the Ittu and Annya, who were partly Islamised but retained a large number of traditional African rites and practices (Trimingham 1976: 207). Frequent military campaigns were conducted during the Egyptian occupation of Harar, particularly against the Babile, Bursuk, Nole and Oberra groups, at which times their villages were burnt to the ground and their menfolk killed (Demissie Gebre Michael 1974: 22).

When the Egyptians left in 1885 and the Emirate was briefly restored under Emir Abdullahi of the Ali-ben-Dawud Dynasty, a new danger threatened from the west. The King of Shoa, the late Emperor Menelik II wished to gain access to the Red Sea. Although he initially launched unsuccessful attacks from Shoa on the Itu groups in the Chercher area in 1883, 1884 and 1885 he finally defeated the Emir's armies at the Battle of Chelenqo on 7 January 1887. After the occupation of Harar, on 29 January of that year, a two-day offensive was waged against the Babile group, whose cattle were stolen to feed Menelik's army (Caulk 1971). Hararghe was again declared the property of the Ethiopian Crown and reforms were subsequently introduced in numerous areas. The Amhara expansion which began during this period and which was only interrupted by the brief Italian occupation during the Second World War, has had important consequences for society in the area. This process of pacification, or *Pax Amharica* as it is known, therefore needs to be examined more closely.

Babile was originally a farming community. During the Egyptian occupation, because of its favourable location between Hararghe and the Red Sea it became a part of a reinforced regional network of local markets and caravan stations in the Eastern Highlands. From the turn of the century onwards, as groups of Amhara migrants entered the area from the west, the local pattern of settlements changed considerably as Amhara military and political centres (Am. *katama*; Or. *magalaa*) spread throughout the conquered territory. These settlements have been described in detail by Kuls (1958) and Alula Abate (1969) among others, who both refer to *politisch-militärischen Zentralorten*. Originally, the *katama* (Am.) were established primarily as permanent military camps to provide the emperor or governor with accommodation and military protection as they travelled about the empire. They were simple fortifications on the edge of inaccessible mountain formations (Am. *amba*). However, some of the *katama* were located in existing villages and hamlets which were important in political, military and, in particular, economic terms. Many of these existing communities already had local agricultural produce and cattle markets which flourished after the advent of the Amhara. At these markets the Oromo and Somali were able to exchange their products for goods which merchants brought from the larger towns. When the road network was later improved and extended, the *katama* along the caravan routes grew in importance in relation to other local markets and craftsmen and traders of different origins began to settle there. The population of Babile expanded rapidly at this time. The settlement became an independent sub-district (Am. *wereda*) within the administrative framework of the province and subsequently a church, a primary school, a telephone post, an administrative building and a clinic were also built.

These historical developments are clearly reflected in the present geographical structure of Babile. The community developed from a simple sedentary farming hamlet with a local market, favourably located between two rivers and on an important caravan route to the Red Sea, into a major political and military centre in the district of Gursum. Around the buildings, which have already been referred to, there are several modern rectangular dwellings, shops and coffee bars, chiefly owned by Amhara, Arabs and Harari. On the edge of the community, around the market place, there are still some traditional Oromo and Somali houses with conical roofs (*tukul*). The heterogeneous nature of Babile – which is discussed later in this chapter in connection with its social structure – increased considerably, largely because of the arrival of the Amhara and the establishment of *katama*. Map 4.2 shows the distribution of *katama* settlements in Hararghe which spread throughout the highlands as outposts of the central authorities. This resulted in decisive political, social, cultural and economic changes in the local society and the accompanying migration of Amhara and Tigray considerably enhanced ethnic variety.

In general, terms such as 'town' and 'village' do not really apply to the settlement and lifestyles of the various population groups in the highlands of Ethiopia. Historically speaking, towns of a singularly urban character (of the type frequently found elsewhere in Africa, Arabia or Latin America) are rare, in view of the fact that settlements of the present-day were established in times of war when the peasant population sought refuge in the steep and inaccessible mountain areas (Nas 1981). Also the Amharic term *katama* literally means a permanent encampment. The large towns such as Harar, Gondar and Aksum, which are exceptions to this general pattern, have religious origins or were inspired by foreign influences.

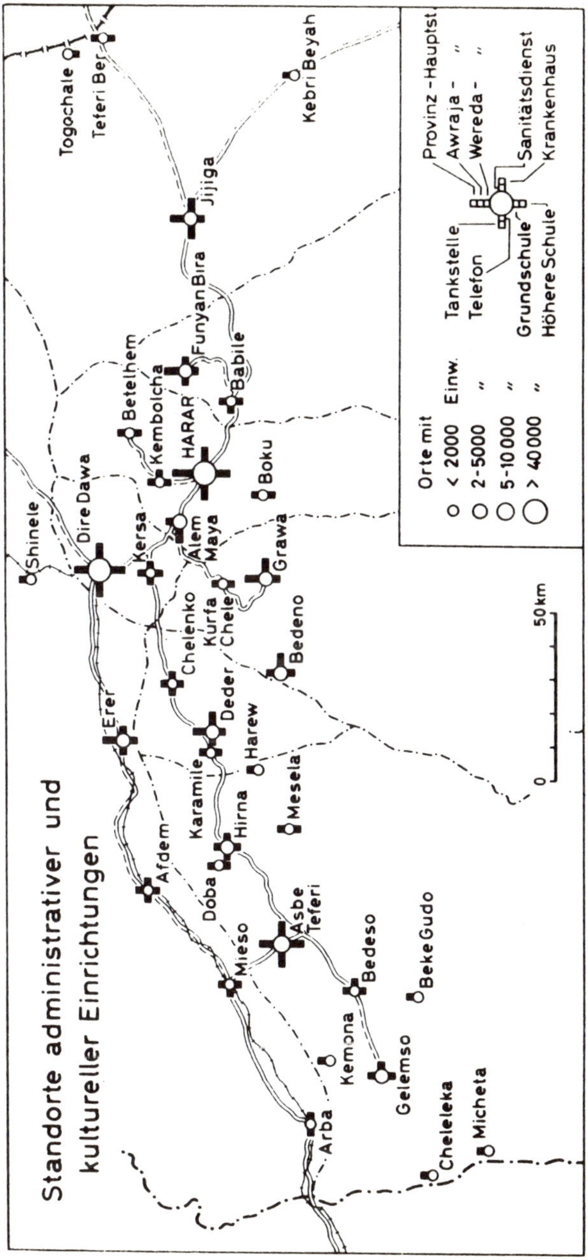


Map 4.2: *Katama settlements in the Administrative Region of Hararghe (Alula Abate 1969, App. N)*

The dominant settlement pattern among local groups in Hararghe – as elsewhere in Ethiopia – is the village community (Or. *ganda*) made up largely of Oromo who are mostly dependent on self-supporting, mixed farms of limited size. A *ganda* usually consists of 10 to 50 household groups and includes one or two clans (Or. *gosa*). As mentioned before, in the course of this century a number of rural communities developed in the new provinces, for example, from existing local market places, with a population of between 2,000 and 5,000 and these form a separate category between the large towns and the numerous *ganda*. Despite differences in ethnicity, religion, economic life and political organisation, the inhabitants of these groups retain their own identity and sense of unity in relation to other communities. In this context, Hunter and Whitten (1975: 84) refer to the wider meaning attributed to the term 'community' by sociologists: *'The concept of the term "community" is used quite loosely by sociologists to characterise a wide range of groups whose members share a sense of identity, specific interest, values, and a role definition with respect to each other'*. Galjart (1978) stresses the 'we' feeling of local groups which determines the boundaries of a local community. Boer (1981: 7) uses the following working definition: '. . . *a group of people living within a relatively small geographic area, sharing at least some economic and social institutions, having at least some interaction among themselves and feeling that they together belong to the same local community'*. In the light of this definition, Babile can be analysed as a multi-ethnic community in the rural area of the Horn of Africa, the internal social structure of which is central to the present study.

Ownership of land in the Oromo *gosa* (Or.) was originally governed by the *gadaa* system which regulated the entire social order, in particular the political and military organisation, a phenomenon which is observed in all Oromo groups in Ethiopia (Haberland 1963: 17). The *gadaa* system was based on classes of age groups succeeding one another at eight year intervals and assuming responsibility for military, economic and ritual tasks and duties from the previous generation (Asmarom Legesse 1973). In the Babile area, the *gadaa* system has lost much of its original significance.

The administrative system of the Emirs of Harar, to which Babile belonged in about 1850 as an 'outlying territory' (Am. *gaffa*), had four important political functions: the *dogin*, the Harari governor who was responsible for the outlying provinces of the Emirate, whose subalterns were the *damina*, the local tribal chief, the *gerada* or clan leader and the *malak*, the neighbourhood chief. In the research area, the position of leader (Or. *abbaa bokkuu*) who was part of the original collective Oromo leadership still exists. When the province became part of the Ethiopian Empire in 1887, the positions of *abbaa bokkuu* and *gerada* were incorporated into the new administrative system as local land agents to collect rents and taxes. The farming land in the region was allocated under a principle of land tenure (Am. *rist*) as private property to soldiers, officials and churchmen who were loyal to the regime. Within this feudal system (Am. *gabar*), local Oromo farmers were employed as tenant farmers. Alula Abate (1969) describes this situation as follows: *Das den Amhara zugewiesene Land wurde fast ausschliesslich nicht von diesen selbst bewirtschaftet, sondern von den dort ansässigen underworfenen Galla. Diese waren als Gabar den Soldaten, Melkegna und Geistlichen zugeteilt worden, d.h. als Hörige, die verpflichtet waren, die Grundherren mit Lebensmitteln und Geld zu versorgen und Frontdiensten zu leisten.*

After the arrival of the Amhara migrants and as a result of the temporary Italian occupation, a very effective and powerful administrative system was introduced in which thousands of Amhara public servants and soldiers came to occupy positions at the provincial, district and sub-district levels.

The administrative system used by the current revolutionary government is still proving difficult to introduce in this area, particularly as far as land reform, the nationalisation of firms and banks and the collectivisation of farms are concerned. It has, however, added a new institution to the existing socio-political structure in Babile, viz. the peasant association, which is primarily concerned with vigorously implementing the principles of *Hebretesabawinet* or 'Ethiopian Socialism', and the closely associated reforms of central authority. Despite the announcement of such measures as the *Rural Land Reform Proclamation* (1975), the *Zemecha Campaign* (1975), the *All Ethiopian Peasant Association* (1977) and the *Socialist Farmers Cooperation Proclamation* (1979) an acceptable programme of reform for the region still has to be drawn up and implemented (Yemane Tekle Mariam 1981).

As a result of the slow progress of agricultural reforms and democratisation in Babile – which came briefly under Somali influence during the 1977 – 1978 Ogaden war – the socio-political system has undergone few fundamental changes. The complex relationships and tensions present in the community have in no way lessened in the post-revolutionary era and in some respects contrasts have become stronger.

The social hierarchy of Babile is largely based on the prestige of local and regional officials who can be divided into four categories:

1. Non-indigenous, mainly Amhara, high-ranking civil servants and party officials who represent the central authorities in the community. They include the holders of the official positions of administrator, army commander, head of the police, district head, and the representative of the Commission for Organising the Party of the Working People of Ethiopia (COPWE) and members of the peasant associations and neighbourhood councils (*kebele*).
2. Traditional leaders of local ethnic groups and religious and secular leaders of the different groups and sects in Babile. These are mainly Oromo and Somali members of the local elite.
3. The semi-urban class of traders, merchants and small industrialists (often non-indigenous), who control most of the money economy in Babile. The people in this category are from different areas and ethnic groups (Harari, Gurage, Arabs, Somali, etc.).
4. The recent category of intellectuals, including students, teachers, campaign leaders, modern health care staff and leaders of development projects. The latter are largely from the capital, Addis Ababa, where they have been trained and educated. In Babile, they account for most of the new opinion leaders who can make a major contribution to socio-political development.

A comparison of the present social structure with the hierarchy in rural communities before the 1974 revolution shows that, despite a major upheaval of the national political system, there have yet been hardly any essential changes in the socio-political organisation. It is true that a significant impetus has been given to the introduction of administrative reforms, but in fact all that has happened is that former Amhara district heads and administrative officials have been replaced by new revolutionary party officials and administrators. Local chiefs and religious leaders have lost their land but have managed to obtain privileged positions for themselves in revolutionary bodies within the political framework of the new regime. The class of traders, merchants and small entrepreneurs has not undergone any change to speak of while an intellectual elite has emerged on a modest scale.

### *4.1.2 Research setting and sample surveys*

Before reviewing the socio-anthropological fieldwork material collected in Babile, the methods used in this study will first be briefly discussed.

The fieldwork linked up to the previous research project, Rural Health in Ethiopia, and was carried out in Babile between 1976 and 1982. It comprised a qualitative and a quantitative part, which, during the various stages of the research, intermingled.

Primarily, the method used was that of participant observation, based on staying and working in the community for extended periods of time, together with conducting interviews and discussions with key informants and representatives of the various ethnic groups in Harar and Babile. Quantitative material was assembled also by means of a questionnaire which had been drawn up and tested in advance. Questionnaires were then completed by local interpreters during household interviews with the help of previously selected heads of household and members of their families. The socio-graphical material was assembled using existing literature, statistical sources and reports, supplemented with field observations. To obtain specific data on the complex relationship between illness, illness behaviour and health care utilisation on the part of the target group, the research was approached from two different perspectives: *community-based* and *institution-based.*

#### Community-based: from the actual population of the community itself

Data on background characteristics of respondents and members of their families, their illness episodes during the twelve months of the fieldstudy together with use of medicines, and utilisation of the traditional, transitional and modern medical systems were collected by means of health interview surveys.

#### Institution-based: from the existing medical systems

The different medical systems were closely examined by means of quantitative and qualitative surveys in order to obtain a better understanding of their functioning and service to the population groups.

As a result of this approach, the following categories of data could be collected:

1. socio-graphical data on the community – the *base-line survey;*
2. data concerning medical services, specifically the medical systems and their staff – *the operational survey*;
3. data concerning illness behaviour and health care utilisation by people in the sample who reported themselves ill during the twelve month period and their contacts with the three systems – *the health interview survey*;
4. individual background factors of these patients, grouped according to predisposing factors (socio-demographic, social and psychological variables) and enabling factors (socio-economic variables) – *the household survey*;
5. data concerning the perceived morbidity of the people in the sample who reported themselves ill – *the health interview survey*;
6. data concerning the different medical institutions present in the region – *the institutional survey.*

Since it was possible in this research to make explicit use of prior knowledge of a number of characteristics of the different ethnic groups in Babile, it was decided to take a stratified simple random sample. The total population was divided into a number of sub-populations using ethnicity as a criterion for stratification. The elements for the sample were then chosen at random from the sub-populations or strata and drawn proportionally so that the sample ratios were the same for all the strata[2].

Official estimates give the number of inhabitants of Babile at the time of the research as roughly 4,000, consisting of approximately 50% Oromo, 35% Amhara, 10% Somali and 5% other ethnic groups (Abdullahi 1976). Table 4.1 shows the total number of people in the sample, according to ethnic group.

It is clear from these figures that more than half of the people in the survey were Oromo and more than a third Amhara. Somali and other ethnic groups make up a much smaller percentage of the population. This ties in with the description given earlier of the *katama* which evolved from market settlements inhabited largely by Oromo and a few Somali households and where Amhara migrants settled at a later date.

Table 4.1 *Number of respondents and households in the sample in Babile, according to ethnic group.*

| | number of households | | number of people | |
|---|---|---|---|---|
| | N | % | N | % |
| Oromo | 176 | 52.2 | 716 | 53.0 |
| Amhara | 130 | 38.6 | 519 | 38.4 |
| Somali | 24 | 7.1 | 88 | 6.5 |
| others | 7 | 2.1 | 28 | 2.1 |
| Total | 337 | 100.0 | 1351 | 100.0 |

In accordance with the theoretical orientation of the system's approach both with regard to the process of seeking and obtaining medical help and to the components of the analytical model, as described in Chapter 2, the data concerning background characteristics of respondents, reported cases of illness and the utilisation of the different medical systems were compiled on the basis of health interview surveys, combined with field observations during illness episodes. In practice, appointments for interviews in the mornings or evenings produced the best results. The houses in the sample were given a number so that the members of the team could return at a later stage, if necessary, for more information, to make corrections or for repeated interview surveys.

The interviews took about two hours per household group and were conducted with a questionnaire which had been tried out and adopted in advance from the previous 'Rural Health in Ethiopia' project (Buschkens and Slikkerveer 1976). Many of the questions were pre-coded to facilitate quantitative analysis. The questionnaire opened with a general section of questions concerning the composition of the household and the background characteristics of all its members. One important section contained questions relating to perceived morbidity and etiology and ensuing illness behaviour exhibited and reported during the previous twelve months by the people who stated they had been ill. Their behaviour was traced per illness episode on the basis of a comprehensive treatment chart in which data were collected concerning the different forms of medical treatment received, together with information about the place and nature of the therapy used, the cost of treatment, and the result of the provision of medical care. A section was also included with opinion- and knowledge-questions concerning local etiology, perceptions, values, ideas and practices which play a role in the illness behaviour of the various groups. Finally, the questionnaire contained a number of questions designed to elicit understanding of illness and utilisation behaviour and existing expectations with regard to improving rural health care in the region. The questionnaire was introduced with the cooperation of the administrator of Babile, who explained it in a series of meetings with village elders, and ethnic and religious leaders from the various local groups. Permission of the *kebele* was also kindly granted and the research team were pleased to note that they aroused great interest and received considerable cooperation from the population during the survey.

The decision to conduct the health interview survey retrospectively over the past twelve months was based, among other considerations, on the expected variation in the pattern of illness and the accompanying utilisation of existing medical systems as a result of seasonal influences[3]. In combination with field observations of management of illness episodes, this method provided a picture of the community relating to the pattern of complaints, illness behaviour and the utilisation of health care by the various members of household groups. At the same time, it enabled a recording of opinions, knowledge and practices in relation to illness and health. In addition to the inhibiting psychological effect of standardised questionnaires when used for medical-sociological and anthropological research, a further problem was created by respondents' under-reporting in a number of cases. The limitations were kept to a minimum by means of repeated interviews and refinement of the definition of physical complaints, treatment practices and the duration of perceived illness (Blum and Blum 1965).

To summarise, the material collected in the field during the various surveys was compiled by the use of four basic research techniques. In the first place, qualitative information was gathered by means of spontaneous discussions with members of various groups and classes. Additional data were then obtained by means of participatory observation during the research team's stay in Babile. The third technique consisted of the health interview surveys using standardised questionnaires to conduct formal interviews with households selected in advance. This technique enabled the measurement of the spread of phenomena among different strata. Finally, an action-based research experiment was conducted in specific cases of illness where a number of patients in the community were provided with medical help and advice by members of the research team. In this way it became not only possible to obtain a better understanding of how patients progress through the various medical systems but also to quantify multiple use of services. At the same time, contacts with doctors, nurses, administrators, traditional healers, religious leaders and members of the local elite groups were intensified and extended.

The previous section has already explained that the community of Babile consists of a number of different ethnic groups, amongst whom a stratified random sample was taken. The presence of people descended from original groups with different ethnic, cultural, religious and linguistic backgrounds indicates that the inhabitants of Babile live in groups in which ethnicity is the dominant, binding element of the social order. Since the socio-cultural differences between these groups is greater than, for example, the feeling of unity within socio-economic classes such as civil servants, soldiers, farmers and traders, it is legitimate and methodologically convenient to describe Babile as a plural community in this part of the Horn of Africa (Van Lier 1977: 8).

## Demographic and ethno-religious composition

As has already been stated, the total population of Babile consists of approximately 4,000 inhabitants among whom a survey was conducted comprising 1,351 individuals from 337 households. The age pyramid of the sample population is asymmetrical with marked differences in specific age/sex categories. The 1,351 individuals in the survey consisted of 671 men and 680 women, which produces a sex ratio of 98.7 (Figure 4.1).

A closer examination of the sample according to age and sex, shows a relatively low man-woman ratio in the 20 – 24 age group (41.0%) confirming the findings of similar studies conducted elsewhere in Ethiopia (Freij *et al.* 1973: 38; Buschkens and Slikkerveer 1982: 61, 62). The stucture of the sample population according to age and sex is set out in detail in Table 4.2.

The low man-woman ratio in the 20 – 24 age group is explained by the fact that men of marriageable age often spend time in the large towns earning money to save for a dowry. The preponderance of women in the population pyramid in the 20 – 30 age group can also be attributed to such factors as polygamy. According to Islamic custom, men are permitted to have several wives if they have the

Table 4.2: *Age and sex of respondents in the sample production*

| Age group | Men | | Women | | Total | |
|---|---|---|---|---|---|---|
| | N | % | N | % | N | % |
| 0 – 4 | 137 | 10.1 | 137 | 10.1 | 274 | 20.3 |
| 5 – 9 | 142 | 10.4 | 115 | 8.5 | 256 | 19.0 |
| 10 – 14 | 75 | 5.6 | 72 | 5.3 | 147 | 10.9 |
| 15 – 19 | 33 | 2.4 | 44 | 3.3 | 77 | 5.7 |
| 20 – 24 | 21 | 1.6 | 50 | 3.7 | 71 | 5.3 |
| 25 – 29 | 64 | 4.7 | 99 | 7.3 | 163 | 12.1 |
| 30 – 34 | 52 | 3.9 | 60 | 4.4 | 112 | 8.3 |
| 35 – 39 | 58 | 4.3 | 40 | 3.0 | 98 | 7.3 |
| 40 – 44 | 25 | 1.9 | 15 | 1.1 | 40 | 3.0 |
| 45 – 49 | 30 | 2.2 | 14 | 1.0 | 20 | 3.3 |
| 50 – 54 | 12 | 0.9 | 8 | 0.6 | 20 | 1.5 |
| 55 – 59 | 13 | 1.0 | 13 | 1.0 | 26 | 1.9 |
| 60 – 64 | 2 | 0.1 | 10 | 0.7 | 12 | 0.9 |
| 65 + | 7 | 0.5 | 3 | 0.2 | 10 | 0.7 |
| Total | 671 | 49.7 | 680 | 50.3 | 1351 | 100.0 |

funds for their purchase and support. This is found sporadically among the Eastern Oromo.

The same table shows that approximately half of respondents in the sample survey (50.2%) consisted of people below 15 years of age and that slightly less than half (48.4%) were part of the economically active group aged 15 – 60. The age structure of the sample population largely corresponds to the usual pattern in developing countries of a 'young' population and in particular confirms the findings of previous demographic studies conducted elsewhere in Ethiopia on population structures (Alula Abate 1969; Statistical Abstract of Ethiopia 1975; Buschkens and Slikkerveer 1982).

Table 4.3 shows the structure of age and sex of the two most important population groups in the survey, the Oromo and the Amhara (N = 1,245) in order to enable a comparison to be made with the age structure of the total population.

Clearly there are very few Amhara men aged 20 – 24 (4 Amhara; 15 Oromo). This can be explained by the fact that young Amhara men are more likely to have the opportunity of going to the larger towns in the west to earn money for dowry. In the 25 – 29 age group, Oromo women are the greatest single group, which is connected with the Islamic system of polygamy.

Table 4.1 presents a total picture of the sample population and shows that, numerically speaking, the Oromo are in the majority

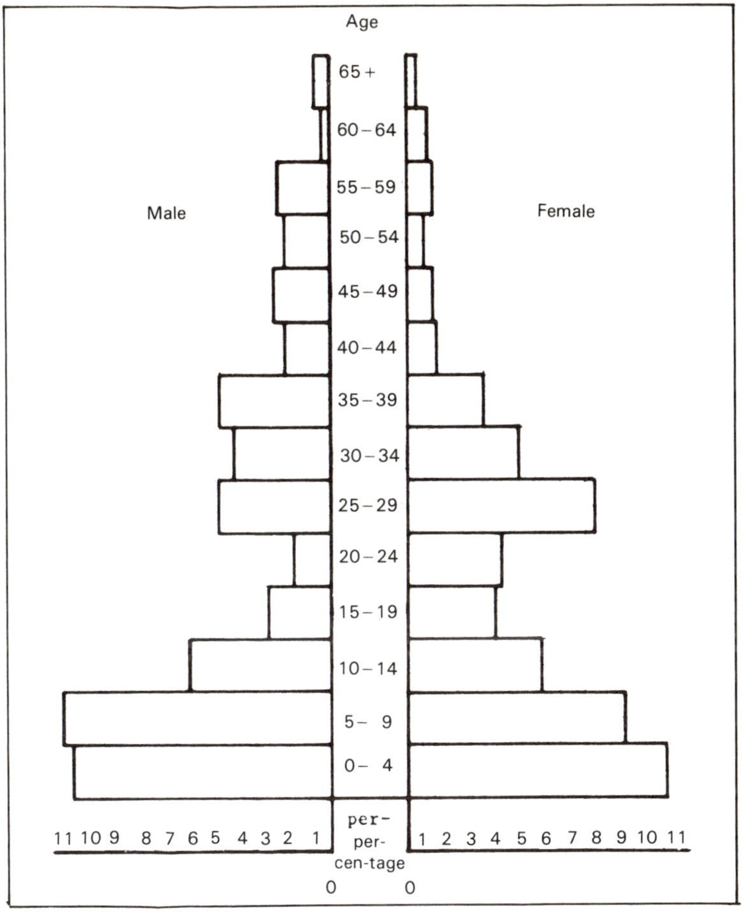


Figure 4.1: *Age pyramid of the sample population in Babile, according to sex, expressed in percentages (N=1,351; 671 men and 680 women)*

(52%). The Amhara form the second largest ethnic group (38.4%), followed by the Somali (6.5%). Although the inhabitants of Babile identify in the first instance with the community as a whole and only exhibit a special sense of unity and identity within their own ethnic groups, these groups will now be briefly described in relation to the religious systems concerned.

Table 4.3 *Age and sex of members of the Oromo and Amhara groups in the survey (N = 1,245)*

| Age group | Oromo | | | Amhara | | | Average subtotal |
|---|---|---|---|---|---|---|---|
| | men | women | sub-total | men | women | sub-total | |
| 0 – 4 | 77 | 71 | 148 | 45 | 51 | 96 | 244 |
| 5 – 9 | 81 | 63 | 144 | 54 | 44 | 98 | 242 |
| 10 – 14 | 40 | 37 | 77 | 33 | 29 | 62 | 139 |
| 15 – 19 | 14 | 20 | 34 | 19 | 15 | 34 | 68 |
| 20 – 24 | 15 | 38 | 43 | 4 | 18 | 22 | 65 |
| 25 – 29 | 34 | 56 | 90 | 21 | 34 | 55 | 145 |
| 30 – 34 | 30 | 32 | 62 | 16 | 24 | 40 | 102 |
| 35 – 39 | 33 | 21 | 54 | 19 | 17 | 36 | 90 |
| 40 – 44 | 14 | 7 | 21 | 8 | 7 | 15 | 34 |
| 45 – 49 | 11 | 6 | 17 | 18 | 7 | 25 | 42 |
| 50 – 54 | 5 | 3 | 8 | 7 | 4 | 11 | 19 |
| 55 – 59 | 4 | 4 | 8 | 5 | 9 | 14 | 22 |
| 60 – 64 | 0 | 6 | 6 | 2 | 3 | 5 | 11 |
| 65 + | 3 | 1 | 4 | 4 | 2 | 6 | 10 |
| Total | 361 | 365 | 726 | 255 | 264 | 519 | 1245 |

## Oromo

The Oromo in the research area are of Eastern-Cushitic origin and belong to the Barentu, one of the two main Oromo groups in Ethiopia. The other main group, the Boran, are found chiefly in the south and the west of the country. The Oromo in Hararghe consist of seven tribal groups (Or. *gosa*) which have settled in the Eastern Highlands. From east to west they are the groups of Babile, Jarso, Nole, Ala, Oberra, Annya and Ittu (Demissie Gebre Michael 1974). The *gosa* are further divided into patrilinear clans which are also called *gosa*. The term *gosa* usually means clan but may also have wider associations. At any event, all the members of a particular *gosa* believe that they are descended from the same founding father and are therefore brothers. The complex structure of the different Oromo groups all over the country is also reflected in the division of the groups encountered during the course of the research in Babile. It should be added, that in addition to the seven Oromo groups east of Harar, there are several mixed groups, namely the Geri-Jarso and Geri-Babile, in the border area with Somalia. Some scholars such as Haberland (1963) and Lewis (1955) regard these groups as belonging to the Somali. Other authors, such as Azais and Chambard (1931) and Huntingford (1955) classify them as Oromo. Since the members

Table 4.4 *Clan origins of heads of Oromo households in the sample survey, divided over the seven* gosa *in the region.*

| *Tribal groups (gosa)* | *Number of household heads* | |
| --- | --- | --- |
| | N | % |
| Babile | 98 | 55.7 |
| Jarso | 34 | 19.3 |
| Nole | 24 | 13.6 |
| Ala | 6 | 3.4 |
| Oberra | 2 | 1.1 |
| Annya | 1 | 0.6 |
| Ittu | 2 | 1.2 |
| Non-Eastern Oromo | 9 | 5.1 |
| Total | 176 | 100.0 |

of these mixed groups in the Babile area clearly identify themselves as Oromo they will be included in the Oromo groups of the study. The location of Babile in the middle of these mixed groups is shown in Map 4.3.

The number of Oromo in the sample survey consisted of 715 individuals from 176 households. To obtain an impression of the clan origins within the group, the *gosa* of all the household heads in the sample survey has been recorded. This is shown in Table 4.4.

The table shows that 98 households (55.7%) came from Babile *gosa*. Within this group, the Wara Maya, the Wara Maru and the Geri-Babile are the most import *gosa*. The 34 households in the Jarso group mainly come from the Wara Danka, Wara Walabu, Wara Sayo and Geri-Jarso *gosa*. The third *gosa*, the Nole, consists mainly of households from the Mana Abu and Halele *gosa*. The remaining *gosa* consist of 6 households from the Arsi group, 2 from the Raya group and 1 from the Akitchu group. These are Non-Eastern Oromo, in other words, Oromo from other parts of Ethiopia.

This picture of the clan origins of the Oromo in the research area corresponds to the earlier findings of Demissie Gebre Michael (1974: 31) who describes Harar as: '. . . *the meeting point of Babile, Jarso, Nole and Ala*'.

Of the total Oromo group of 716 individuals in the survey, 667 (93.2%) said they were Muslims. (The remaining 49 were Christians; they were mainly members of households of low-ranking Oromo

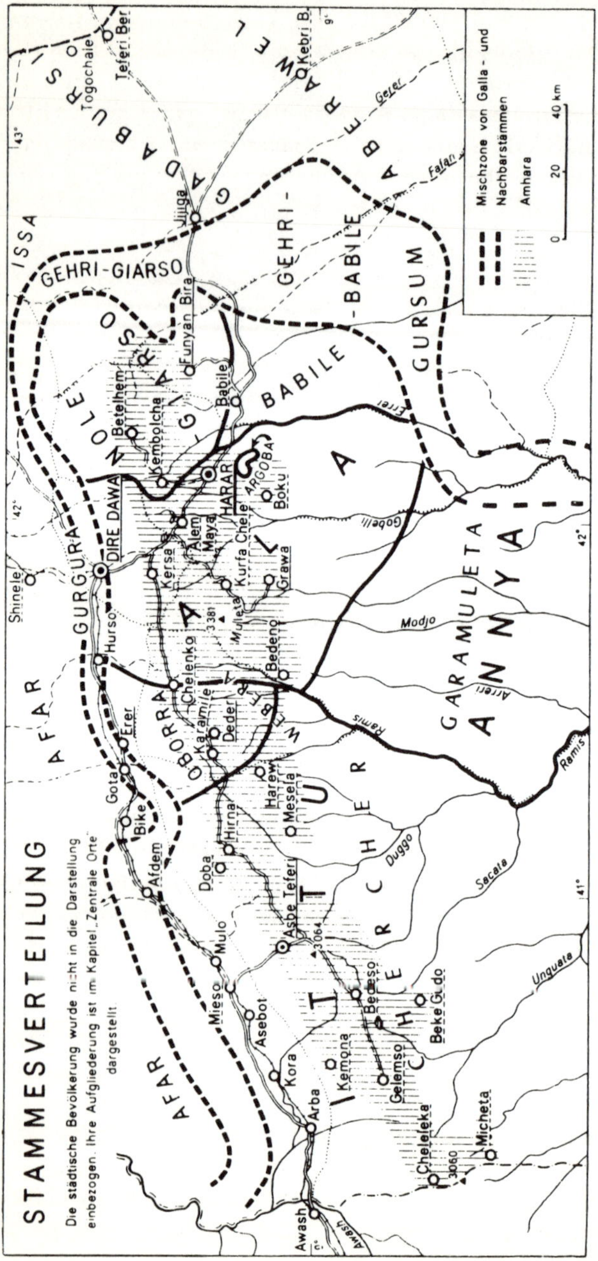


Map 4.3 *Geographical distribution of ethnic groups in the Highlands of Hararghe (Alula Abate 1969)*

public servants and soldiers who had been converted to Christianity. The tribal origins of 9 of the 49 were in the Non-Eastern Oromo groups from other parts of Ethiopia. Three of these cases involved a mixed marriage with an Amhara woman. The religious life of the Oromo in Babile is guided by two imams and the focal point of the way of life is the large mosque where religious gatherings are regularly held.

## Amhara

The Amhara and Tigray, who form the dominant ethnic group in Babile, belong to the semitised segment of the population. As indicated earlier, the Amhara migrated from the central Ethiopian Kingdom in the Western Highlands to Hararghe during the reign of Emperor Menelik II, towards the end of the last century. Military leaders, members of the clergy and public officials who had served the emperor well, formed a privileged class and were rewarded with pieces of fertile Oromo land in the conquered area. As the occupational structure will show, many Amhara soldiers in Babile used until quite recently to own land which was often tilled later on for them by Oromo tenants (Am. *gabbar*). Since the revolution – which was still in progress while the research was being conducted – this situation has gradually changed, a development the tenants have generally welcomed with enthusiasm.

The sample survey of 1,351 persons included 519 Amhara from 130 households, that is more than a third (39.4%) of the total. As will be shown later, when considering the pattern of settlement of the inhabitants of Babile, these people came originally from the western and central parts of Ethiopia, namely Gojam, Gondar and Shoa. All 519 Amhara belonged to the Ethiopian Church which has been a strong presence in Babile. The influence of Christianity, counteracting that of Islam, has been an important element in the process of 'Amharization' of Hararghe.

## Somali

The Somali in the sample who, like the Oromo, belong to the Eastern Cushites, have mixed to a large extent with the Oromo in Babile and indeed have adopted a similar lifestyle and agricultural techniques. This group consisted of 88 individuals, from 24 households belonging to a number of patrilinear clans (Som. *reer*) which have settled over the years in the community.

Table 4.5 *Clan origins of Somali heads of households in the sample survey*

| | Number of households |
|---|---|
| | N |
| Marihana | 9 |
| Ogaden | 6 |
| Melingur | 2 |
| Schejkash | 2 |
| Habra Aual | 2 |
| Gada Bursi | 2 |
| Reer Usman | 1 |
| Total | 24 |

The clan origins of these Somali households in the survey are indicated in Table 4.5.

All 88 Somali from the 24 households were Sunni (Orthodox Muslims) observing the Shafi'ite Islamic legal system. The Islamic Qadiriyah Order (Ar. *tariqa*) which in Eastern Ethiopia centres on the city of Harar, is represented in Babile by a sheikh of the Gada Bursi clan. The Somali are the most devout of the ethnic groups in Babile and Islam plays a dominant role in their entire lives.

## Other ethnic groups

The ethnic origins of the remaining 28 people in the sample are as follows: 17 Gurage, 5 Harari, 2 Kambata and 4 Arabs. The Gurage settled in the towns and rural communities as traders and shopkeepers and made up three households in the sample. The two Harari heads of household had originally moved to Babile as itinerant traders and later settled permanently with their families. The Arabs in the sample also emigrated to Babile as traders, in their case from Berbera. The Kambata head of household had been sent to Babile as an official in the Ethiopian government service. The Gurage are Christians as are the Kambata, whereas the Harari and Arabs are Muslims.

To summarise, the ethnic and religious origins of the various population groups in the sample seem to overlap with one another to a large extent. For instance, all members of the Amhara group belong to the Ethiopian Christian Church as do two-thirds of the members of the other ethnic groups (67.9%). More than nine-tenths of the Oromo (93.2%) are Muslims as are the Somali, Harari and

Arabs. The next section examines the extent to which this classification of ethnic and cultural groups is reflected in language, place of birth, kinship system and the pattern of settlement.

## 4.2 Culture and Socio-Economic Status

In addition to the aforegoing description of the demographic and ethno-religious composition, this section will present an outline of the cultural and socio-economic context of the community in which the medical ideas and practices will be studied in the following chapter.

### *4.2.1 Language, kinship and housing*

The various languages and dialects spoken in the community belong to the two families of languages found in Ethiopia: Semitic and Cushitic. Particularly in this area, linguistic heterogeneity exists, which generally divides along ethnic lines in Babile.

The language of the indigenous population was Oromifa, a Cushitic language which is known as the Eastern-Oromifa dialect because of the geographical area in which it is spoken. Oromifa is spoken by the Oromo and the Somali – with whom they have mixed – as the first language both within and between the groups. Amharinya or Amharic, which is written in the Sabaean alphabet, is spoken in the research area by the Amhara in the first instance. It was introduced at the end of the last century by Amhara migrants as the *lingua franca* and today it is the official language of Ethiopia. As both groups are also fluent in Amharinya as their second language, they can – like most other ethnic groups – be regarded as bilingual.

Amharinya is also the first language of a number of Oromo groups who have mixed with the Amhara while it is the second language of the Oromo, Somali and the other ethnic groups. Harari, the special South-Ethio-Semitic language of the inhabitants of the nearby city of Harar is written in Arabic script. It is spoken by the other groups as the language of trade. Somali, which like Oromifa is an Eastern Cushitic language, has marked similarities with Oromifa and is spoken by Somali who have settled in Babile.

A variety of languages and dialects have come into being through the interaction of various Cushitic and Semitic speaking groups in the area. As a result, different languages are often spoken within groups, while Amhara is spoken between groups, particularly by people wishing to make use of government services. The consequences of these different uses of language whereby Amharic, the official language is identified particularly by non-Amhara with the dominant Amhara elite in Babile, can be seen in social problems such as lack of communication, opposition and even conflict.

The kinship system among the different ethnic groups is, generally speaking, characterised by the fundamental unity of the family (Or. *warra*). The nuclear family is the dominant form in the structure and composition of all the groups in question. Unlike the Amhara, who are monogamous, the Oromo and Somali regard polygamy as the ideal form of marriage. In practice, however, it remains something of an exception because of the depressed economic situation in rural areas. Four Oromo household heads and one Somali in the sample had two wives. The social organisation of the Oromo is largely determined by a system of patrilinear kinship relationships. The Oromo in the sample were members of a number of patrilinear clans in which exogamous marriages were preferred. Partners may be chosen from the same ethnic group but not from the same *gosa*. Respondents expressed a slight preference in this connection for marriageable women from the surrounding mountain villages. There was no instance in the sample of levirate or of cross-cousin marriages which are found elsewhere among certain Oromo groups (cf. Huntingford 1955; Markakis 1975; Buschkens and Slikkerveer 1982). This also applied to the Somali group in Babile.

All groups practise circumcision of both boys and girls (clitoridectomy) despite increasing opposition from progressive young men and women. Several cases of infibulation were reported of girls in the Nole clan of the Oromo and among the majority of the Somali in the sample. Both practices are carried out between the ages of nine and twelve. De-infibulation takes place immediately before or after marriage.

In both Islamic groups, men seem to occupy a more important position than women and generally speaking take the important decisions concerning the day-to-day affairs of their household group, including health care.

The social system of the Amhara, which ties in with important institutions of the neighbourhood, household group and the land

Table 4.6 *Composition of households in the sample survey according to ethnic group*

| Member of household | ethnic group | | | | |
|---|---|---|---|---|---|
| | Oromo | Amhara | Somali | Other | Total |
| | N | N | N | N | N |
| head of household | 176 | 130 | 24 | 7 | 337 |
| partner | 130 | 97 | 18 | 5 | 250 |
| son of household | 211 | 149 | 16 | 10 | 386 |
| daughter of head of household | 172 | 123 | 25 | 6 | 326 |
| brother of head of household | 3 | 5 | — | — | 8 |
| sister of head of household | 4 | 3 | — | — | 7 |
| son of partner | — | 2 | — | — | 2 |
| daughter of partner | — | 1 | — | — | 1 |
| father of head of household | — | — | 1 | — | 1 |
| mother of head of household | 6 | 2 | 1 | — | 9 |
| grandson of head of household | 2 | — | — | — | 2 |
| grand-daughter of head of household | 7 | 1 | — | — | 8 |
| other relationship | 3 | 2 | 1 | — | 6 |
| unrelated | 2 | 4 | 2 | — | 8 |
| Total | 716 | 519 | 88 | 28 | 1351 |

ownership, is also governed by kinship relations. However, the institutional complex of kinship and tribal origin does not play such an important role among the Amhara as it does among the Oromo and Somali. Kinship relations are only of definitive significance in relation to marriage and land-ownership. Exogamous marriage is characterised by a predominantly patrilocal and in some cases by a neolocal pattern of settlement.

Some understanding of the distribution of the indigenous and non-indigenous populations of Babile can be gained from the reported birthplaces of the 1,351 respondents consisting of 671 men and 680 women. This confirms the patrilocal principles: a larger percentage of women than men (49.3% as opposed to 42.5%) were not born in Babile.

Evidently, the basic unit within all ethnic groups is the nuclear family, often as part of a large household group, made up of one or more relatives living together with the family. The following section considers the composition of all households in the sample survey by ethnic group.

A comparison of the households in the sample shows that the nuclear family is the dominant form among all ethnic groups. Only 27 Oromo (3.8%), 20 Amhara (3.8%) and 5 Somali (5.7%) did not belong to this type of household. Among the other ethnic groups the nuclear family is the only type of household. In the majority of cases, the people who are not members of the nuclear family are the mothers of household heads. In Hararghe it is usual for the widowed mother of a household head to live with the family of the eldest son (cf. Table 4.6).

The average size of all households in the sample is 4.0 persons. The size of households in relation to ethnic groups is shown in the following Table 4.7.

Table 4.7 *Size of household groups in the sample survey according to ethnic group, together with the total number of members of household groups.*

| number of members of household group | ethnic group | | | | total number of members of household group |
|---|---|---|---|---|---|
| | Oromo | Amhara | Somali | Other | |
| | N | N | N | N | N |
| 1 | 13 | 17 | 2 | — | 32 |
| 2 | 23 | 19 | 3 | — | 90 |
| 3 | 29 | 26 | 7 | 3 | 195 |
| 4 | 39 | 20 | 7 | 3 | 276 |
| 5 | 30 | 20 | 2 | — | 260 |
| 6 | 23 | 18 | 2 | 1 | 264 |
| 7 | 10 | 3 | — | — | 91 |
| 8 | 8 | 4 | 1 | — | 104 |
| 9 | — | 1 | — | — | 9 |
| 10 | 1 | 2 | — | — | 30 |
| Total | 176 | 130 | 24 | 7 | 1351 |

Table 4.7 shows that the Oromo have the greatest average household consisting of 4.2 persons, followed by the Amhara and the other ethnic groups, both of which have average households consisting of 3.8 persons. Somali households are the smallest with an average of 3.6 persons.

Almost all of the houses in Babile share the same basic functions, despite differences in outward appearance. They serve as the central place for the household group where food is stored and prepared, where the members of the household eat and sleep and also where domestic animals and cattle are housed and looked after.

There are two basic types of house in Babile:

1. the traditional, round, thatched houses (*tukul*) found throughout the Eastern Highlands among the peasant population, and
2. the rectangular houses with corrugated iron roofs, built in recent years, particularly in larger marketplaces and towns.

   This latter type is increasingly common in mountain villages. The first type of house is inhabited by Oromo farmers in rural areas and can be seen in groups of 5 to 50 in the middle of agricultural land. The walls consist of a strong lattice construction made of wooden poles and branches covered with a sort of mortar (Am. *chika*), made from a mixture of clay, straw and cow dung. The conical roof consists of tree trunks covered with bundles of thatch resting at an angle against a central vertical pole (cf. Buschkens and Slikkerveer 1982: 70, 71). The houses of the more prosperous farmers often have brick walls faced with white plaster. In some cases, the wealthy farmers have built bigger rectangular houses for themselves with a corrugated iron roof (Or.: *qorqorroo*). Rectangular houses dominate the larger marketplaces and *katama* to an increasing extent.

The differences between the two types of house are largely external. As elsewhere, living quarters, sleeping accommodation and the areas for cooking food, storing supplies and housing cattle are similar. The social significance of a particular type of dwelling is reflected mainly in the prestige from living in the newer type of house. For the neighbourhood it is an indication of the level of prosperity of the household in question.

In Babile, the most important buildings along the main road can be recognised by their rectangular form and brick walls as can the

Table 4.8 *Type of house of household groups in the sample, according to ethnic group*

| type of house | ethnic sub-group | | | | | | | | Total | |
|---|---|---|---|---|---|---|---|---|---|---|
| | Oromo | | Amhara | | Somali | | Other | | | |
| | N | % | N | % | N | % | N | % | N | % |
| round | 40 | 11.9 | 2 | 1.5 | 1 | 4.2 | — | — | 43 | 12.8 |
| rectangular | 136 | 40.4 | 128 | 38.0 | 23 | 6.8 | 7 | 2.1 | 294 | 87.2 |
| Total | 176 | 52.3 | 130 | 39.5 | 24 | 11.0 | 7 | 2.1 | 337 | 100.0 |

shops, restaurants and bars round the marketplace. Public officials, soldiers and other representatives of central government also tend to live in the rectangular type of house. Residential areas consisting of round, thatched houses occupied mainly by Oromo and Somali families are grouped between these more recent dwellings. The various ethnic groups can, broadly speaking, be identified by their pattern of settlement and certain residential areas are grouped along ethno-cultural lines. For example, the Amhara in particular live around the administrative building and along the main road. The Oromo and Somali live in family groups round the old marketplace (Or. *magalaa*) and on the edge of the community. The distribution of two types of dwelling in the sample among the main ethnic groups in the community is set out in Table 4.8.

From this table it can be seen that only 43 (12.8%) of the household groups in the sample live in a round type of house. These are mainly Oromo farmers from Babile who account for 40 household groups (11.9%). The rectangular houses are predominantly occupied by Oromo (40.4%) and Amhara (38%), generally belonging to the 'well-to-do' social class. In 107 households (approximately 30%) the inhabitants slept – instead of in bed – on skins on the floor; 52.9% of them were Oromo.

The types of house described above in which farmers and their animals often share sleeping accommodation and where sanitary facilities, sewers and potable water supplies are usually non-existent, increase the danger of spreading infectious diseases, a number of which are dealt with in section 4.3.

## 4.2.2. *Economic life, level of prosperity and occupational structure*

The economic life of the inhabitants of Babile depends first and foremost on agriculture (37.4%). The services sector provided by government comes second with only a slightly smaller share, while almost one fifth of the population is involved in economic activity connected with trade (18.7%). The remaining 7.7% of economic life is made up of other occupations (craftsmen and artisans) and local religious services. Closer examination reveals that particular occupations are closely associated with certain ethnic groups which earn their living in different economic sectors.

For example, Table 4.9 shows that more than half of the Oromo household heads (54.5%) work as arable or cattle farmers while more than two-thirds of the Amhara (67.7%) work in government service or in the army. The table also shows that trade is the most important occupation of the other ethnic groups and, to a much smaller extent, this applies both to the Oromo and Somali. The other ethnic groups comprise mostly Harari and Arab merchants.

The picture becomes clear if the pattern of economic activity in Babile of each ethnic group is placed in the historical framework which has already been described. The area originally inhabited by

Table 4.9 *Type of economic activity of household heads in the sample according to ethnic groups**

| economic activity | ethnic group | | | | | | | | Total | |
|---|---|---|---|---|---|---|---|---|---|---|
| | Oromo | | Amhara | | Somali | | Other | | | |
| | N | % | N | % | N | % | N | % | N | % |
| agriculture & live stock | 96 | 54.5 | 15 | 11.5 | 14 | 58.3 | 1 | — | 126 | 37.4 |
| trade | 35 | 19.9 | 17 | 13.1 | 7 | 29.2 | 4 | — | 63 | 18.7 |
| government and army service | 32 | 18.2 | 88 | 67.7 | — | — | 2 | — | 122 | 36.2 |
| other occupations and various services | 13 | 7.4 | 10 | 7.7 | 3 | 12.5 | | — | 26 | 7.7 |
| Total | 176 | 100.0 | 130 | 100.0 | 24 | 100.0 | 7 | — | 337 | 100.0 |

*In this and following tables — means that no percentage is stated as fewer than 20 cases were reported (N 20)

Table 4.10 *Occupational structure of the sample according to type of economic activity and ethnic group*

| | | ethnic groups | | | | |
|---|---|---|---|---|---|---|
| Economic activity | occupation | Oromo | Amhara | Somali | Other | Total |
| arable and | farmer | 75 | 13 | 3 | — | 91 |
| livestock | labourer | 1 | 2 | 7 | 1 | 11 |
| farming | shepherd | 20 | — | 2 | — | 22 |
| | livestock | — | — | 4 | — | 4 |
| | owner | — | — | — | — | — |
| trade | trader | 28 | 16 | 3 | 3 | 50 |
| | shopkeeper | 7 | 2 | 2 | 1 | 12 |
| government | civil servant | 7 | 21 | — | 2 | 30 |
| army and | road builder | 3 | 6 | 1 | — | 10 |
| civil | soldier | 21 | 52 | — | — | 73 |
| service | policeman | 1 | 5 | — | — | 6 |
| | teacher | — | 4 | — | — | 4 |
| religious | sheikh | 1 | — | 1 | — | 2 |
| functionaries | imam | 1 | — | — | — | 1 |
| and local | demina | 1 | 2 | — | — | 3 |
| authorities | debtara | — | 2 | — | — | 2 |
| other | weaver | 2 | 1 | — | 1 | 4 |
| free | tailor | 2 | — | — | — | 2 |
| occupations | potter | 1 | — | — | — | 1 |
| | shoemaker | — | 1 | — | — | 1 |
| | blacksmith | 1 | — | — | — | 1 |
| | driver | 1 | — | — | — | 1 |
| | barkeeper | — | 3 | — | — | 3 |
| | beggar | 3 | — | — | — | 3 |
| Total | | 176 | 130 | 24 | 7 | 337 |

the Oromo gradually came to play an important role at the turn of the century as a marketplace along the major caravan route to the east and a thriving trade developed. After the Amhara occupation of Hararghe, a large number of military and administrative representatives of central government moved into the area because of its major strategic and military importance. As noted before, the process of 'Amharisation' was accompanied by substantial migration of Amhara families who settled permanently in the community. Table 4.10 shows the occupational structure of the sample population classified according to the type of economic activity and the various ethnic groups.

Table 4.10 shows that more than half (55%) of all household heads in the Oromo group earn their living as farmers, often from mixed farming. A number of them have a second occupation for example as a woodworker, wood carver or basket weaver. All respondents who said that their main occupation was that of farmer, owned a piece of land, while the agricultural labourers worked for the Oromo or Amhara farmers.

The three main products grown in this area are millet, peanuts and sesame seeds. To cope with the problems of drought, crop failure, and soil exhaustion, the Oromo in the area use a system of interplantation, combining cultivation of a main crop with a number of other crops or vegetables. In the area around Babile, a field rotation system has been developed which is known as the *durra complex* (Brooke 1956: 211). Durra or grain sorghum (*Andropogon sorghum*) under the generic name 'Bishinga' is grown in combination with peanuts, sesame seed, maize, beans, peppers, melons and vegetables. Peanuts and sesame seed form the two major cash crops in this system and are sold to traders at the market in Babile.

*Chat* (Or. *jimma*) is grown on the high mountain slopes and the irrigated terraces north of Babile. Popular among the Muslim population in particular, it is increasingly competing with coffee as a high-income crop. Because it is so profitable, it often occupies the best areas of irrigated land around the mountain villages. The bundles of twigs are sold for high prices at local markets or exported to Djibouti and the Arabian Peninsula (Buschkens and Slikkerveer 1982: 65). Because of the low rainfall in this area and the increasing popularity of *chat*, coffee, which used to be an extremely important crop in the area round Babile, has now become rare.

The less important crops grown in the area include potatoes, bananas, melons, oranges, pomegranates, guava and various local herbs and spices. Often the Oromo keep a few cattle and poultry largely for their own consumption. Distinctive local beehives are also found under the eaves of houses or in nearby trees producing wild honeycombs for domestic use and applications in traditional medicine.

Twenty Oromo household heads were shepherds. They looked after herds of sheep and goats along the mountain slopes around Babile, often helped by their children. Because of the relatively high level of production of cereals, peanuts and cattle products, a number of farmers have become cereal and dairy produce merchants who earn a living by supplying produce from the market at Babile to the nearby cities Harar and Dire Dawa. Twenty-eight heads of household in the survey practised this occupation. The

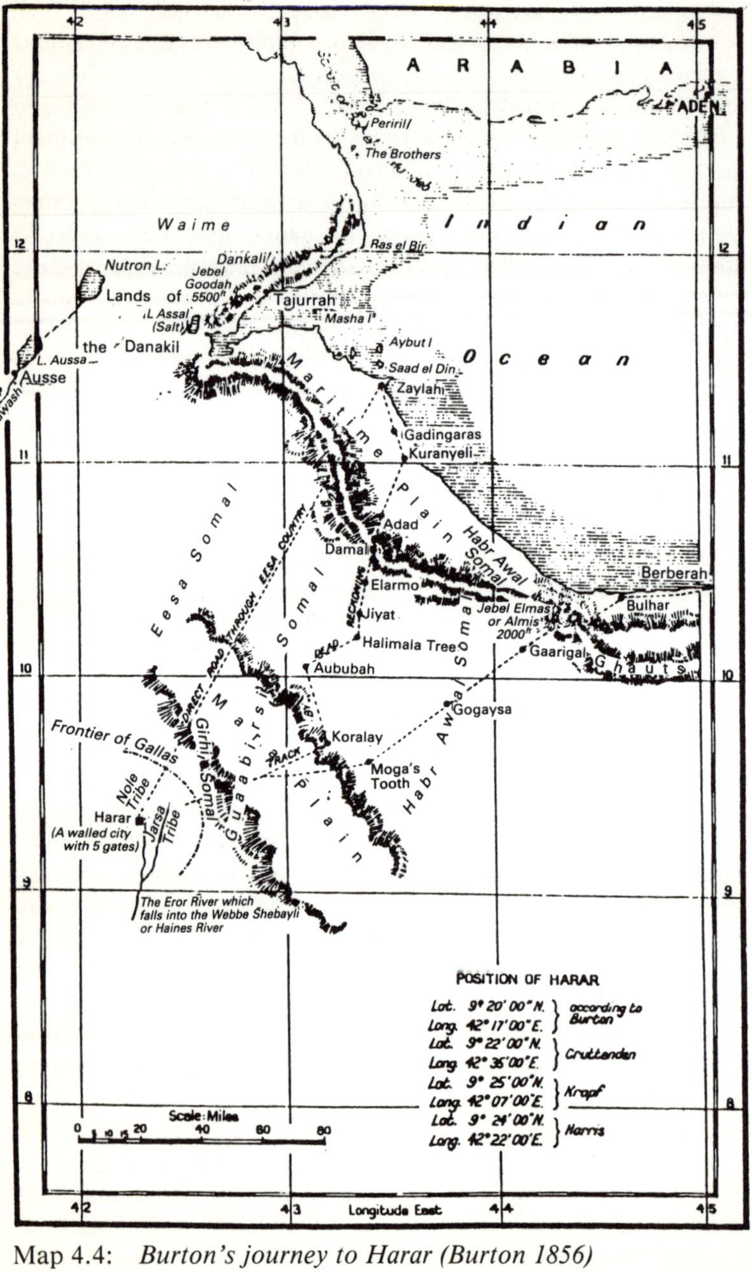


Map 4.4: *Burton's journey to Harar (Burton 1856)*

seven Oromo shopkeepers all owned small shops selling goods such as ironmongery, household articles, salt, kerosene and cotton cloth.

Only seven Oromo heads of household in the sample were tax officials working for the Ethiopian government. Twenty household heads were professional soldiers with the Ethiopian army, mainly in the lower ranks. Three Oromo household heads worked for the Highway Authority and one was employed at the police station. One sheikh and one imam from among the group were responsible for the spiritual welfare of the Muslims while the *demina* performed the largely ritual function of local leader of the various Oromo clans in Babile. Finally, the group included eight self-employed craftsmen including potters, tailors, weavers and blacksmiths. This group also included three beggars who attempted to earn a living by begging at the market in Harar.

As far as the occupational structure of the Amhara household heads in the sample is concerned, just over one-tenth (13%) were independent farmers. They owned and worked their own land and used the same production system as the Oromo and Somali farmers. Two Amhara were employed as agricultural labourers. The sixteen Amhara grain merchants in the sample, like the Oromo dealers, arranged the sale of agricultural products to the larger towns in the east of the country.

Table 4.9 also shows that a large proportion of the Amhara household heads in the sample were in government service. Two-thirds of them were either civil servants or members of the armed forces (67.7%), including fifty-two soldiers, twenty-one government officials, six road builders, five policemen and four teachers. In total, the group represented more than one-third (36.5%) of the government sector within the community. There were also two priests (Am: *debtara*), three bar keepers, one shoemaker and one weaver.

The majority of twenty-four household heads of the Somali group in the sample, like the Oromo household heads, earned a living as arable or livestock farmers. They included three farmers each with their own farm and seven agricultural labourers working on their employers' farm. Even more than among the Oromo household heads, livestock farming plays an important role in the economic life of the settled Somali in Babile. This is probably because the Somali used to be nomads and still derive considerable prestige from owning cattle. Six Somali household heads in the sample stated that their main occupation was that of livestock farmer; they sold their daily products on the market in Babile. In addition, six were shopkeepers. The two remaining household heads in the group included one religious leader and one daily worker. The household heads from the other ethnic groups were occupied chiefly outside the agricultural sector. Two Gurage had settled as shopkeepers in Babile; one Harari, one Gurage and one Arab household head were traders and two Gurage were low-ranking officials in the government service. Finally, it was found that Oromo and Somali farmers in particular often have a second trade, for example as a leather worker, potter, woodworker, weaver or traditional healer in addition to their main occupation.

Although the process of implementing the post-revolutionary measures in the social, political and economic sectors had started during the time the research was being carried out and local committees, peasant associations and neighbourhood councils (Am. *kebele*) had been set up in Babile, implementation of the *Rural Land Reform Proclamation* was proving more difficult and agricultural production was continuing in the traditional manner. The delay in reorganisation had partly been caused by the opposition of landowners and because of the lack of administrative control in the border area. In view of the fact that prosperity in rural areas is not exclusively associated with ownership of land, but also with tenant rights and the ownership of cattle, the pattern of distribution of farm land and the number of cattle owned by the various ethnic groups will now be examined in detail.

Table 4.11 shows land utilisation by household heads in the sample, classified according to size of arable land and ethnic group. The table clearly indicates that almost half the Oromo household heads (47.7%) own a certain area of agricultural land as do more than a quarter of the Amhara (27.7%). As a result of the rural land proclamation of 4 March 1975, which established public ownership of all rural land in Ethiopia, many Amhara landowners had moved to the towns and land redistribution to farm families had started. It is also clear from the table that almost two-thirds of farmers in the sample (60.3%) own less than 100 square metres of land while roughly a third (36.5%) farm an average of 5,500 square metres. This means an average ratio of approximately 1.25 acres per household group and confirms the widespread practice in the highlands of *shebeta* (Ethiopian unit of 3.3 hectares) where four or

Table 4.11 *Size of agricultural land per household in the sample, according to ethnic group*

| size of arable land | ethnic group | | | | | | | | Total | |
|---|---|---|---|---|---|---|---|---|---|---|
| | Oromo | | Amhara | | Somali | | Other | | | |
| | N | % | N | % | N | % | N | % | N | % |
| no land | 92 | 52.3 | 94 | 72.3 | 20 | 83.3 | 5 | — | 211 | 62.6 |
| 1,000 sq. metres | 46 | 26.1 | 26 | 20.0 | 3 | 12.5 | 1 | — | 76 | 22.6 |
| 1,000 – 10,000 sq. metres | 34 | 19.3 | 10 | 7.7 | 1 | 4.2 | 1 | — | 46 | 13.6 |
| 10,000 + sq. metres- | 4 | 2.3 | — | — | — | — | — | — | 4 | 1.2 |
| Total | 176 | 100.0 | 130 | 100.0 | 24 | 100.0 | 7 | — | 337 | 100.0 |

five families make communal use of one piece of land (Demissie Gebre Michael 1974: 73).

Table 4.11 shows that the Oromo dominate all three categories of land ownership. Twenty-six of the thirty-six Amhara household heads in the sample farmed on their own land; the remaining ten pieces of land worked by the Amhara originally belonged to Amhara landowners who had been given land as soldiers or public officials. Under the new Land Reform Act, it was conveyed to Oromo or Somali farmers as well as to the Amhara farmers who had previously rented the plots.

Although Oromo and Somali in particular originally derived prestige from owning cattle, for economic reasons this phenomenon has declined considerably because of the absence of suitable pasture. A number of farmers also keep sheep and goats in addition to cattle. Donkeys are often used as means of transport by both farmers and merchants. The research into livestock ownership in the area shows that two-thirds (66.2%) of all households do not own any sheep or goats, partly due to increasing scarcity of land. The largest number of households which still keep sheep or goats – 62 or 22.3% – were Oromo. This includes some ten households which are economically dependent to a large extent on keeping small livestock. The picture with regard to cattle is the same: approximately three-quarters of the sample households did not have any cattle. The largest number of households which owned on average more than one cow were Oromo. Only one-tenth of all households in the sample could afford to keep one or more donkeys. Here, too, the Oromo household heads were in the majority.

Previous research and observation in the field make it possible to assess the annual per capita income of the population in the community as between 200 and 500 bir (1 Ethiopian bir = 0.50 US $) which falls into the category of lowest incomes in Third World countries. A number of problems confronting the population in the area, particularly farmers, created this situation, despite the availability of potential resources. As mentioned before, such factors as drought, failed harvest and disease, together with social and political constraints, have contributed significantly to a situation of actual poverty in which a number of households in the research area, despite recent reforms, still find themselves.

In addition to these external threats, certain factors within the community – such as religious feast days, excessive fasting and imprudent use of *chat* – sometimes aggravates the difficult situation for many people.

Despite the frequent spells of poverty, various categories of income can be distinguished. By incorporating a number of objective indicators of prosperity in the questionnaire such as income, type and state of repair of the house, size of land and number of cattle and pack-donkeys and by means of a subjective estimate of the welfare of the households by the trained interviewers, it was possible during the quantitative processing of the material to use factor analysis to divide the households into three types of socio-economic status (SES): *well-to-do, average* and *poor*. The distribution of these three socio-economic classes among the ethnic groups is set out in Table 4.12.

The table shows that less than one-tenth (8.6%) of all households in the sample belong to the well-to-do class. There is a slight difference between the Oromo (7.4%) and the Amhara (10.8%) but there are hardly any Somali in this category. A comparison of the three socio-economic classes within the Oromo and Amhara groups shows that although the number of households in the well-to-do class is almost the same, there are major differences in the other two classes. Almost three times as many Oromo fall into the poor class compared with the Amhara: 31.8% against 13.8%. The largest number of Somali households were also found in the lowest socio-economic class (13).

Generally speaking, the socio-economic structure in Babile

Table 4.12 *Socio-economic status of households in the sample according to ethnic group*

| socio-economic status | ethnic group | | | | | | | | Total | |
|---|---|---|---|---|---|---|---|---|---|---|
| | Oromo | | Amhara | | Somali | | Other | | | |
| | N | % | N | % | N | % | N | % | N | % |
| well-to-do | 13 | 7.4 | 14 | 10.8 | 1 | 4.2 | 1 | — | 29 | 8.6 |
| average | 96 | 54.5 | 98 | 75.4 | 10 | 41.7 | 5 | — | 209 | 62.0 |
| poor | 67 | 38.1 | 18 | 13.8 | 13 | 54.1 | 1 | — | 99 | 29.4 |
| Total | 176 | 100.0 | 130 | 100.0 | 24 | 100.0 | 7 | — | 337 | 100.0 |

corresponds to the hierarchical system described above. The composition of the local elite differs from group to group. Unlike the Oromo, among whom the ownership of land and cattle largely determines socio-economic status, the Amhara attach most prestige to positions within the armed forces or government service. The poor among the Oromo and Somali, who account for 31.8% and 54.1% respectively of the two groups, consist largely of the landless households in Babile which lead a marginal existence. The effect of socio-economic status as an important background variable in relation to the illness behaviour of patients will be dealt with more fully in the analysis of the process of health care utilisation behaviour.

## 4.3 The Regional Pattern of Illness and Health

Before describing and analysing the processes of illness behaviour and health care utilisation, it is necessary to examine the present pattern of morbidity in the Eastern Highlands. Using the scarce medical studies (objective morbidity surveys) conducted in the region, an attempt will be made to present a profile of the most common types of illness. This section links up with the theoretical orientation of the study explained in Chapter 2 which stressed the importance of perceived morbidity (PM) as a major determinant of health care utilisation and subsequently describes the pattern of reported illness from the subjective morbidity survey in the community.

In comparisons of the available medical studies in Ethiopia by such authors as Russell (1958) and Schaller and Kuls (1972), Buschkens and Slikkerveer (1982: 77, 78) came to the conclusion that the majority of illnesses in Ethiopia – as in the majority of Third World countries – are caused by infectious diseases, poor diet and malnutrition and infant mortality (approximately 106 – 108 per 1,000 inhabitants).

Average life expectancy is very low (35) while infant mortality (up to the age of 14) is estimated to range from 175 to 385 per 1,000 inhabitants. Generally speaking, malaria is the single most registered disease in Ethiopia but typically 'western diseases', such as heart and vascular ailments, are almost relatively uncommon. The twelve most common infectious diseases or groups of illness as recorded in the epidemiological studies of 1961 of the Ministry of Public Health and published by Schaller and Kuls (1972) are as follows:

1. malaria
2. parasitic skin diseases
3. helminthiasis
4. infectious eye diseases
5. syphilis
6. dysentery
7. gonorrhea
8. pneumonia
9. tuberculosis
10. influenza
11. typhus
12. leprosy

Information concerning the pattern of illness in Hararghe is primarily contained in three studies carried out in hospitals and health centres in the towns of Dire Dawa and Harar. Having compared these studies, Buschkens and Slikkerveer (1982: 80) come to the conclusion that '. . . *there is no marked divergence in the pattern of diseases in this province as a whole'*. The most important problems in public health terms are caused by malaria, tuberculosis, intestinal parasites, venereal diseases, eye and skin diseases, schistomiasis, leprosy, anaemia and liver diseases.

As far as health in the rural areas of Hararghe is concerned, the only studies available are those by Schneider (1975) and Buschkens and Slikkerveer (1982). The former is a medical study of a sample of 1,721 persons in the community of Dogu and the surrounding area, consisting of 83% Oromo, 16% Amhara and 1% Somali. Dogu is in the Gara Mulatta district in the southern part of the Eastern Highlands.

Schneider (1975) recorded the following twelve diseases as the most frequent in the following order:

1. intestinal parasites
2. trachoma
3. other forms of conjunctivitis
4. scabies
5. tuberculosis (presumed)
6. serious wounds
7. tuberculosis (confirmed)
8. bronchitis
9. fungal infections
10. pyoderma
11. urethritis
12. unilateral blindness

The second research was carried out in two peasant villages in the districts of Harar Zuria and Woberra, both in the central part of the Hararghe Highlands – ganda Helele and ganda Ebro Mohammed – where a total of 326 people were examined. The results of this research by Buschkens and Slikkerveer (1982) can be arranged in the following order:

1. intestinal parasites
2. infectious intestinal diseases
3. trachoma
4. diseases of the oesophagus, stomach and duodenum
5. disease of the oral cavity, salivary glands and mandible
6. anaemia
7. pneumonia
8. ear infections
9. eye infections
10. tuberculosis
11. skin diseases
12. scabies

Compared to the situation elsewhere in Ethiopia it is immediately noticeable that malaria is not among the twelve most common illnesses in either health survey. This is because the malaria mosquito (*anopheles*) is rare in the Eastern Highlands at more than 2,000 metres. Schistomiasis, which is a serious problem elsewhere in Ethiopia, hardly occurs at all in the area (cf. Akilu Lemma 1973; Polderman 1975). Otherwise the pattern recorded in the two studies is broadly similar to the general pattern of illness in Ethiopia.

A comparison of the results of the medical research in Dogu, ganda Helele and ganda Ebro Mohammed shows that, inter alia, illnesses of the oesophagus, stomach and duodenum and of the oral cavity, salivary glands and mandible are very frequent. They are attached by some researchers to high consumption of *chat* by the local population of this area. Besides a feeling of well-being or excitement this stimulant also results in loss of appetite and loss of weight (Buschkens and Slikkerveer 1982: 65 – 67).

To summarise, the picture of morbidity in the rural areas of Hararghe is largely determined by the frequent occurrence of parasitic and infectious diseases which are largely attributable to poor hygiene. The large number of complaints and illnesses affecting the digestive tract frequently found in the rural areas of Hararghe can be ascribed to the high consumption of *chat*.

The following section examines the extent to which the above pattern of illness is reflected in the perceived morbidity by the population itself and in the accompanying pattern of complaints by respondents in the survey.

## 4.4. Indigenous Oromo and Amhara Disease Classifications

During the qualitative research it became clear that when a resident of Babile is affected by illness, he or she first attempts to discover its cause. Knowledge concerning the causes of illness is regarded as a significant aid towards finding a cure. During the household interviews, efforts were made to register the explanation for the disease, supplied by the respondent in every reported case of illness. Although this was not easy to begin with, it gradually became clear that illnesses are usually explained in terms of two indigenous categories of concepts: 'daily life' and 'spiritual life'.

The first group of illnesses and causes which Foster (1983) refers to as 'naturalistic' diseases originate to a large extent in local conditions, lack of income and inadequate hygiene. Local conditions mentioned by respondents were unemployment, poverty, malnutrition and poor diet, too much work, poor housing, etc. However, the majority of respondents were familiar with the concept of a contagious disease (Am. *talalafi basheta*; Or. *hogamishii*) and associated it with the transfer of illness or disease in everyday life. Although the concept was only associated with a limited number of diseases such as bronchitis, leprosy, food poisoning and scabies, it did have an effect on behaviour. Specific measures taken to prevent illness which is regarded as contagious involve avoidance of physical contact with infected persons, not sharing food with them and devoting special attention to hygiene. Occasionally, the concept was used in the sense of an individual being 'infected' with a 'personalistic' disease by a supernatural being (Or. *jiinii*), for example in the case of snake bites, wasp stings and diseases caused by insects (ear infection), rabies and 'bodily fluid from a spider' (skin rash).

The illnesses and causes of illness in the 'personalistic' category

Table 4.13 *Indigenous classification of perceived illnesses in Babile. Names are in English, Amharic and Oromo, together with traditional causes and/or symptoms*

| Name of disease | | | Indigenous cause and/or symptoms | |
|---|---|---|---|---|
| English | Amhara | Oromo | Amhara | Oromo |
| haemorrhoids | kintarot | huduu fora | swelling | idem |
| adenoiditis | angar | bofa | swollen glands | idem |
| amoebic dysentry | yadan taqmat | albaatii | diarrhoea | idem |
| ascaria | wasfat | mukurtii | 'worms in the stomach' | — |
| nose bleed | afincha damma | funuuna | — | caused by *jiinii* |
| cholera | cholera | cholera | — | — |
| diabetes | sukkur bemmam | d'ukkuba sukkura | — | — |
| intestinal disorders | qurtat | mar'umaan | 'sharp pain in the stomach | idem |
| eczema | lams | roobbii | sometimes associated with leprosy | caused by Allah |
| gastritis | yechabtanyal | singiggoo | stomach cramps | idem, after eating *chat* |
| heart disease | yalebb dekam | d'ukkuba onnee | — | — |
| pertusis | sal | qufa | — | — |
| headache | ras matat | d'ukkuba mataa | 'hit on the head' | sometimes caused by *jiinii* |
| influenza | gunfan | dufkaka | umbrella term for colds and 'flu | idem |
| cancer | yanaqarsa baxta | hola | | caused by Allah |
| whooping cough | tektek | qakkee | sometimes not regarded as an illness | 'children's disease' |
| fever | teqwesat | lagda | umbrella term for fevers | idem |
| liver disease | gubbat | tiruu | swollen liver | — |
| tapeworm | shut | metoo | through eating raw meat | idem |
| malaria | waba | busaa | fever like 'fire' | fever |
| migraine | feltat | hurgunoo | periodic headaches | sometimes caused by *budaa* |

Table 4.13 *(continued)*

| Name of disease | | | Indigenous cause and/or symptoms | |
|---|---|---|---|---|
| English | Amhara | Oromo | Amhara | Oromo |
| nausea | aglasallasa | hogisa | through eating food which is 'off' | idem |
| ear infection | yayoro homan | d'ukkuba gura | caused by flying insect | — |
| rabies | ebd | d'ukkuba saree | dog disease | idem |
| ringworm | chefe | roobbii | itchy rash | caused by *jiinii* |
| back pain | yagarba hemen | bukuu bimudi | back pain through heavy work | idem |
| scabies | — | ekaka | chito | itchy skin |
| muscular pain | gwaya sabbaraw | c'eekuu | caused by contact with a certain crop | caused by cold |
| roundworm | tel | raammoo | — | through eating meat |
| boils | begunj | d'ullaa | especially in the throat | caused by *jiinii* |
| tonsilitis | qemo | araba laga | — | — |
| trachoma | ayn maz | d'ukkuba ijaa | disease of the eyelids | idem |
| chicken-pox | kuffeni | guftii | not regarded as a disease | 'children's disease' |
| ulcers | yaqalla | madaa | caused by *jiinii* | idem |
| abscess (hand/foot) | ebach | goffla | — | swelling in older people, often caused in youth |
| anaemia | — | — | — | caused by *jiinii* |
| fracture | tesabbara atent | lafee c'abe | caused by *jiinii* | idem |
| 'evil eye' | buda | budaa | possession by an evil spirit | idem |
| epilepsy | yabuda basheta | gegeba | illness caused by *budaa* | — |
| lumps or swelling on the head | ebtat | iitoo | — | caused by *jiinii* |

Table 4.13 *(continued)*

| Name of disease | | | Indigenous cause and/or symptoms | |
|---|---|---|---|---|
| English | Amhara | Oromo | Amhara | Oromo |
| gonorrhoea | chabat | c'op'too | caused by urinating in sun or moonlight | idem |
| leprosy | qumtenna/ qommata | juzama | the great illness caused by God | caused by Allah |
| pneumonia | yasamba mec | kuku/ qilleensa | 'afflicted by the wind' | caused by *jiinii* |
| smallpox | fantata | maree | attributed to *jiinii* | idem |
| rheumatism | qurtemat | d'ukkuba c'ap'sanoo | caused by *zar* | — |
| syphilis | werde | baajee | caused by *jiinii* | idem |
| tuberculosis | naqresa | somba | caused by *jiinii* (in the form of a red snake) | idem |
| food allergy | magenya | bira | — | caused by *jiinii* |

would only be fully identified and described after some time. Apparently people are more willing to provide information about illnesses caused by God (and hence in the realm of religion) than about those with magic origins. Most 'religious' diseases were explained as the punishment of God or Allah and only rarely were spirits such as *zar* (Am.) or *jiinii* (Or.) mentioned. Included in this category are anaemia, skin diseases, rachitis, allergies, paralysis, abscesses, fractures and rheumatism. The general assumption within the community is that the majority of these diseases cannot be treated by modern health care personnel trained in the west.

Table 4.13 sets out the traditional classification of perceived morbidity among respondents in the two largest ethnic groups, the Oromo and the Amhara. As far as possible, opinions on the cause and perceived symptoms have also been recorded (cf. Messing 1972; Buschkens and Slikkerveer 1982: 89 – 95).

It shows that, in so far as it is possible to speak of a specific condition, the local population discern almost twice as many naturalistic illnesses as personalistic illnesses. In a number of cases, the relationship between a category and perceived morbidity was not straightforward: a number of illnesses or symptoms are attributed to a naturalistic as well as a personalistic cause. This is the case, for example, with certain types of snake bite and abortion. Children's diseases, which are often not regarded as a specific physical condition, also fall outside the classification in numerous cases. They include measles, chicken-pox, whooping cough, dysentery and German measles. The number of reported personalistic diseases among the Oromo is greater than among the Amhara; they also mentioned more often *jiinii* as the cause of illness.

The way in which the inhabitants of Babile experience and respond to illness will be dealt with in more detail in the discussion of the opinions and practices relating to the different components of the plural medical system in the area. Knowledge of the human body, hygiene and methods of preventing illness and treatment will also be given special attention.

In conclusion, it is clear that as far as health of the population is concerned, particularly with regard to the pattern of morbidity, there is hardly any difference between the national and the local pattern in Babile with the exception of one or two specific diseases. On the other hand, perceived morbidity and indigenous classification of disease among the two main ethnic groups do show some variation as regards both symptoms and etiology. In the course of the analysis of illness behaviour the study will focus on the way in which differences in traditional etiology go hand in hand with the pattern of health care utilisation. The next chapter examines the extent to which the plural character of the community is reflected in the complex medical configuration in this part of Africa.

## Notes

1. Almost half the inhabitants of Hararghe consist of Oromo, most of whom are Muslims. The Oromo from this region, the Eastern Oromo, belong to the Barentu, who together with the Borana form the two largest Oromo groups in Ethiopia. Trimingham (1976: 206) has identified the links

between the various groups (including the four sons of Kallo: Oberra, Nole, Babile and Ala) as follows:

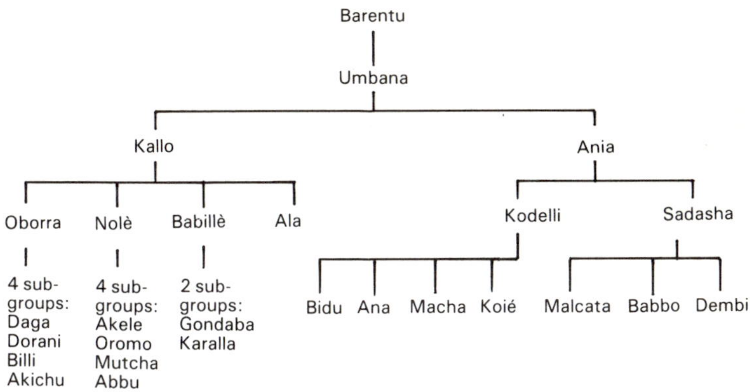


2. In using the stratified simple random sample, the total population was divided into a number of sub-populations where ethnicity was used as a stratification criterion. The elements for the sample were chosen in a random fashion from the sub-populations or strata. The elements were drawn proportionally so that the sample fractions were kept the same for all strata. In this way it was possible to make generalisations about the whole population of Babile without any re-weighting. Stratified sampling has been used in the study because of the possibility that the various characteristics may vary per ethnic group (Segers 1975: 104 – 106; Moser and Kalton 1979: 85).
3. Most utilisation studies conducted in the west and in developing countries use the retrospective method where the behaviour is established of people who have already sought medical help and have received treatment. Although it is sometimes difficult for respondents to remember aspects of their illness behaviour over a long period of time in the past and to recall it correctly, a period of twelve months is the best way of finding out about aspects such as chronic illness and the accompanying range of illness behaviour decisions (cf. Blum and Blum 1965; McKinlay 1970, 1972).

# 5

# The Plural Medical System in Babile

## 5.1 Multisystemic Configurations of Medicine

Further to the previous description of the complex, plural character of Babile as a result of processes of acculturation and transculturation in the Horn of Africa, this chapter considers the extent to which knowledge, practices and behaviour within the community concerning illness, diagnosis and treatment exhibit a similar, plural character.

Broadly speaking, the social, cultural, ethnic and historical aspects of health, illness and healing constitute a complex system of various medical traditions within the community. However, there is such a wide range of medical concepts, attitudes, beliefs and practices among various population groups that it seems appropriate to speak of a pluralistic medical configuration. Similarly, the institutional and organisational aspects of the treatment of various forms of illness in the area do not constitute one comprehensive system. The different ways in which the medical services operate and the large number of medical practitioners and consultants in Babile also call for an approach in terms of a diversity of medical systems rather than a single one. For example, ancient medical traditions still survive as an essential part of the current cultural pattern, alongside modern medicine which central government has promoted since the beginning of the century. Recent studies show that although western-oriented medicine has been successful in combating a large number of epidemics and treating several infectious diseases, so far it has been ineffective in the peripheral areas of the country (cf. Van der Mark 1971; Statistical Abstract of Ethiopia 1975; Schneider 1975; Comprehensive Health Service Directory 1977; Buschkens and Slikkerveer 1980; 1982; Slikkerveer 1982).

On the basis of Dunn's definition (1977) of a medical system referred to in Chapter 2, the pattern of medicine of Babile will be regarded as a complex network of social and cultural traditions and institutions which for generations have enabled the community to deal with crises of illness and death, variously expressed in beliefs and practices among both medical specialists and the local population. Because of the importance of acculturation in the development of medicine in this part of the Horn, the concept of the medical system will be placed within the historical context of the region. In examining the complex range of medical traditions in the research area it would be an oversimplification to speak of a traditional and a modern medical system. The wide range of perceptions and etiologies of illness and the different cultural, religious and ethnic aspects of medical practice, together with the ways in which different population groups use a variety of specialists necessitate a multiple perspective. Moreover, a division into a traditional and a modern system would ignore the dynamic character of the different medical traditions which have been subjected to change over the centuries. The interaction between co-existing systems would also be overlooked. Nevertheless, a study of the various types of medical specialists and practitioners shows that many of their curative techniques are not always based on any one clearly defined medical system; nor can they be categorised as such. Some practitioners use typically local methods while others resort to Islamic or Christian practices. In some cases, modern, pharmaceutical medicines are even used in various traditional forms of treatment. However, the study shows that the practitioners operating in the different systems adopt similar attitudes and employ comparable techniques.

The fact that in view of such variety the concept of a dual medical system previously employed in anthropology cannot be applied to analyse existing medical ideas and practices in Babile has significant implications for research into health care utilisation patterns of the population groups concerned. The 'new' ethnomedical approach in anthropology referred to in Chapter 2 offers a more realistic assessment of the ideological and cultural bases of all medical systems in

Babile, including the official system of cosmopolitan medicine (cf. Press 1980). The use of such holistic perspective to analyse the different medical systems – rather than a 'scientific model' which regards all 'non-scientific' traditional medical systems as irregular and therefore deviant – also means that a number of sub-systems can be distinguished and described within the traditional medical system. This approach allows for pluralism in terms of the diversity of knowledge and perceptions regarding illness, diagnosis and therapy, lay and professional healers, institutions and services, all of which are dealt with below.

In Eastern Ethopia, there are a number of complex medical traditions of diverse size and origins which operate in different ways alongside one another and in conjunction with the modern, cosmopolitan system. As far as the Eastern Highlands of Hararghe are concerned, Buschkens and Slikkerveer (1982: 53—55) introduced an analytical differentation in their research into the functioning of government health care facilities among the culturally homogeneous groups of the rural Eastern Oromo, distinguishing a traditional and a modern system, with a transitional system of pharmaceutical medicine operating in between.

By contrast, the ethnomedical study of culturally heterogeneous community of Babile requires a more complicated differentiation in medical systems in order to examine the various ways in which patients of different ethnic groups seek and obtain medical treatment. Such differentiation should be based on the geo-historical developments in the area accommodating different medical ideas and practices of the population.

Not surprisingly, these medical traditions have evolved in parallel fashion to the historical process of transculturation which has taken place between local and regional cultures with distinct traditions. As far as the development of the culture in this part of Africa is concerned, Redfield's comparative study of cultural systems (1956) offers a useful tool to differentiate between the 'great tradition' and the 'little tradition' which he describes as : '... *the separation of culture into hierarchic and lay traditions, the appearance of an elite with secular and sacred power and including specialised cultivators of the intellectual life and the conversion of tribal peoples into peasantry.*' Redfield (1956: 77-78) goes on to explain the interdependence of these two traditions: *'Great tradition and little tradition have long affected each other and continue to do so.'* He describes them as '... *two currents of thought and action, distinguishable yet ever flowing into and out of each other.*'

From this standpoint, the traditional medical system in Babile may be described as a persistent system '... *comprised of little and great traditions which have interacted in the past and which are still interacting today*' (Redfield 1956: 86). The great and the little traditions function in conjunction with one another. In the African context, the 'great tradition' of medicine could indeed refer to the important traditions of written theory and practice of Graeco-Arabic medicine and Amhara-Christian medicine as well as to recent cosmopolitan medicine, while the 'little tradition' refers to the local Cushitic medicine of the Oromo and the Somali.

If the geographical, historical and socio-cultural features of the Babile area are added to this classification, an even more refined typology of medical systems can be distinguished:

- a *a local medical system* which encompasses traditional Cushitic medicine, i.e. Oromo and Somali traditions;
- b the *regional medical systems* of the major Arabic and Amhara traditions; and
- c the *cosmopolitan medical system* recently introduced by the central government into the area.

If the local system under a. and the regional system under b. are grouped together as the traditional medical system and c. is taken to be the modern system, there is a third system operating in the area which provides the local population with specific medical treatment: the transitional medical system. It is not exclusively Ethiopian nor, strictly speaking, are the 'specialists' part of either the traditional or the modern system. It consists of application on a large scale of commercially available medication which has been provided in Hararghe since the end of the last century, as the result of the development of the European pharmaceutical industry. Figure 5.1 shows a simplified model of the plural medical system in the Highlands.

## 5.2 The Traditional Medical System

The traditional medical system in Babile consists of a conglomeration of overlapping elements, which have enabled the local

| | | |
|---|---|---|
| Plural Medical System | Traditional medical system | Local medical (sub) system of Cushistic medicine<br>Regional medical (sub) system of Arabic medicine<br>Regional medical (sub) system of Amharic medicine |
| | Transitional medical system | Medical system of commercial pharmaceutical medicine |
| | Modern medical system | Medical system of cosmopolitan medicine |

Figure 5.1: *Simplified model of the plural medical system in Eastern Ethiopia (Slikkerveer 1982: 1862)*

population to cope with illness over the centuries. A number of these elements in terms of popular medical beliefs, conceptions and practices and methods of treatment used by the practitioners and institutions can be distinguished by analysis and then grouped under the appropriate medical (sub) system.

To begin with, local medical traditions obviously did not develop in a vacuum. Traditional methods of treating illness and beliefs about its causes developed in the indigenous local culture, within which both personalistic and naturalistic interpretations of illness and health were an important element. In the course of time these traditions have been subjected to various influences and have changed as the result of contacts with other cultures; beliefs and practices have been assimilated and transformed. In some cases, this has been accompanied by changes in the cosmology or religion of particular groups. In accordance with Koumaré's (1983: 25) observation that: *'Traditional medicine caters for most of the health needs of at least 80% of the African population'*, a similar segment of the present population in this part of Africa does not have access to modern medicine. So it is clear that the complex traditional medical system still provides the only regular source of the medical needs of the local population. The functional approach towards the provision of services enables the researcher to identify and analyse many of the elements of the diverse systems which have survived to the present day. In addition, recent studies into the effectiveness of official medical services confirm that modern health care only reaches a small proportion of the population in the peripheral areas of Ethiopia. Outside the Horn of Africa, traces of old medical systems have not only survived to the present day but in certain cases have even undergone a particular form of re-evaluation, often as a part of a wider socio-political movement. In this context Crozier (1977: 341) in his study of Chinese medicine mentions a number of forms of 'medical revivalism' in contemporary China, while Slikkerveer (1985) observes a recent process of 'reculturation' in traditional medicine in South Sulawesi, Indonesia.

In the research area, the existing traditional medical system can be conceived as a number of overlapping (sub) systems:

1 local Cushitic folk medicine which came about in the area in the sixteenth century at the time of the great Oromo migrations. Traces of this system are still recognisable in the culture of the Eastern Oromo and Somali groups in Babile;
2 Arabic medicine which spread throughout the area with the process of Islamisation from the Arabian Peninsula. This process which later evolved gradually from the major Muslim centre in the East, the Emirate of Harar, from the eighteenth century onwards, eventually resulted in the Egyptian occupying forces imposing their traditions on local population groups in the second half of the nineteenth century;
3 Amhara medicine which was introduced into the area at the end of the nineteenth century after the conquest of Harar by Emperor Menelik II. The process of *Amharisation* which followed throughout the province of Hararghe, helped Amhara medical traditions to spread.

Although it is difficult to make a clear distinction between these three (sub) systems in Babile, an attempt is made to describe them in terms of relevant perceptions, practices and various types of healer.

### *5.2.1 The local Cushitic medical (sub) system*

This includes local medical traditions, a number of elements of which are still found among certain population groups in Babile. They derive from the old, pre-Islamic and pre-Christian medicine of the indigenous Cushitic (Oromo and Somali) inhabitants of the region and belong to that part of the culture which Redfield (1956: 70) describes as the '... *little tradition of the unreflective many* ...' which, as he goes on to say, '... *works itself out and keeps itself going in the lives of the unlettered in their village communities.'* Before examining the sources available to describe this local system in more detail, it is useful to establish how a large number of its elements managed to survive and adapt despite far-reaching acculturation. Assuming the interactions and relations between the 'little tradition' and the 'great tradition', as described above, an ongoing process of development can be traced as regards the culture elements in the period before Islamisation and Amharisation. The following factors play a role in the process of 'cultural persistence' of elements of indigenous Cushitic folk medicine.

First, the Oromo, and the Somali who have mixed with them, form the largest ethnic group in Babile (approximately 60%). Both groups exhibit a predominantly Oromo culture pattern in the community, by contrast with the Amhara (approximately 38%) who emigrated to the area at a later date. It should also be remembered that Babile is situated in a largely Oromo area of Hararghe where the rural Oromo are dominant.

Second, compared with other culture areas outside Africa (such as China and Iran), the research area has only recently come under the influence of the major Arabic and European cultures, largely as already mentioned, because of its isolated geographical position. The pastoral Oromo – who settled in the fertile Eastern Highlands in the sixteenth century – resisted repeated attempts by the Emirate of Harar to subjugate them (cf. Muhammad Hassan 1973). It was not until the eighteenth century that they increasingly came into contact with Islam (cf. Trimingham 1976: 107). Towards the end of the nineteenth century and in the early twentieth century the area then came under the influence of Egypt, the Kingdom of Ethiopia and Italy in rapid succession. Finally, recent attempts by the modern Ethiopian Republic to establish a system of modern medicine have not eliminated local medical traditions.

Third, despite the influence of the Harari, Egyptians, Amhara and Italians, the indigenous Cushitic groups have managed to retain their original identity, a phenomenon reported elsewhere among the population of rural areas (cf. Buschkens and Slikkerveer 1982). In addition to this historical explanation, two social institutions have specifically enabled the Oromo to retain their own identity despite acculturation: the Oromo family system and the Oromo class system. The traditional patrilinear family system is still found among the Oromo. Levine (1974: 129) attributes this among other things to their historical resilience: *'The Oromo family is much more stable than the Amhara family.'* This is reflected at the present time in a number of social activities which revolve round the Oromo family; other activities are still undertaken within the wider family or neighbourhood (Or. *ollaa*) which includes a number of local kinship and class groups. Traces of the *gadaa* system are still encountered among the Eastern Oromo in the Horn. The Oromo political system based on *gadaa* was weakened by the Amhara conquest of Hararghe towards the end of the nineteenth century, and now only survives in a small number of religious and ritual ceremonies.

This significance of the religious and ritual elements of the *gadaa* system which still survive in the local medical system is often expressed in the strong cosmic link between religion, magic and medicine. This type of link has been demonstrated in a large number of non-Western cultures in the early socio-anthropological and historical literature (cf. Paul 1955; Read 1966; Gelfland 1964; King 1966; Buck *et al.* 1970; Morley 1976). Sigerist (1951: 209) noted that traditional attitudes often make no distinction between medicine, magic and religion: *'In primitive medicine, magical, religious and empirico-rational views and practices are blended so as to form an inseparable whole . . .'*; in many cultures, the local religion has provided a framework in which mysticism, magic and medicine are combined. Apart from the empirical context, a number of Oromo still attribute this kind of inter-relationship to the local deity (Or. *waaqa*). The pre-Islamic Cushitic religion was characterised by an important animistic component. Bruce (1790) and Burton (1856) mentioned *Sabaism* as the oldest monotheistic religion present in pre-Islamic Eastern Africa. In connection with the views of the Oromo who later converted to Islam, Paulitschke (1893) observed that sabaism was created and spread throughout the area by travelling prophets (Or. *ambiota*) in the distant past. He noted on its continued existence: *'Dieser alte Monotheismus, ein reiner und einfacher Theismus mit animistischer Grundlage, schimmert noch bei vielen Stämmen in seiner Originalität leise selbst unter der Islamitischen Decke hervor . . .'*. Despite Islamisation, Muslim traces of sabaism which have retained their ritual function alongside the worship of Allah can still be found among the Shafi'ite segment of the Muslim population of Babile.

In old Cushitic medicine, personalistic and naturalistic elements were generally regarded as one within the cosmic system (Foster 1983). Later on, however, a split probably occurred in local etiology between 'magico-religious' illness and 'empirico-rational' illness as it did in several old medical systems outside Ethiopia (Sigerist 1951). Within the context of this local medical system, people still seek to explain the majority of common illnesses in such personalistic terms and accordingly consult mystical practitioners such as sorcerers, exorcists, snake charmers, soothsayers and magicians for treatment.

The illnesses caused by naturalistic elements are then treated by means of counter-irritation (Or. *gubaa*), cauterisation (Or. *koobuu*) and bonesetting. These practices were used largely by pragmatic specialists with considerable skill and knowledge of fractures, domestic remedies and medical plants. However, there are still magical elements in their treatment, so that there is an overlap between the two categories in specific cases. Messing (1972: 245) speaks in this connection of 'medical interdigitation' between mystical and rational elements in the treatment provided by traditional practitioners in Ethiopia. This concept, which stresses the cosmic inter-relation between religion, magic and medicine, is practised in Babile by some traditional healers. In the research there are a number of traditional healers who can be regarded entirely or partly as typical representatives of the local Cushitic medical (sub) system.

The sources which have been consulted to form an impression of the Cushitic medicine will now be indicated briefly. There is only a limited amount of information in the literature since the majority of authors describe the various cultures in the context of the period after the Islamisation and Amharisation of Eastern Ethiopia. However, a reasonably clear picture can be obtained from early publications by Paulitschke (1893), Cerulli (1922), Piovano (1942) and Messing (1972). Several old local manuscripts – chiefly containing lists of traditional medicinal plants – form an important source for the reconstruction of the *corpus medicorum* of the local medical system. Non-medical manuscripts and books also yield important information on medical practices from the standpoint of patients and the elevation of local healers by members of the community. For instance, old manuscripts from Harar occasionally refer to local medical perceptions and practices among the population groups living around this cultural centre.

Another source consists of oral traditions which play an

important role in handing down indigenous medical knowledge. The absence of detailed written records of medical practices from the pre-Islamic period emphasises the importance of the oral tradition, traces of which can still be found in the area. It is not only the most important way of transferring knowledge from father to son and from mother to daughter among local traditional specialists, but also enables medical concepts and practices of folk medicine to survive for many generations. Folk medicine comprises the traditional home remedies (Or. *dawwaa mana*) often used by the mother or grandmother to cure members of the family.

On the basis of information of the above sources combined with the qualitative and quantitative data from the research in Babile, a description follows of elements which belong to the present local medical sub-system. As is to be expected, these are mainly found among the Oromo and Somali groups in the form of perceptions concerning a number of illnesses, their traditional remedies and of curative techniques used by the local healers. In addition, a classification is given of the various types of practitioners in the local system.

## Perceptions and practices

The results of research into the local medical sub-system show the cosmic link between religion, magic and medicine in a number of traditional views held by the Oromo and Somali concerning the causes of illness. For example the Oromo concept of *qoolloo* refers to an ancient cosmology aimed at the use of natural elements and products without disturbing the equilibrium. These may vary from stone or wooden building materials and tools to local medicinal plants or other natural products from which remedies can be prepared.

During conversations with a number of Oromo and Somali household heads in Babile, it was discovered that *qoolloo* often manifest themselves in the region as mountain and river spirits to whom animals must regularly be sacrificed (Or. *qalma*) in order to ensure health and good luck. The *qoolloo* can be traced back to the old Cushitic pantheon of sabaism in which the deity or creator (Or. *waaqa*) is surrounded by an army of good spirits (Or. *ayyaana*) and demons (Or. *jiinii*). The *jiinii* still play a role today in explaining the origins of predominantly personalistic illnesses including the 'evil eye' (Or. *budaa*) as the cause of epilepsy, paralysis and hysteria.

The term *budaa* creates such fear that the majority of respondents would not even use it and refused to give a direct answer when asked about it. The diseases generally associated with evil spirits include serious conditions such as leprosy, venereal diseases and tuberculosis. Sudden deaths, accidents and murder are also attributed to *budaa*. The 'evil eye' can be magically transferred to other people, for example by an old woman, as a result of which the victim may suffer from certain mental disorders. The symptoms of this type of illness always start with absent-mindedness, loss of appetite, apathy, and unconsciousness and the patient may eventually die. *Budaa* may also affect a family's harvest if one member of the family is envious or jealous of the beauty or the wealth of a relative or neighbour.

*Jiinii* (Or.) can also cause illness if taboos are contravened. Impotence (Or. *falijii*) for example, can be caused by failing to wash the sexual organs after intercourse. Gonorrhea (Or. *c'op'too*) can be caught by looking at the sun while urinating. Leprosy (Or. *juzam*) is often seen by the local population to be the result of breaking the taboo on sexual intercourse outside the house (Or. *segitan*). During the household interviews, only a small number of respondents could bring themselves to mention *jiinii* (Or.) as the cause of illness. As far as local etiology is concerned, the Oromo also believe in *kadara* (Or.) a specific spirit which brings illness. If a household is visited by a *kadara* – which may stay for any length of time – the health of the members of the group is endangered and a peace offering will often be made by slaughtering a black ox or a female sheep in ritual fashion at a special site (Or. *hojubaa* or *mijuu*). The ritual involves eating and throwing away part of the animal's flesh. On the same day coffee is mixed with butter in a small bowl (Or. *killa*), thrown three times into the fire (Or. *tachasu*) and drunk by the whole group. Butter (Or. *qabee*) is also smeared on the patient's forehead as a form of protection. Sacrificial sites are to be found on the edges of the villages and under several old trees inhabited by spirits. It is forbidden to approach such places at night.

In addition to the personalistic elements in the perceptions of the local population, there are several empirical elements in which the method of treatment is defined as naturalistic. This can be the case with fractures, wounds, throat complaints and slight internal complaints. The treatment of these illnesses is not primarily determined by supernatural or magical principles but by using the rational knowledge and skills of local healers and the empirical effect of natural products and medicinal plants. However, sometimes magical and religious rituals may be included in the way these remedies are administered. For example, the plants concerned are picked in a special manner, often at specific times and the medicines are prepared and administered in a particular fashion.

In Babile, particularly among the Oromo, a number of curative medical practices are used within the household or family, often by the mother or grandmother. These traditional home remedies form an important part of the local medical sub-system in terms of their pragmatic character and the specific category of illness they have been used to treat over generations. They usually consist of a mixture of ritual and rational practices, such as administering medicinal plant extracts within the home and slaughtering sacrificial animals, in combination with practices such as shaving the hair of the patient and rubbing oil, powder, butter and potash on the affected parts of the body. Medical knowledge varies from simple recipes to the appropriate treatment for a number of illnesses and forms an important part of the oral tradition within the local medical system. Illnesses treated in this way include so-called 'non-Western diseases' which many Oromo assume cannot be treated by outsiders such as doctors trained in the modern system, e.g. anaemia (Or. *alati*), fractures (Or. *lafee c'abe*), the 'evil eye' (Or. *budaa*), abscesses (Or. *goffla*) pneumonia (Or. *qilleensa*), skin disease (Or. *sibijii*) and swelling of the temples (Or. *dankaboi* ). In addition to sacrificing animals, other non-curative elements consist of prescribing and wearing *dumuga* (Or.) and *megira* (Or.), two special types of amulet, which unlike *kartasa* (Or.) and *ketab* (Am.) do not have any connection with Islam or Ethiopian Christianity. They offer protection against several supposedly personalistic illnesses such as swellings on the head (Or. *itaweh*) and on the temple (Or. *dankaboi*).

## Practitioners

It is not easy to classify the varied and extensive range of traditional healers within the local system into distinct categories on the basis of specialisation and the methods of treatment used by these local healers. For example, some only treat naturalistic illnesses in an empirical manner, while others use predominantly personalistic elements both in presenting cures and medicines to patients and handing out amulets. A number of local practitioners can be grouped according to the following criteria: a) the category of local illness they treat; b) the part-time nature of their vocational practice; c) their limited formal education; d) the way of entry into the system and their specialisation; e) the way they are remunerated or reimbursed by patients for the treatment provided.

Linking up with the practice of using home remedies and the special knowledge of how to treat several common diseases by non-professional healers, such as farmers, potters and blacksmiths, who are assumed to possess specific knowledge of the properties of one or more medicinal plants and make this knowledge available to their fellow villagers (often without expecting any form of payment), the practitioners in the Cushitic local medical sub-system can be divided into the following categories:

the *qaalluu* Or.) or *qaallica* (Or.), the local spiritual healer;
the *ogeesa* (Or.) or *wogessha* (Or.), the local pragmatic healer;
the *ogeettii* (Or.), the local midwife.

The original Cushitic titles of these functionaries, as well as the medical concepts and practices they use, confirm their association with the local system.

## The qaalluu or qaallica

The Oromo and the Somali who have mixed with them treat the *qaalluu* (or *qaallica*) with a great deal of respect, often regarding them as holy men who are in direct contact with the spiritual world of *ayyaana* (Or.) and *jiinii* (Or.). The respect is expressed in the form of address or title *qaalluu* (Or.) which means 'Master of the Spirits'. The majority of these mystical healers have their own individual spirit which needs to be worshipped every year with sacrificial ceremonies. Spirits play an important role in making the diagnosis of the illness and in determining the appropriate treatment for patients. The *qaalluu* is mainly concerned with treating personalistic diseases caused by the 'evil eye'. The treatment of these almost always involves ritual exorcism by means of spells and fumigation or by flagellation. Providing amulets, *dumugaa* (Or.) and *megiraa* (Or.) are among the important non-curative tasks of these healers. To prevent swellings on temples, *dankaboi* (Or.), several dried stalks of a tall local grass are rubbed over the chest and neck of the patient, split in two, plaited and then hung round the neck in ritual fashion as *megiraa* (Or.).

To prevent swellings on the head (Or. *iitawe*), the *qaalluu* gives patients an amulet (Or. *dumugaa*) made from the woodlike stem of a mystical bush. Sometimes these practitioners treat somatic illnesses by giving patients medicines such as plant extracts mixed with honey and butter. For example, patients with fevers are given a drink made from wild honey and melted butter while swelling infections are treated by massaging butter and animal fat into the affected part of the patient's body. Milk, butter and camel urine are among the curative ingredients in remedies used by the *qaalluu*.

Payment for this kind of treatment is regarded as essential if the medicine is to have a positive effect. A gift of nature for example in the form of a medicinal plant, should be compensated by a simple offering of coffee, tobacco or *chat* in order to restore the natural balance of the cosmos. *Qaalluu* take up their vocation either as a result of inheriting knowledge and skills from their father or mother, or because they have been inspired by spirits, dreams or visions. They often live a simple and retired existence and are not united in any form of brotherhood or local elite. A distant attitude also characterises their relations with the other members of the community and patients; the *qaalluu* never touches his patients and may not himself be touched or have his hand shaken. In some cases he may only be addressed through an intermediary or assistant.

## The ogeessa or wogessha

This is a pragmatic specialist in fractures, tumours and wounds. The title *ogeessa* means 'someone who soothes' in Oromifa and his medical practices involve a number of techniques and instruments geared to treating mainly naturalistic illnesses. Often the *ogeessa* is a skilled surgeon with wide knowledge of medicinal plants and traditional remedies which he grows himself or gathers from special places in the mountains.

In addition to fractures and wounds, the *ogeessa* also treats haemorrhoids, abscesses, ulcers, headaches, swellings on the head, ear infections, muscular cramps, lumbar complaints and various forms of cancer. His methods of treatment range from counter-irritation by means of singing, cauterisation and having patients inhale the smoke of burning leaves (Or. *ulacuu*) to operating and cutting out infected wounds, removing the uvula, bleeding and removing the tonsils. There used to be several very famous *ogeessa* in the Babile area who, according to informants, even carried out amputations and trephinations successfully. Among the present *ogeessa* there are also skilled traditional dentists who are capable of carrying out surgery on the jaw. In Babile, the *ogeessa* carry out circumcision of boys (Or. *d'agnaqaba*) most usually among the Oromo and Somali groups (See Plate 9).

The wide range of instruments used by these specialists include a number of modern tools, disinfectants, oils and kerosene indicating their pragmatic orientation. They use a cow's horn (Or. *koobaa*) to suck out blood from wounds, etc., horse hair to carry out tonsillectomy and to remove the uvula, and a razorblade for incisions, circumcision and blood-letting. Formerly, these operations used to be carried out with a stone blade made from obsidian. They also use pincers, screwdrivers, scissors and tweezers for a number of forms of dental treatment. Although the *ogeessa* conduct their diagnosis and treatment largely on empirical and rational grounds, traces of magico-religious practices can sometimes be detected in their practices. Like the *qaalluu* they obtain ingredients from medicinal plants and associate restoring the natural balance with certain mystical rituals which have their origins in ancient Cushitic cosmology. As noted before, this phenomenon has been encountered elsewhere in Ethiopia as medical interdigitation (cf. Messing 1972).

Like the *qaalluu,* the *ogeessa* receives payment for medical treatment consisting primarily in an act of 'compensating nature', seldom taking the form of money. Millett, coffee, tobacco and *chat* are the most common gifts which they receive from their patients. Although there are one or two part-time *ogeessa* in Babile, the level of specialisation and professionalism of the majority is high; it is confirmed by the special position they occupy. Some of them – either men or women – originally took up the occupation as illiterates because of personal gifts or a sense of vocation, intially as simple traditional osteopaths or herbal doctors. Many of them have developed into famous healers because of their ambition and willingness to learn from other medical systems. Certain *ogeessa* do not confine themselves to the oral transfer of indigenous medical knowledge but try to learn more about Arabic, Amhara and cosmopolitan medicine. Particularly in the larger cities of Eastern Ethiopia, there are several *ogeessa* who have been trained by an Islamic healer (Ar. *'ulamā'*) and have officially sworn an oath (Har.

*tuftii*) (cf. Buschkens and Slikkerveer 1982: 40, 41). Unlike the *qaalluu,* therefore, the *ogeessa* maintain contacts with other traditional healers from the region. They are constantly receptive to innovation and as will be indicated later, in some cases they refer patients to other traditional practitioners.

## The ogeetti

The *ogeetti* is the often illiterate, traditional midwife who forms part of the local medical sub-system in Babile. This occupation is often conducted on a part-time basis by women from the Oromo and Somali groups who hand down knowledge from mother to daughter. Medical knowledge and practices are transmitted mainly via the oral tradition as are their specific treatment techniques. The latter are often accompanied by a blessing ritual (Or. *eebba*) at which the *ogeetti* is responsible for the natal and post-natal care of women in the community, mainly Oromo and Somali, and for carrying out clitoridectomy (Or. *absumada*) among young girls. They also conduct a number of ritual duties connected with death and marriage which are not directly connected with their role as a midwife. Most births take place under the supervision of an *ogeetti* who often applies special massage techniques. After birth, the *ogeetti* cuts the umbilical cord, ties it up and then buries the placenta behind the door of the parent's house. In cases of complicated births she always confers with the *ogeessa.* The *ogeetti* carry out clitoridectomy and infibulation on the same day, usually on girls aged 9 and 10 and sometimes 11, who are then wrapped in a special bandage from the hips to the knees (Or. *sabbataa*). After three days it is cleaned by the midwife herself. In the first week the girls are not allowed to move and are cared for by their mothers or older women in the community.

The rewards for the traditional midwife as for the *qaalluu* and *ogeessa* usually consist of coffee, *chat,* millet, tobacco, etc., and eating a kind of porridge (Or. *suro*) with the patient's family and chewing *chat* in a special ceremony known as *ujuraa* (Or.). There are still one or two midwives among the *ogeetti* in Babile who can also treat a number of diseases in addition to performing the duties mentioned above. These include children's diseases, women's diseases, ear and eye infections, and stomach complaints which they treat mainly by means of medicinal plants. The social position of the *ogeetti* within the Oromo and Somali groups is very important. They are invited together with the *ogeessa* to virtually all the important events and festivities in the community and are often asked for advice.

Generally speaking, the high level of social interaction and two-way provision of services between the Oromo and Somali inhabitants of the community on the one hand, and practitioners in the local medical sub-system on the other, together with the method of payment for traditional medical services by means of simple gifts, confirms the cooperative arrangements usually found among these groups. The functioning of groups '... *to the pursuit of corporate interests through cooperative endeavours ...*' which Levine (1974: 140, 141) calls the 'solidaristic association' of the Oromo, is therefore not only reflected in surviving traces of the old *gadaa* system and the duties within the *olla,* but also in the way the local medical sub-system operates.

### *5.2.2 The regional Arabic medical (sub) system*

This major traditional (sub) system includes the medical knowledge and practices of Arabic medicine originating from the Middle East and around the Mediterranean. It is the 'great tradition' of Islamic scholars recorded in manuscripts and books often used by learned specialists from elite groups. It developed largely in the Middle East and reached Ethiopia from the East when Islam spread throughout the Horn of Africa. It was originally introduced into the research area as a transplanted medical system being a part of the process of acculturation, but later it rapidly became established as the dominant medical system within the existing culture pattern of the Islamised Cushitic population groups, as a result of the powerful process of Islamisation. Large parts of the local medical system were incorporated and, finally, regional Arabic medicine developed into an important component of traditional medicine in the area.

As indicated in Chapter 3, the first systematic spread of Islam in the Horn of Africa from the Arabian Peninsula took place between the tenth and the eleventh centuries, cutting off the Abyssinian Kingdom from the Red Sea. During the twelfth and thirteenth centuries, a number of powerful Muslim states were established in the Somali coastal region and in the interior as far as the eastern and southern borders of the Eastern Highlands. At this time, the *hinterland* came more and more under the influence of Islam. However, it was not until the last quarter of the nineteenth century (1875-1885) that the Egyptians attempted the mass subjugation of the Oromo and Somali settlers in the highlands. The Egyptian occupation of Harar and the surrounding district was only temporary but it had serious repercussions, mainly for the spread of Islam. In this connection, Trimingham (1976: 121) points out the role played by the teachers of the Koran or *faqih* (Ar.): *'Fekis were encouraged to travel in all directions to teach the social discipline of Islam and the performance of the Islamic prayer was made obligatory under penalty of confiscation of property.'* The fact that the Oromo and Somali eventually converted to Islam can largely be attributed to the way in which the system adapted to the local African culture. Cecchi (1886: 342) underlines this: *'Islam for these people ... is a religion which better than Christianity had adapted itself to their way of life.'*

The interaction between and co-existence of these major Islamic and Cushitic cultures in the Eastern Highlands was more or less hierarchical. In his study of the relationships between Islamic doctrine and Islamised local cultures, Von Grunebaum (1955) states that: *'... one of the two patterns is recognised as the more advanced; it is assumed to make authority; it is almost exclusively represented in the writings as well as the public actions of the elite; social prestige is dependent on its adoption. In the dar al-Islam, the Islamic pattern is in general in the position of the great tradition. In contrast the little tradition is the catchment of the popular undercurrent. Its effectiveness is still felt by the intelligentsia but officially it will be denied or depreciated. Where the hypotheses of the great tradition are considered beliefs, the hypotheses of the little tradition will be considered superstitions'.*

Von Grunebaum (1955) regards the process of acculturation between the two cultures as a process of accommodation by the two traditions: *'... as when the Islamic teachers recognise the popular tradition as the religion of the ignorant or tolerate local practices which might have been considered heretical'.* He makes a distinction between a process of integration and incorporation of the local culture within the Islamic tradition: *'The expanders of hierarchic Islam may integrate the local belief or practice with orthodoxy by interpretations of doctrine that provide a sanction for it.'* The process of transculturation mentioned in Chapter 3 also applies to this process of mutual acculturation between local and regional cultures (cf. Ortiz 1970).

During this period, the Arabic sciences (Ar. *'ulum al-'Arab*) of historiography, literature, astrology, law and medicine spread throughout the area. Medical specialists, usually known as *hakīm* (Ar.), who practised Arabic medicine, settled in Harar and several larger rural communities in the area. To begin with they concentrated on providing medical care primarily for the local elite. Arabic medicine belongs to the part of culture to which Redfield (1956: 70) refers as the: '. . . *great tradition of reflective few . . . cultivated in schools or temples*'. It is chiefly the tradition of the educated elite with whom the local culture first came into contact: *'The tradition of the philosopher, theologian, and literary man is a tradition consciously cultivated and handed down ...'* Education and training within this process chiefly involved knowledge of Arabic and of Islam as a religion. The Koran schools (Ar. *madrasah*) played an important role in the spread of Islam. Trimingham (1976: 142) notes: *'Although teaching may be confined to little more than the recital of passages of the Qur'an and the prayer formulae, this system of educational concentration upon religion is one of the factors which helped Islam so much to dominate the life of the peoples it has converted.'* In the Horn of Africa, for a long period schools were only found in Harar and the Somali coastal towns. It was not until the second half of the nineteenth century that the area was involved in an Islamic revival and subsequently the teaching of the Koran spread rapidly. Trimingham (1976) describes this process as follows: *'Teaching sheikhs of all kinds started schools in Muslim centres, especially in the kingdoms around Gibe, in the Harar region, throughout Eritrea and Somalia and in the Jabarti and Yamanite colonies.'* Today there are still a number of Koran schools throughout the Highlands of Eastern Ethiopia. The education system to which they belong is described in more detail in the section dealing with the training of practitioners in the Arabic medical system. Before describing the elements of this important regional system in Babile, it is useful to consider the historical development of Graeco-Arabic medicine and the way it spread to this part of Africa.

Traditional Arabic medicine originally developed as a result of the conflict between the old folk medicine of the Bedouins and the classic Hellenic medical sciences. Hellenic Sciences reached their culmination during the mass translations of the Greek medical handbooks and manuscripts into Arabic under the caliphs of the

Abbassid Dynasty, in the second part of the eighth century. Ancient Arabic medicine of the Bedouins in the pre-Islamic period mainly consisted of treating illness with magical ceremonies for which there was virtually no theoretical or empirical basis. The practices were based on limited anatomical knowledge and were restricted to a few forms of medication and some simple surgery, the most important aspects of which were blood-letting and cauterisation (cf. Ullmann 1970: 16). Here, the magical element occupied a particularly important position in the form of ritual sayings and formulae. Despite the advent of Islam in the seventh century, this situation did not change very much. Ullmann (1970: 27) notes: *Das Auftreten des Propheten Muhammad brachte hinsichtlich der medizinischen Verhältnisse weder praktisch noch theoretisch eine wesentliche Änderung mit sich. Im Koran, in dem sonst so viele Lebensprobleme der Menschen angesprochen sind, werden der Arzt und die Medizin nirgends erwähnt.*

Although, as far as medicine is concerned, the Prophet confined himself to comments about hygiene and diet and stressed the medical properties of natural products such as honey, grain, milk, etc., his ideas had a major impact on the development of Islamic medicine. Most importantly, the view of the Prophet later became an effective tool used by the growing religious counter movement led by a number of orthodox Koran scholars and traditional zealots. This movement developed into a major component of Arabic medicine as 'prophetic medicine' (Ar. *aṭ-ṭibb an-nabawī*).

When the Arabic Empire expanded to include Syria, Egypt, Palestine, Persia and North Africa during the period of the first four caliphs, the direct successors of the Prophet, the Arabs in Damascus under the Ummayad Dynasty in 661 came into closer contact with classical Greek medicine, or the Galen medical system. This was based on the humoural pathology of the school of Hippocrates of Kos, and subsequently adapted by Aristotle and by the school of Pneumatists and incorporated by Galen into a considered rational medical theory of the balance of the four bodily fluids (Greek: *eukrasis*). Initially, the concepts of this new medical science were only slightly absorbed by Arabic medicine because of the language barrier, but this changed when the Greek texts were translated on a large scale. Ullmann (1970: 25) stresses the significance of this work for the development of Arabic medicine:

*Als die 'Abbasidenkalifen' und ihre Minister in der zweiten Hälfte des achten Jahrhunderts griechische medizinische Werke in grossem Massstab ins Arabische übersetzen liessen, leiteten sie eine kulturgeschichtliche Entwicklung ein, deren Bedeutung und Auswirkungen nicht leicht überschätzt werden können.*

Especially in the course of the ninth century, Greek medical texts by Hippocrates, Galen, Diocles, Erasistratos, Archigenes, Kriton, Rufus and others were translated into Arabic and the Galenic system was adopted almost wholly by the Arabs. Translations were also made at this time of a number of Indian medical manuscripts which resulted in Indian pharmacology being incorporated into Arabic medicine. In this way the Galen medical system formed the basis of Arabic medicine which flourished during the next three centuries. In this period the humoural theory of medicine was formulated in Arabic documents and Syrian Arabic doctors began to practise the new rational medicine. The golden age of Arabic medicine lasted from the tenth to the twelfth centuries; after that the system ceased to develop and a period of decline set in (cf. Ullmann 1970: 108).

As mentioned above, however, within orthodox Muslim circles, there was growing antipathy among non-medical traditionalists, lawyers and historians to the Galenic system of medicine. Eventually this reaction, which became more and more prominent under the name of 'prophetic medicine', involved the re-evaluation in religious terms of pre-Islamic Bedouin folk medicine, based on sayings attributed to the Prophet (Ar. *hadīth*). Thereupon, prophetic medicine was eagerly accepted by the Islamic population who preferred the authority of the Prophet to that of the 'heathen' Hippocrates. Astrology, magic and folk beliefs were thus elevated to the level of medicine. Ullmann (1970: 185) comments on this development: *'Auf diese Weise wurde alter medizinischer Volksbrauch, Aberglaube und Amulettzauber religiös geweiht und übertüncht und mühsam in den Rang einer "Wissenschaft" erhoben.'*

Despite criticism from within Arabic medical circles, 'prophetic medicine' gained momentum as a religious movement as can be seen from more than a thousand documents, manuscripts and books. Subsequently it became an important part of the Arabic medical system introduced and adapted into conquered territories in combination with the other Arabic sciences as part of the whole process of Islamisation. In this way Arabic medicine was introduced from the Arabian Peninsula into East Africa as part of Islamic expansion. At the beginning of the sixteenth century it gradually spread among the population of Eastern Ethiopia from the important Muslim outpost of the Emirate of Harar. As indicated before, this development reached its climax in the research area during the Egyptian occupation of Harar in the second half of the nineteenth century when the Oromo and Somali were almost completely subjugated and subjected to the influence of Islam. As the following section shows, Arabic medicine finally developed into a dominant regional medical system in Babile.

## Perceptions and practices

The Islamic inhabitants of Babile – who make up two-thirds of the total population – have a number of perceptions and practices relating to illness and health which are closely associated with Islam. More than one-fifth of the Oromo and Somali households in the survey perceive 'punishment of Allah' as the major cause of illness while about three-quarters of them regard death as the work of Allah.

Magic and a belief in the 'evil eye' as the cause of illness have been completely incorporated into Muslim culture in Babile and are essential elements of the Arabic medical system. Recognition of *budaa* and of possession by spirits (*jiinii*) illustrates how local cultural elements have been incorporated into Islam. This also applies in the way in which an otherwise strictly monotheistic religion tolerates local Oromo and Somali saints to whose tombs the sick and the underpriviledged frequently make pilgrimages. Von Grunebaum (1955) speaks in this connection of '*... the justification within the framework of orthodoxy of the cult of the saints*'. As mentioned before, astrology and magic constituted substantial elements of 'prophetic medicine' which was introduced in Eastern Ethiopia as a key feature of Arabic medicine. Astrological concepts in traditional prevention of illness and in diagnosis can be recognised in Babile in the taboo forbidding certain types of action during a full moon and the ban on sexual intercourse on Islamic rest days such as Monday and Friday, non-observance of which may produce venereal diseases. The significance of astrology for prognosis and therapy are dealt with in more detail in the following account of the practitioners operating within the Arabic sub-system.

The rules of Islam can be recognised in the belief that people are vulnerable to illnesses at certain times of the day, such as during the period of afternoon prayer (Or. *sa'attii asri*). Nevertheless, the habits of regularly saying prayers to Allah to prevent people and cattle from being affected by illness and to ward off accidents and crop failure, which the Oromo and Somali call *sijara amatah* (Or.), can be traced back to the emphasis Islam places on frequently quoting the Koran. The Islamic protective saying *'bismillah'* is found throughout the whole of the Horn of Africa. The majority of heads of households attempt to model their lifestyle on the laws of Allah and the rules of the Prophet are forcefully applied. The tolerant attitude shown by the Oromo and Somali to the sick, invalids and crippled and their resistance to any form of birth control also reflect the strong influence of Arabic medicine.

The belief in the medical power of Islamic amulets (Or. *kartasa*) made of quotations from the Koran written on paper or parchment rolled up in a reddish-brown leather bag and worn round the neck is a clear form of an Arab way of prevention which is described in many Islamic medical texts (see Plate 15). It ties in with regularly quoting the Koran during the day which Muslims are encouraged to do from childhood. The passages are mainly chosen to provide protection against illness and accident. The use by the Oromo and Somali in Babile of home remedies also shows strong evidence of the influence of Arabic medicine. The practice of using natural products for certain diseases, as described in the Koran, is widespread among Muslims. It includes the preparation of honey drink (Or. *illii*) for internal disorders, the use of water (Or. *bisaan*) for ritual cleansing during medical practices and dissolving plant extracts to make medicinal drinks to be administered to patients. The ritual collection and consumption of spices which derive from Arabic medicine by non-specialists also has its origins in the Islamic pharmacopoeia. Spice gatherers are usually farmers, blacksmiths and potters who make the knowledge they have inherited from their father or mother available to the members of their group, and in some cases they consult Arabic lists of medicinal plants which have been translated into Oromifa and adapted to the local flora (cf. Figure 5.2).

## Practitioners

The practitioners who belong to the regional Arabic medical (sub) system differ from the specialists in the other traditional systems

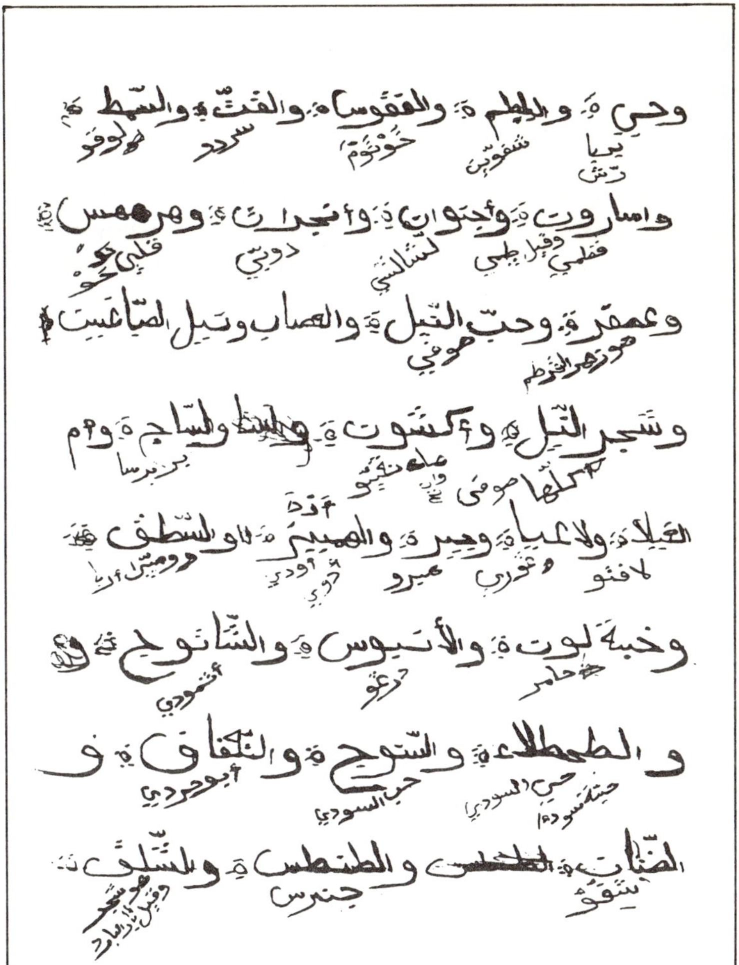

Figure 5.2: *Arabic–Oromifa list of medicinal plants*

mainly as regards their knowledge and utilisation of Arabic medical texts and the teachings of Islam. Most belong to the local elite groups of Koran scholars, lawyers, astrologers and healers who have settled in the towns and the larger communities in Eastern Ethiopia. They are members of the educated class, the bearers of Muslim culture, who have played such an important role in the process of Islamisation. These healers treat various diseases and

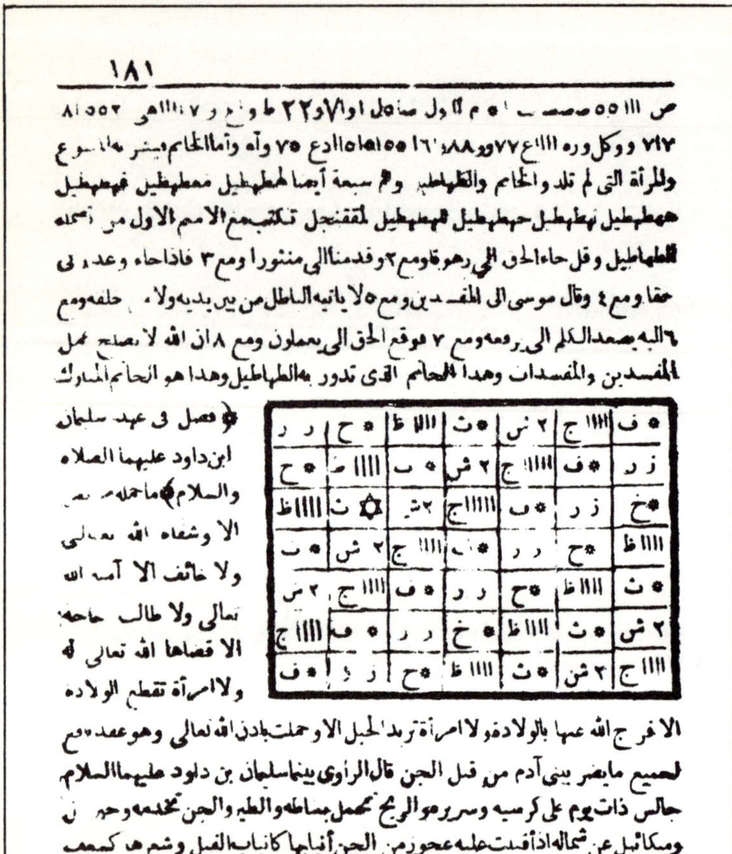


Figure 5.3: *Astrological quadrant from a recent reprint of the medical textbook of Jalāl-ad-Dīn as-Suyūtī (1505)*

although they use both religious and pragmatic techniques, Islam is central in their approach to illness. In the majority of cases they are full-time specialists with high social status in the community and they are paid or rewarded in a discreet fashion for their services. Some famous healers in this category are accredited with sacredness and widely known as local Muslim saints (Or. *awlia*).

In Babile, the following types of practitioners operate within the Arabic regional medical (sub) system:

the *kabira* (Or.) or *kabir* (Har.), the learned Islamic healer;
the *sheikh* (Or.) or *saygha* (Har.), the Islamic medical teacher.

## The kabira or kabir

The most important Islamic healer in the area is known as *kabira* in Oromifa and *kabir* in Harari which literally means 'religious teacher, indigenous doctor who heals by means of amulets'. It comes from the Arabic word *kabīr*. The *kabira* are usually men who have been trained in the theory and practice of Arabic medicine after having been educated at a traditional Koran school. They prefer to treat accidents, internal complaints and mental illnesses and place health and disease entirely within the context of Islam. They interpret the case of illness as a punishment for contravening the Islamic rules laid down by Allah. In specific cases, certain illnesses are attributed to possession by spirits (Or. *jiinii*). The 'evil eye' (Or. *budaa*) which also occurs in the local medical system is explained in most cases as the result of magic rituals by enemies.

The theoretical recognition of rational elements in etiology such as cold, spoiled food, neglect of hygiene, poisoning and accidents reveals the influence on Arabic medicine of the Greek medical tradition of Hippocrates. Pragmatic treatment of the patient based on Greek medicine is often elevated to a form of magico-religious medicine within the religious context of Islam. Although strong rational theories concerning hygiene, diet, infection and anatomy are recognisable in the medical practices in the *kabira*, healing is made dependent on the instructions in the Koran and in Arabic medical texts.

In making their diagnosis, some *kabira* consult a *kitab* which is also known as *kataba* in Oromifa. It is a book in Arabic which explains the origins of diseases, often linking them with the days of

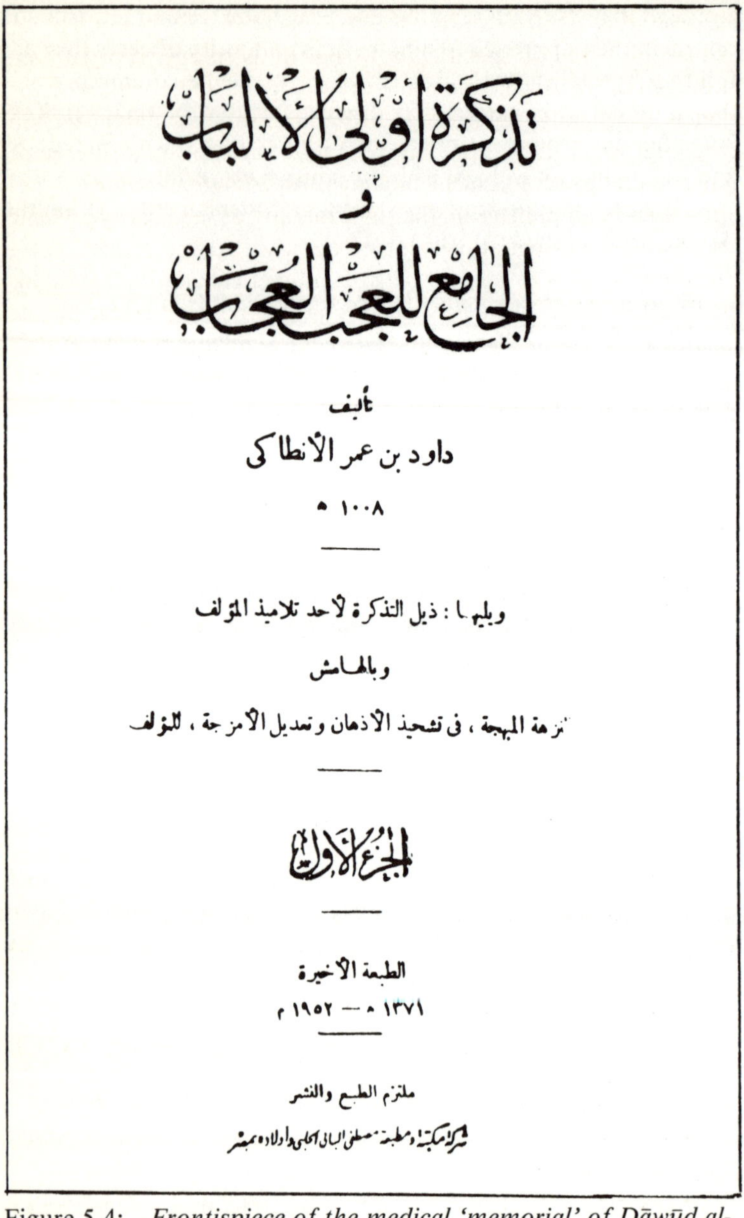

تذكرة أولى الألباب

و

الجامع للعجب العجاب

تأليف

داود بن عمر الأنطاكى

١٠٠٨ هـ

ويليها : ذيل التذكرة لأحد تلاميذ المؤلف

وبالهامش

النزهة المبهجة ، فى تشحيذ الأذهان وتعديل الأمزجة ، للمؤلف

الجزء الأول

الطبعة الأخيرة

١٣٧١ هـ — ١٩٥٢ م

ملتزم الطبع والنشر

شركة مكتبة ومطبعة مصطفى البابى الحلبى وأولاده بمصر

Figure 5.4: *Frontispiece of the medical 'memorial' of Dāwūd al-Anṭākī (1579)*

the week on which a disease first occurs. The technique of divination, based on specific knowledge of astrology, is often used in diagnosis. In Arabic medicine knowledge of the position of the planets is generally regarded as being necessary for diagnosis and prognosis which can ultimately be traced back to the influence of Galen and Hippocrates (cf. Ullmann 1970: 255). Such knowledge is often used in administering the right therapy or medication. Magic also forms an essential element of curative practices: the *kabira* cures certain diseases with the help of a numerical quadrant from his medical textbooks, which is said to have a positive effect on the treatment. (Figure 5.3 shows the astrological quadrant in question.)

The specific tasks of the *kabira* in Babile include reciting Islamic texts or prescribing amulets of written Koranic texts on paper or parchment aimed mainly at preventing illness and accidents. Manipulation with written-out Koranic texts also forms part of his therapy. For example, he may write out the texts in ink, dissolve them in water and then serve the resulting solution as a beneficial drink to his patients. Inhaling the smoke of burning Koranic texts or burning texts behind the house of the patient are other techniques used by the *kabira.* In addition to the water, milk and honey, etc. used for medicinal purposes, extracts of medicinal plants – most of which derive from the Arabic pharmacopoeia – play an important role in his arsenal of medication. The *kabira* often uses recipes from Arabic handbooks. Plant extracts are prepared in large bowls using various finely chopped ingredients. The *kabira* himself usually grows and collects the medicinal plants he uses.

The *corpus medicorum* used by these traditional healers consists of a number of Arabic medical books in addition to the Koran. They are often copies or reprints of sixteenth-century Arabic medical manuscripts which deal with the establishment of medical practices and the composition of medicines. In the research area, a number of practitioners use the 'memorial' of Dāwūd al-Anṭākī (1579) which was reprinted in Cairo at the turn of the century (Figure 5.4). In addition to recipes for medicinal drinks such as a fruit drink with honey (Or. *roba*), a mint drink (Or. *juleb*) and syrups (Or. *sjorbaa*), the book explains magical numerical quadrants and formulae. Figure 5.4 shows the frontispiece. Another medical text book used by several Arabic healers in the area is a reprint of a manuscript of Jalāl-ad-Dīn as-Suyūṭī which deals with well-being and wisdom as aspects of the human condition. It contains primarily prophetic medical texts and instructions (cf. Ullmann 1970: 188).

The medical treatment provided by the *kabira* (Or.) is generally regarded as an act of piety towards Allah which can only increase the skill and fame of the healer. In many cases, however, his services are rewarded by secret payments of *chat,* coffee, millet or tobacco. The size of the remuneration oftens depends on the resources of the patient and the skill and reputation of the *kabira.*

The training of the *kabira* largely consists of long and intensive study of Arabic writings and texts from the Koran. Promising young men are supported by their families or communities to attend a Koran school in the area. Joint financial support for study purposes (Or. *qaarija*) may sometimes be provided for years and is also regarded as an act of piety. As a rule, students return to their villages on completion of their studies to take up positions in the community as men of learning. As noted before, many Koran schools were set up around Harar under a teacher (Ar. *'ulamā*) as a result of the spread of Islam during the second half of the nineteenth century. Traditional Koran schools are still found in rural areas and in several large towns in Hararghe. After attending a Koran school, where they learn Arabic script and recite Koranic texts, a number of students go on to specialise in Arabic sciences (Ar. *'ulūm al-'Arab*). Suitable students then attach themselves to a famous traditional Muslim scholar who has the honorary title of *sheikh* (Or.). The decision to specialise in Arabic medicine based on the hereditary 'power of healing' (Har. *tuftii*), which is reserved for a limited number of families, is usually motivated by divination or divine calling to the office by revelation in visions or dreams. During the training in Arabic medicine, much emphasis is placed on the religious aspect of diagnosis and therapy. In addition, theoretical subjects such as anatomy, diet, pharmacology, sexual hygiene and the healing power of natural products and medicinal plants are dealt with. Phenomena such as 'evil eye' and possession by spirits are also dealt with, as are protection and healing using amulets, numerical quadrants and specific Koran texts.

To conclude their training the *kabira* receive a ritual blessing (Or. *ijarza*) from their master, allowing them to serve as medical practitioners within the community. The *kabira* are hereby formally recognised as having the power of healing (Har. *tuftii*) which is also expressed in the rituals used to treat patients. For example, the *kabira* chew *chat* and then ritually spit it out at patients while

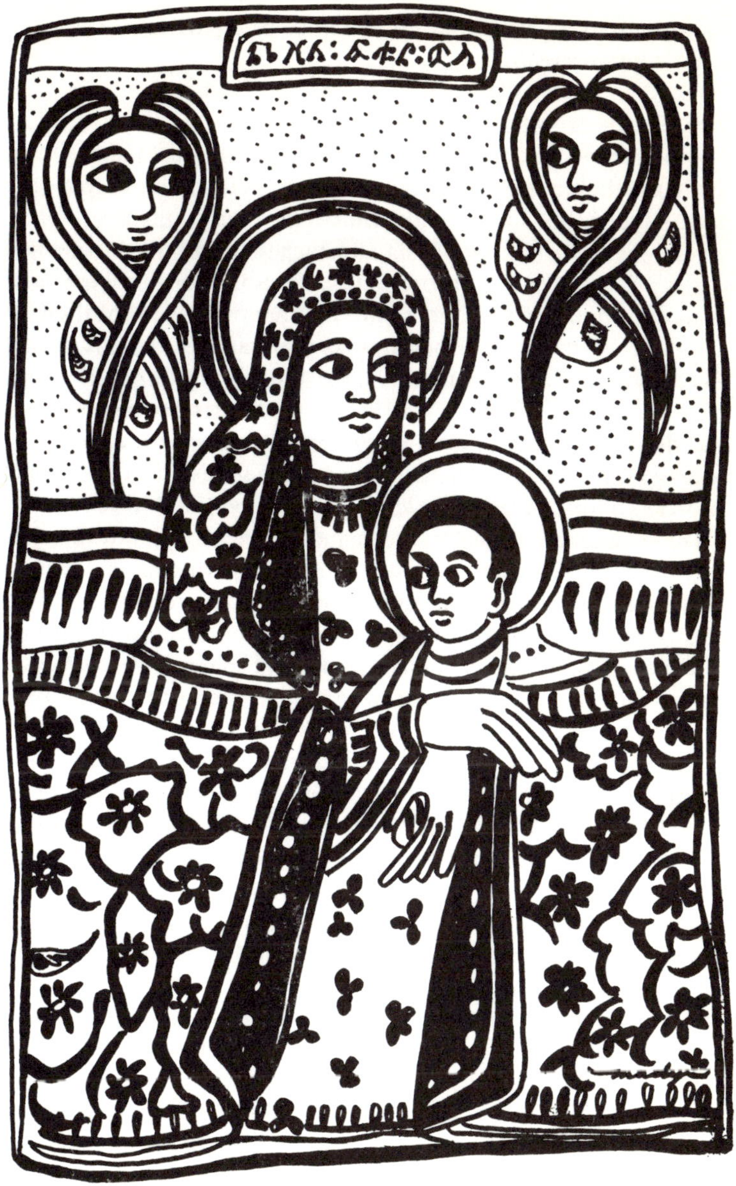

Figure 5.5: *Icon from Tigray depicting the Holy Virgin with Child, often worshipped for the preservation of health and the healing of disease.*

quotations from the Koran are read out or a particular remedy is being administered.

## The sheikh or shaykh

The honorary title of *sheikh* in Oromifa literally means 'local scholar in the traditional sciences' and comes from the Arabic word *šayk̲*. Among the Muslim population of the community it is reserved for the highest category of Islamic teachers in the Arabic medical system. The *sheikh* (Or.) are sometimes famous healers who possess an aura of holiness and, when they die, are revered as local saints. Their graves are visited by pilgrims from a wide area. Tombs of local *sheikh* saints are found around Harar and west of Babile along the main road (see Plate 6). These regional scholars belonging to the traditional elite have the exclusive right to confer the power of healing (Har. *tuftii*) on the *kabira* who conclude their training with the 'sheikh' during a ritual blessing ceremony or *eebba* (Or.).

These rather elitist healers are mainly concerned with the magico-religious aspects of Arabic, prophetic medicine and hand down the knowledge and power of healing to younger generations. Over the ages, the *sheikh* have been the guardians and protectors of medical knowledge contained in sacred books and manuscripts, which is made available by the *kabira* and *sheikh* brotherhoods to the glory of Allah and for the benefit of the Muslim community. They lay down traditions and, most interestingly, record the complete genealogy of teachers and their pupils sometimes as far back as *sheikh* Hippocrates, *sheikh* Pythagoras, *sheikh* Galen and *sheikh* Aristotle (cf. Buschkens and Slikkerveer 1982: 38). Their patients are often members of the rural and urban elite who frequently undertake long journeys to be treated by a famous *sheikh*. Even more so than among the *kabira,* the medical practices of a *sheikh* reveal the dominating influence of religion linked to a knowledge and application of the texts of the Koran. Rational considerations are often submerged under a plethora of applications of the sayings of the Prophet and medical texts by the old Islamic practitioners of 'prophetic medicine'.

To summarise, in the research area, the regional Arabic medical system originally spread from Harar among the communities in the highlands, including Babile. As a result, a more sophisticated form of medicine – particularly concerned with internal and mental illnesses – became available to Islamic patients, usually from the higher social strata. The important place occupied by the magico-religious elements of 'prophetic medicine' within this regional medical system can be explained by the willingness shown by the Oromo and Somali not only to adapt to Islam but also to interpret phenomena of health and healing in the light of their new religion.

### *5.2.3. The regional Amhara medical (sub)system*

After the conquest of Harar in 1887 by Emperor Menelik II, Hararghe was annexed as a Province of the Ethiopian Empire and the process of Amharisation of the region began. With the advent of new rulers, Babile developed from a regional marketplace east of Harar into an important political and military settlement (Am. *katama*) in the border area with Somalia. When Amhara settled in the area with their families, economic life flourished and the local population came into contact with Ethiopian-Christian culture. The influence of this new culture on the Muslim groups in the Eastern Highlands, however, was not deeply rooted and even today there are numerous differences between the two groups. The distance between the Christian Amhara and the Muslim Oromo and Somali has not become any less since then and only a small number of Oromo and Somali has converted to Christianity, or mixed with the Amhara. As a result, components of the regional Amhara medical system have only been adopted to a very small extent by the indigenous inhabitants of Babile and have largely remained the preserve of the Amhara who now form approximately one third of the total population (38%).

The medical knowledge, perceptions and practices which spread in the research area as a result of the expansion of the central Ethiopian Empire constitute the regional Amhara system. This includes the medicine of the Ethiopian-Christian healers whose theories and practices are recorded in numerous medical manuscripts and textbooks. Like Arabic medicine, classical Amhara medicine has been considerably affected by external influences. Written sources include handbooks from Morocco and Egypt and even manuscripts from Jerusalem (cf. Rodenson 1967: 54). The earliest medical texts are in *Ge'ez,* the classical language of the Ethiopian Empire; the more recent handbooks on the other hand date from the eighteenth century and are written in Amharic. Foreign doctors traditionally enjoyed considerable prestige in Ethiopia. One of them, the Greek Giyorgis, who had come to the country as a

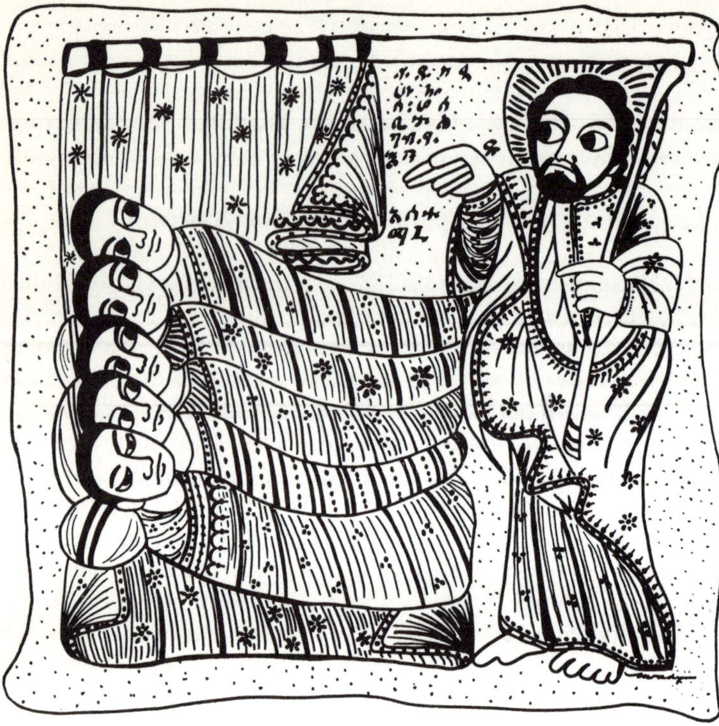

Figure 5.6: *Saint Peter commiserating with the sick (Ethiopian miniature on parchment)*

soldier in about 1865, later became an important healer and magician, fully conversant with Greek and Amhara magic (Rodenson 1967).

As in Arabic medicine, illness and death in Amhara medicine are explained both in terms of personalistic and naturalistic forces. However, the Ethiopian-Christian religious perspective concerning the prevention and treatment of illness dominates magical and rational elements within Amhara medicine. Pankhurst (1968: 40) notes: *'great reliance was placed on application to God, prayers being composed against either illness in general or specific complaints.'* In the traditional literature of Amhara medicine there is often a mixture of magico-religious and empirico-rational views and practices which can be attributed in part to the influence of indigenous medical concepts of folk medicine. For example, a medical text book published by Griaule (1930) which contains instructions on how to treat epilepsy, fever, syphilis, rabies, etc., also contains numerous magical formulae to fend off the 'evil eye' (Am. *budaa*), conquer demons and evil spirits and to resist the dangerous influence for conditions which are not really illnesses at all; for example, a medical manuscript by Gerazmac Gäbräwäld published by Teshai Berhane Selassie (1971) explains not only rational methods of treating illnesses using herbs and potash (in Amharic) but also a number of magic prayers (in *Ge'ez*) against theft, poverty and lack of human love.

In his account of traditional Amhara-Tigray medicine, Messing (1972: 243) observes a: '. . . *syncretisation of mystic and pragmatic beliefs* . . .' expressed in a cosmology aiming at the manipulation of natural products used in therapy without fundamentally changing them. The incorporation of indigenous Semitic traditions within the regional Amhara system can also be seen in the *qole* complex in the Amhara-Tigray culture which has marked similarities with the indigenous Cushitic belief in *qaalluu* (Or.). It consists of a belief that every individual has a personal spirit or *qole* (Am.) which can easily be insulted by neglect or mockery. When this happens, the person concerned becomes extremely susceptible to certain physical and mental complaints (cf. Messing 1972: 244). If the individual indeed falls ill, this must first be demonstrated in the form of symptoms of possession by a spirit, so that his environment will accept him as a patient. Often treatment can only be obtained through the *zar* cult which developed over the years in the centre of Ethiopia, particularly in the town of Gondar. Here many *zar*-doctors have their headquarters and are surrounded by a large number of patients and followers. Later on, several *zar*-doctors settled in various parts of the country as a result of the expansion of the old Abyssinian Kingdom. There are several *zar*-doctors in Hararghe (cf. Young 1982: 21-42).

The success of the treatment provided by the mystical healers from the Amhara system depends largely on the power of their personal spirits which are demons or *zar* spirits. If their 'own' spirit is more powerful than that of the magician who has bewitched the patient, the healer will be capable of driving out the evil spirit and of curing the illness (cf. Young 1975; Reminick 1977).

Amhara medicine also includes a large number of rational practices to prevent or cure illness. During the great epidemics of the past, Bruce (1790) and Wurtz (1898) mentioned patients being isolated and people being forbidden to travel to infected areas. The practice of inoculation was well-known in Ethiopia long before the nineteenth century. The traditional pharmacopoeia contains an extensive number of medicinal plants and intensive use was also made of animal products such as honey, butter and sheep fat to treat smallpox, malaria and a number of other diseases (cf. Pankhurst 1968: 637). Traditional Amhara healers regularly used techniques such as counter-irritation (Am. *matakos*) in order to treat rheumatism and internal diseases, cauterisation (Am. *wagemt*) to treat snake bites, infections, etc. and blood-letting to relieve headaches. For a long time they have used thermal baths and springs to treat fevers, venereal diseases, rheumatism, leprosy and skin diseases. Pragmatic elements within traditional Amhara medicine consist of surgery, the setting of broken limbs and basic dental care.

## Perceptions and practices

The Amhara population in Ethiopia have certain perceptions and practices regarding illness and treatment which can be grouped within the Amhara medical system. Some members of the group regard a number of illnesses and diseases as the punishment of God. These include abscesses, fractures, epilepsy, gonorrhoea, pneumonia and tuberculosis. The Amhara generally try to prevent illnesses of this kind by making pilgrimages such as the mass annual pilgrimage to St Gabriel's Church at Kulubi. Traditional preventive measures in the system include the wearing of Christian amulets (Am. *metab*) and being re-baptised or sprinkled with holy water by a religious healer. The amulets consist of Ethiopian-Christian texts in Ge'ez or Amharic, written on rolled pieces of parchment and worn round the neck on a silk cord. Most of these amulets are dedicated to Jesus, St Sebastian, St Peter or King Solomon. Also, silver Coptic crosses on a necklace are worn as amulets for protection of good health. Icon veneration is another preventive method among Amhara groups. The Amhara pray to the Virgin Mary (*Maryam*) portrayed on ancient icons not only to prevent illness and misfortune but also to cure predominantly personalistic illness (Figure 5.5). Usually in such circumstances they also pray to St Peter as the protector and healer of the sick (Figure 5.6).

Possession by *zar* (Am.) is regarded particularly by Amhara women in Babile as causing increased susceptibility to apathy, paralysis, insomnia and sterility. There are several *zar* societies whose members not only consist of married women but also of the chronically sick or mentally disturbed. *Zar* societies fulfil an important social role: they admit women, who generally feel discriminated against by the traditional refusal to allow them to enter the buildings of the Ethiopian Church and members of other ethnic and religious groups and people from the lower social classes. For example, the *zar* cult in Babile includes several non-Christian Somali and Oromo. The 'evil eye' which, according to several informants, lives in a number of local blacksmiths with evil powers who can turn themselves into hyenas at night, usually manifests itself in epilepsy and hysteria. *Budaa* can also manifest themselves in misfortune, crop failure or serious accidents. Possession by spirits can only be treated by practising *zar*-doctors in the area. As with Arabic medicine, the Amhara strongly believe in the influence of astrology on illness and recovery. A number of Amhara informants were convinced that the positions of the stars (Am.*hebra kokab*) determine the time of recovery and the nature of the correct medicine. Under these circumstances, patients prefer to consult the traditional Amhara astrologer-healer described in the following section.

As far as the transmission of infectious diseases is concerned, a large number of Amhara adheres to the indigenous concept of infection (Am. *talalafi basheta*) where personal contact with patients suffering from these illnesses is usually avoided. This corresponds to a large extent with the Cushitic idea of *hogamishii* (Or.) and ties in with the belief that the best protection against leprosy is to drive lepers away from the family or the community. The important role played within the regional Amhara system by natural products such as plant extracts and animal products can be seen in the use of home remedies against, for instance, internal illnesses, children's diseases, headaches, gastritis and skin diseases. They are usually administered by Amhara women within the family or the kinship group. They always involve empirical considerations relating to the rational elements of Amhara medical tradition and are often successful in treating less serious complaints.

## Practitioners

The medical specialists who operate in Babile as part of the traditional Amhara system have extensive knowledge of Amhara medical texts and Ethiopian-Christian doctrine which they translate into practice. Like the educated Islamic healers they belong to the local elite and practise mainly in the towns and the large rural communities in the Eastern Highlands in which the Amhara and Tigray settled in the course of the present century. They are usually full-time specialists who enjoy considerable prestige as members of the brotherhoods of educated Amhara and are sometimes also heads of large communities. An excellent account of the structural relationships between and among practitioners and their clients in terms of medical knowledge and practices of the Amhara medical system has been presented by Young (1982). The following types of practitioner operate in Babile as part of the Amhara regional medical (sub) system:

the *dabtara* (Am.), the learned Christian healer;
the *meshaf-gelach* (Am.), the Christian astrologer;
the *zar*-doctor (Am.), the mystical spirit exorcist;
the *woggesha* (Am.), and *medehani tenija* (Am.), the pragmatic healers;
the *tanqway* (Am.), the soothsayer-magician.

## The dabtara

*Dabtara* (Am.), literally means a non-ordained clergyman who is well versed in the rituals, literature and the Holy Scripture of the Ethiopian Church and refers to the religious healers within Ethiopian Christianity. Sometimes referred to as lay priests, they treat both somatic and mental illnesses, mainly by prescribing amulets, arranging sacrificial offerings and advising patients to make pilgrimages. Amulets (Am. *ketab*) containing religious texts in Amharic are prescribed for both preventive and curative purposes. In some cases, the method of treatment used by the *dabtara* includes dissolving ink-written formulae in water and then administering the resulting solution as a medicinal drink to patients, thereby establishing a link between the spirit of the formula and the body of the patient. In certain cases, the *dabtara* will also advise praying to a saint portrayed on an icon. The sacrifices to combat, for example, venereal diseases and internal disorders consist of the ritual slaughter of a black sheep or black goat, whereupon the flesh of the animal is eaten by the patient and his close relatives. Sometimes pilgrimages are made to holy places and springs on the recommendation of the *dabtara*.

There are also rational elements in the usually religious treatment methods of the *dabtara* such as inoculation, counter irritation, the prescription of medicinal plants and administering of charcoal. Treatment with *koso* (Am.) a traditional medicine made from the crushed dried flowers of a local shrub dissolved in water, is a tried and tested remedy against tape-worm but, in view of its side-effects, far from safe (cf. Pearce 1972: 41, 42). Holy water is also used as a medicine either in drink or to baptise or re-baptise patients.

The medical-religious services to the community are carried out for 'the glory of God'. Payment by patients often depends on the nature of the treatment and the patient's own financial resources. The education and training of *dabtara* includes the formal mastery of Amharic script and Ethiopian literature, including a thorough knowledge of the Bible. Together with the Ethiopian Christian priest (Am. *qes*) and the Islamic *sheikh*, the *dabtara* belong to the local elite and therefore enjoy considerable prestige within the community.

## The meshaf-gelach

The Amhara astrologer, whose main role as a practitioner of the Ethiopian Church is to establish a prognosis for his patients, is called the *meshaf-gelach* (Am.) – literally meaning 'opener of the book'. Using astrological formulae and numerical quadrants from books written in *Ge'ez* he compares the mathematical constellation of the name of the patient with his stars in order to determine the correct remedy in the form of amulets, medicines or pilgrimages. Plate 3 shows two pages of a medical handbook of a *meshaf-gelach*. Like the *dabtara*, the traditional astrologer-healer is usually a member of the religious elite as a scribe of the Ethiopian Christian Church.

## The zar-doctor

The *zar* cult (Am.) is represented in the research area by several communities, each under the leadership of a *zar*-doctor who, in Hararghe, is often addressed by his followers as *sheikh*. He is a mystical healer who is assumed to possess a powerful spirit (Am. *zar*) which can manipulate spirits entering the bodies of patients and even exorcise them. The complaints of patients presented to *zar*-doctors vary considerably and include epilepsy, hysteria, apathy, paralysis, rheumatism, sterility and miscarriages. Patients of the *zar*-doctors also include individuals whose health has suffered as a result of social problems such as unemployment, loneliness, an unhappy marriage or poverty. In general they are usually Amhara, but they also include some Oromo and Somali.

During long nocturnal sessions, *zar*-doctors and their patients go into a trance and spirits are driven out by repeating oaths and in certain cases by expelling demons with the help of the *sheikh*. Gifts from patients in the form of notes, coins, bundles of *chat*, coffee, millet and tobacco are collected in advance in the name of God and later divided among the members of the *zar* cult for joint consumption. The treatment provided by the *zar*-doctors usually takes place in an esoteric atmosphere of prayer and song with abundant use of incense, *chat* and eau de cologne. The *zar*-doctors surround themselves with assistants and dress in expensive garments, decorated with mystical symbols such as crescent moons, stars and hearts.

Several Amhara informants in Babile said they regularly attended the meetings of the famous *zar*-doctor *Sheikh* Taye who had a special building constructed outside the nearby town of Dire Dawa for such sessions. Buschkens and Slikkerveer (1982: 39) give an account of such a nocturnal meeting held by this *sheikh* who originally came from an important *zar* cult centre near the town of Gondar in central Ethiopia.

Although the *zar*-doctors, who are often well-to-do, do not have any official ties with the Ethiopian Church, they are highly regarded by their religious colleagues and by the largely Amhara groups. Like the *dabtara* and the *meshaf-gelach* they belong to the local elite and may reckon many high-ranking Amhara officials among their clients.

### The woggesha and medehani tenija

These pragmatic healers, usually illiterate, whose titles in Amharic literally refer to 'reliever of pain' are traditional osteopaths in the regional Amhara system. In many ways, the *woggesha* (Am.) resembles his Cushitic counterpart, the *ogeessa* (Or.). He uses a number of simple surgical instruments including a razor, scissors and a cow's horn (Am. *wagamt*) to treat fractures, wounds, muscular complaints, boils and abscesses, but he also has a deep knowledge of traditional medicines made from extracts of medicinal plants, roots, fruits, vegetable oils and fats. In a number of reported cases in Babile, the *woggesha* also provided specialist help with the circumcision of Amhara boys and with complicated births.

Like the *ogeessa*, the *woggesha* in Babile have close links with their counterparts in other traditional medical sub-systems in the area. In some cases, there is even a form of referral system between these pragmatic healers.

Some Amhara herbalists who also use pharmaceutical medicines of local and regional origin and who specialise in a number of naturalistic illnesses are known as *medehani tenija* (Am.). They often have their own premises which include a simple pharmacy and examination room. The *medehani tenija* have wide medical knowledge and sometimes consult a number of illustrated traditional medical handbooks in Amharic (See Plate 2).

### The tanqway

The *tanqway* (Am.) is a mystical healer consulted by members of the community chiefly to establish the cause of predominantly personalistic illnesses and to provide patients with appropriate remedies. The *tanqway* have similarities with the Cushtic *qaalluu* and in a wider context belong to the category of African 'medicine men' (Messing 1972). Their main methods of treatment consist of smoking out or exorcising evil spirits (Am. *buda*) from patients with serious symptoms including epilepsy, paralysis, leprosy, tuberculosis and venereal diseases. Their help is also sought in cases of crop failure, theft, accident and apathy. Strikingly, the other types of healer in Babile from the various medical systems generally avoid contact with the *tanqway*. The more educated healers are likely to regard him as a quack and often advise patients not to use his services.

To summarise, it is evident that within the complex traditional medical system in the research area, the historical processes of transculturation at local and regional levels are clearly recognisable in the development of the various local and regional (sub) systems. The etiology, perceptions and practices among the population groups and the different forms of treatment practised by traditional healers can broadly be divided into two types of disease and methods of treatment: personalistic and naturalistic. Although patients seem to make a clear choice for treatment of the majority of illnesses and disorders, in a number of cases there is overlapping and mutual referral among several sub-systems for one illness episode. This is not only observed in the choice of a pragmatic or a mystical healer, but is also reflected in the methods of therapy: 'empirical' medicines are often administered in a magical way or vice versa. Interdigitation, as it is called, is not restricted to the medical system of one ethnic group, but occurs among the Amhara, the Oromo and the Somali. Among Christian and Muslim population groups it represents the expression of a cosmology in which natural components are closely tied up with an all-embracing and predominantly religious system, within which framework the correct diagnosis and treatment are determined and carried out by competent practitioners.

## 5.3 The Modern Medical System

The first contact between Ethiopian Empire and western medicine occurred in the early sixteenth century. Later on, in the course of the nineteenth century, western medicine became increasingly influential as a result of contacts with European travellers, missionaries and doctors. However, it was not until the end of the nineteenth century that the inhabitants of Hararghe came into regular contact with cosmopolitan medicine (cf. Pankhurst 1965). Before describing the elements of the present modern medical system in Babile, the following section presents a brief review of the introduction and development of modern medicine in the research area with a reference to an earlier description in detail by Buschkens and Slikkerveer (1982: 44 – 52). In addition, post-revolutionary developments in health care introduced by central government since 1974 will be briefly described.

Modern medicine was introduced into the area both by the state and private individuals such as Egyptians, Amhara and Italians. During the occupation of the Emirate of Harar by the Egyptians (1875 – 1885), the town underwent a series of reforms relating to trade, administration, the army, education and health care. The inhabitants of Harar and the surrounding areas were introduced to an early form of western medicine largely through army doctors in occupied areas. A number of important sanitary provisions were made and several diseases, including smallpox, were successfully combatted. Ali Pasha, the Egyptian Governor of Harar, was a fervent advocate of western medicine and therefore attempted to eliminate all forms of traditional medicine. When a smallpox epidemic broke out in 1882, he had most medical books and pharmacies of traditional healers destroyed and burnt. He also attempted to reduce by force the excessive use of *chat* by the local population (Paulitschke 1888: 235). Because of the hostile relations between the Egyptian forces occupying Harar and the Oromo and Somali in surrounding areas, however, few elements of western medicine managed to penetrate to the periphery during this period. After the Egyptian withdrawal and the conquest of Harar by the armies of Emperor Menelik II in 1885, a new era dawned and the Amhara spread modern medicine in Hararghe which they had partly taken over at an earlier date. Emperor Menelik II was very interested in technical innovations and was fascinated by modern medicine. He invited an Italian-medical mission to visit the Empire and one of its members, Dr. Nerazzini, stayed permanently in Harar. At the end of the Italian-Ethiopian War of 1895 – 1896, the Italian government sent a medical mission under Dr. De Martini to nurse the Italian war wounded and in the process some medical care was provided for non-Italians. Pankhurst (1968: 644) notes on the mission: '*It established itself in Harar, where it also attended to members of the public, 3,432 people being treated between January and May 1897.*' Several medical missions followed from Italy, Russia, France and England and increasingly they geared their services to the needs of the local population. Modern hospitals were built in Harar and Dire Dawa and with the support of Ras Makonnen, the Governor of Harar, a Capuchin missionary, Jorasseau, established a leper hospital in Harar. This was soon followed by the construction of the Ras Makonnen Hospital which later came under French control with a view to the French colony of Djibouti. The hospital also provided medical care for the local population (Pankhurst 1978: 650). The Tafari Makonnen government hospital was later built in Harar and this was followed by a Swedish pharmacy in Dire Dawa and a French hospital for officials and workmen involved in the construction of the railway from Addis Ababa to Djibouti.

In 1907, the basis of modern government on western lines was established in Ethiopia and health care became the responsibility of the Public Health Department of the Ministry of Home Affairs. A number of public health measures and vaccination programmes were undertaken but health care was still largely restricted to the capital, Addis Ababa, and several larger towns in the provinces. The Ethiopian Red Cross was founded in 1935.

The process of health care development was interrupted by the Italian-Ethiopian war (1935 – 1941). During the Italian occupation, approximately 200 medical doctors were added to the occupation army and provided health care largely for Italian soldiers, colonists and road builders, but they also treated some Ethiopians (Perham 1948: 240 – 421). Mass prevention programmes to combat infectious diseases and public health information campaigns were launched. During this period, as part of preventive health care measures, the Italians set up the first systematic programme of modern health care in rural areas which included 44 clinics and pharmacies in Hararghe. Despite the rapid development of health care, the rural population made relatively little use of the modern institutions and health in Ethiopia barely improved as a result. After the liberation by Allied troops in 1941, a number of Italian doctors stayed on in Ethiopia and continued to practise medicine. The education and training of health care staff was initiated under an English director of medical services and the existing medical institutions were expanded.

At the same time, action was taken from outside Ethiopia by several international organisations and by WHO and the UNRRA. In 1947, the Public Health Proclamation established the legal basis for a modern programme of health care in Ethiopia and the Ministry of Public Health was founded in 1948. Schools to educate and train nursing staff were opened at the hospitals, and in 1954, the opening of the School of Public Health in Gondar heralded an important stage in the history of the development of modern health care. Community health officers, community nurses and sanitarians received their training at the School of Public Health and later went to practise in the health centres in the provinces. Since this time, a network of first-aid posts, health centres and hospitals has developed throughout Ethiopia. In 1964, a Medical School for training doctors and pharmacists was founded at the Emperor Haile Selassie I University in Addis Ababa.

In 1975, a year after the Ethiopian revolution, more than 4 million peasant households were rallied as part of the Development Through Cooperation Campaign (Am. *Zemecha*) in some 18,000 peasant associations and, in the 1977 – 1978 period, the number increased to include 8 million households in 28,583 associations. Under the influence of the international political reorientation of the Provisional Military Administrative Council (PMAC), and internal social, economic and political changes, central government then initated a number of experiments with centrally oriented modern medical services. On the basis of promising results achieved by Ethiopia's new allies, the Soviet Union and Cuba, a model of national health care delivery was chosen, affirming health care as a fundamental human right accessible to everyone under the protection of the state. Under the motto *Ye-Itiopia Hebretesebawinet* ('Ethiopian Socialism', referring to self-confidence, the dignity of labour and victory of common property) the PMAC proclaimed the same year the radical Land Reform Act. Education and health, together with arable farming, livestock farming, communications and infrastructure then became the basic principles of a new ideology of socio-economic growth. The implementation of this new approach, which emphasised large-scale introduction of modern medicine, was later incorporated within the *zemecha*. It encompassed major projects on basic health education, preventive care and environmental sanitation, focussed on the prevention of common communicable and infectious diseases in rural areas, where the general lack of adequate hygiene and frequent malnutrition among children aggravate general health problems (cf. Slikkerveer 1982: 1864). In this way about one million people were provided with health care information and 296 clinics were built, more than one half of the total in Ethiopia; via the *zemecha* more than 1550 midwives were trained, the number of nursing staff increased by 150% and 1¼ million inhabitants of rural areas were vaccinated against infectious diseases such as typhoid, whooping cough, yellow fever, rabies and cholera (cf. Milkias 1980).

However, despite the success of the campaign in increasing the political consciousness of the population, reducing illiteracy and setting up a medical aid programme, the results in relation to improving health care, particularly in rural areas, have been disappointing. Although modest improvements in national expenditure on health care occurred from roughly 5% of the total national budget per year in the period 1970 – 1975 to roughly 5.5% and 6.6% in the period 1976 – 1978, a simultaneous decrease in capital investment in the health care infrastructure almost nullified long-range improvement. After the revolution, the central government

Table 5.1: *Hospitals, health centres and health stations, operating in the disticts of Gursum and Harar Zuriya in 1976, and the number of outpatient visits**

| *district* | *location* | *hospitals* | *outpatient visits* | *health centres* | *outpatient visits* | *first-aid posts* | *outpatient visits* |
|---|---|---|---|---|---|---|---|
| Gursum | Babile | — | — | — | — | 1 | 800 |
| | Gursum | — | — | 1 | 4027 | — | — |
| Harar | Alemaya | — | — | — | — | 1 | 1111 |
| | Aneno | — | — | — | — | 1 | 555 |
| | Bati | — | — | — | — | 1 | 1300 |
| | Bisidimo | 1 | 23.049 | — | — | — | — |
| | Ejersa Goro | — | — | 1 | 9417 | — | — |
| | Fadis | — | — | — | — | 1 | 1500 |
| | Harar | 3 | 11.848<br>27.037<br>16.147 | — | — | — | — |
| | Kersa | — | — | — | — | 1 | 3104 |
| | Kombolcha | — | — | — | — | 1 | 5205 |

*Not including the army hospital at Harar
(cf. *Comprehensive Health Service Directory*, 1977; Buschkens and Slikkerveer 1982)

had decentralised administration of health services to local levels and regional offices of the Ministry of Health initiated assistance to the peasant associations in constructing outlying health centres and health stations, which provided basic outpatient services to the rural population. By 1980, Cuba had sent some 300 Cuban medical technicians (including 100 doctors) to assist local efforts to alleviate Ethiopia's most urgent medical needs in the periphery (Nelson and Kaplan 1981). Since the initial steps towards the recently adopted approach were taken during the still on-going revolutionary process at the time of the research, it cannot yet be demonstrated that fundamental improvement in rural health care has so far solely failed because of a rigid reorientation in the field of medical practice and belief, still disregarding the familiar socio-cultural context of health and disease, and the related enormous manpower resources of traditional and transitional health workers and specialists. Even so, there was a modest improvement in the delivery of modern health care in the post-revolutionary period in Hararghe.

Table 5.1 shows the operational formal health care institutions in the 1976 – 1977 period in the districts of Gursum and Harar Zurya, used by the local population of Babile. It also indicates the number of outpatient visits to each institution in so far as these are available from official statistics.

The hospitals in Hararghe are found chiefly in the large towns. There are two in Dire Dawa, and six in Harar as well as those in the rural towns of Asbe Teferi, Deder and Bisidimo. There were 768 hospital beds in 1976, which means a ratio of 1:2600 inhabitants which is appreciably less than the official standard of 1:250 inhabitants used by the government. Moreover, 96% of all beds are in the two large towns in the administrative region, Harar and Dire Dawa. In 1976, the hospitals in Hararghe had a total of 24 doctors, 2 health officers, and 1 pharmacist (cf. *Comprehensive Health Service Directory* 1976).

Primary health care in the rural areas of Hararghe is currently still being developed, but the 7 health centres and 29 health stations which were operational in 1977 were far from capable of supplying the population with basic health care. Schaller and Kuls (1972: 95) observe that the Ministry of Health has devised a plan for the future which envisages a ratio of one health centre per 50,000 inhabitants and one health station per 5,000 inhabitants. These ratios, however, had not yet been achieved at the time of the research. Buschkens and Slikkerveer (1982: 52) report that the ratios for health centres and health stations in the Highlands of Hararghe are 1: 237.500 and 1: 63.517 respectively which represents 25% of the government's objective. Usually these health centres are headed by a health officer, but because of the desperate shortage of health care personnel in Ethiopia, medical assistants received their qualification after taking a one-year course organised in Hararghe through the government hospital at Dire Dawa. Candidates are admitted after completing eight years of primary education. Junior health assistants can qualify as health assistants after two years' additional practical experience and an additional one-year course.

A number of special health care programmes are being carried out in Hararghe in addition to the establishment and expansion of a network of curative health care facilities based on the principle of the referral system. These include the Malaria Eradication Service, the Smallpox Eradication Project and the Tuberculosis and Leprosy Control Programs (cf. *Health Services in Socialist Ethiopia* 1978). In Bisidimo, a village to the southwest of Babile, a leprosarium called *Ganda Koree* has been established to which a hospital is attached which treats lepers. The centre has been set up by the German Leprosy Relief Association.

Patients in the research area who use the modern medical system usually begin by consulting the health station in Babile which is manned by a junior health assistant. They then consult the health centre in Gursum some 20 km north of the community run by a health assistant. In serious cases, they visit the hospital at Harar which is 45 km away. Only very few, well-to-do, patients are able to attend one of the national hospitals in the capital Addis Ababa at the centre of the Ethiopian referral system.

The perceptions and practices associated with the modern medical system are not well known or accepted by the population of Babile. Only a few informants were familiar with the major principles of western medicine such as bacteriology, antibiotics, the etiology of infectious diseases and viral infections. A number of informants from the predominantly Amhara group were capable of associating the concept of infection (Am. *baguru yamer*) and infectiousness (Am. *talalafi*), which are well-known in Amhara medicine, with modern practices of vaccination, injection (Am. *marfe*) and the use of antiobiotics. In practice, patients tend to resort to these methods of treatment if they are suffering from serious forms of tonsilitis, high fevers and attacks of malaria. There is considerable interest among patients affected by these illnesses in having injections in one of the modern medical institutions in the region. Aspirin is also a generally accepted medicine against headaches, back ache, insomnia and rheumatic complaints.

## 5.4 The Transitional Medical System

There is a third medical system operational in the Eastern Highlands in addition to the traditional and the modern systems. It is a form of commercial, pharmaceutical medicine which has been chosen to conceptualise as the transitional medical system (Slikkerveer 1982; Buschkens and Slikkerveer 1982). This a-typical Ethiopian system can be considered as an intermediate system partly parallel to the traditional and to the modern medical system. It comprises a form of commercial pharmaceutical medicine which has been similarly observed in Asia, Western Europe and the United

States. It is characterised by utilisation on a large scale of commercial products and the sale of domestic and western pharmaceuticals. Taylor (1977: 288) describes a corresponding type of system in the Punjab as: . . . *an underground system of health care that provides the bulk of medical treatment for the people in India.*

He goes on to observe that: *The greatest hazard is the tendency of such pseudo-indigenous practitioners to use the most powerful drugs possible in order to achieve quick results.*

This type of health care has its origin in Europe where different drugs were manufactured as commercial products known as *galenicals*, for the first time in the seventeenth and eighteenth centuries (cf. Leslie 1977: 271). During the nineteenth century, patent medicines spread throughout the world as a result of the activities of businessmen whom Young (1961) has described as 'toadstool millionaires'.

Strictly speaking, the 'specialists' in the transitional system and the practices they use do not belong either to the traditional system or to the modern system. They are often laymen with scant knowledge either of traditional or cosmopolitan medicine who sell pills, capsules, medicinal drinks and injections in shops or as they travel to markets throughout the country. Their practices are often illegal and contravene regulations concerning making up and dispensing prescriptions, but as in many developing countries where facilities are scarce, it is virtually impossible to prohibit these being sold (cf. Buschkens 1979). Important considerations here are the economic and financial interests of the major pharmaceutical industries and the position of intermediaries, together with the absence of any government controls. In addition to the negative effect of the high price of these drugs – which are often adulterated – there is a serious risk that certain strains of bacteria will become resistant if antibiotics and similar drugs are incorrectly used on a uncontrolled scale.

The transitional medical system came to Ethiopia at the beginning of this century. Pankhurst (1968: 136 – 137) describes how this happened as follows: *The penetration of modern medicine prior to World War I was effected not only by doctors and hospitals but also by foreign merchants in the ordinary course of trade. The establishment of Addis Ababa around 1887 – 1991 was followed by the advent of a number of European, Indian and other shops, almost all of which tended to deal in medicines.*

With the establishment of a number of official pharmacies in Addis Ababa and in the large provincial towns, the commercial system of modern medicines – which had largely been in the hands of uneducated Indian and Armenian merchants – declined somewhat. Subsequently, however, it spread throughout the country as a clandestine system. In addition to the official pharmacies, druggists and shopkeepers in rural areas, there are today illegal medicine sellers, quacks, and dealers in traditional medicines with a minimum of pharmacological training, who sell their wares on street corners and at local markets. Kloos (1974: 84) comments as follows on the way these merchants operate in Addis Ababa: *'The illegal drug vendors have a large market among a population that for the most part was born in the provinces and that adheres by varying degrees to traditional disease concepts and methods of healing.'* They include the popular 'injectors' or 'needlemen', who travel from village to village, mainly in rural areas, supplying injections of antibiotics – often diluted in water – to anyone and everyone at a high price (cf. Asfau Desta 1971). The rural population generally perceive these informal functionaries as private, indigenous healers, experienced in the application of certain modern medicines for the cure of specific disease-categories such as malaria, venereal diseases, pneumonia, gastritis and intestinal complaints. Messing (1972) observes: *In addition to preceding traditional attitudes and practices relating to health there is usually also what might be called an 'intermediate level' of infiltration into the rural hinterland by self-styled, unqualified 'dressers' who have equipped themselves with hypodermic needles hopefully filled with some healing liquid.*

In Hararghe, there are four 'official' druggists' shops authorised to sell pharmaceutical preparations, cosmetics, etc., to the general public which do not dispense medical products or distribute medicines containing narcotics. There are also 83 drug vendor shops in the province whose activities are restricted to selling a limited number of medicines and cosmetics manufactured in a standard way. The commercialisation of medicines in Ethiopia is characterised by the excessive use of chemotherapy by laymen and quacks. There are no official figures on the numbers of illegal drug vendors, 'injectors' and 'needlemen' and it is difficult to make an estimate since they are constantly on the move and always work in secret.

The views of the population of Babile concerning the practitioners in this system suggest that the patients generally have confidence in several of their medicines to treat specific diseases such as worms, fevers, skin diseases, eye and ear infections, venereal diseases and headaches. Many of the population turn to the drug vendors if they are suffering from these types of illness, since these dealers use traditional concepts and methods, sometimes in combination with 'clinical' techniques such as injections, examining patients and prescribing medication. During the study, it was extremely difficult to gain access to the practitioners in the transitional system in view of their secret and often illegal practices. However, it was evident that drug vendors obtain the ingredients for their products and medicaments from dealers in the larger towns and then sell them on street corners and at markets, occasionally to traditional healers. In Babile, several 'specialists' operating in this way included a former nurse at the Harar military hospital, a dresser from Addis Ababa who had not finished his medical training and several former soldiers from central Ethiopia. Two drug vendors had originally settled in the area as traditional healers but had decided to concentrate on selling drugs, mainly for business reasons in view of the remarkable results with industrial pharmaceutical products.

Despite the often reprehensible manipulation of traditional and cosmopolitan medical principles and practices, concrete data have supported the idea that practitioners of the transitional medical system have assumed a significant role in health care delivery in rural Ethiopia, where traditional medicine falls short and cosmopolitan therapy is still less accessible to the majority of the population.

In conclusion, the previous sections have established that the complex and plural character of Ethiopian society, in which various ethnic groups with different languages, religions and economic activities coexist, is reflected in the different perceptions and practices of these groups concerning the cause of disease and illness, diagnosis, way of treatment and the type of healer and health care personnel. The social, cultural and historical aspects of illness and health within the medical traditions of these groups present so varied a picture that a pluralistic model is necessary to study and understand the configuration of the medical systems and subsystems in this part of Africa. The following chapters deal with the health care seeking and utilisation patterns of the members of the community and examine the extent to which the response of the population to the plural system has a multiple character, expressed as a plurality of utilisation of the three medical systems.

# 6

# Patterns of Health Care Utilisation

## 6.1 The Process of Illness Behaviour

This chapter examines the process of seeking and obtaining health care by respondents in the survey in the event of illness. Focussing on management of illness episodes including all actions from the moment of symptom perception until complete recovery or death, the chapter describes the range of efforts taken by the highland population when they believe themselves to be ill.[1] This includes self-care and the use of home remedies, consultation within the household group, visits to local and regional healers and treatment in health stations, health centres and hospitals. In accordance with the analytical model described in Chapter 2, it considers utilisation of different medical systems in the highlands as a dependent variable. In view of the transcultural nature of health care in Babile and the complex plural character of the medical system as a whole, utilisation of various medical systems is analysed in order to identify the factors which act as significant determinants in promoting or inhibiting the utilisation process. As the present study is mainly concerned with utilisation of health care and the determinants which affect this process at various levels, the analysis does not include an assessment of the quality and range of health care services provided.

Although self-care is also included in the analysis, the focus is on external action which leads to utilisation of the plural medical system.

After outlining the choices made by respondents in relation to the types of medical treatment available, including the choice not to seek treatment, the chapter goes on to describe the types of action taken in order to achieve recovery. After a description of the overall patterns of health care utilisation of the plural system, the chapter concludes with an assessment of phenomena such as differential-, multiple- and under-utilisation of services.

### *6.1.1 Reported illness and illness behaviour*

This section contains a detailed account of the illness behaviour of respondents as reported in the twelve months preceding the health interview survey. 'Illness behaviour', as explained in Chapter 2, refers to any activity undertaken by a person who feels ill to define his illness and to discover a suitable remedy (Kasl and Cobb, 1966). To obtain a better understanding of the complex nature of the illness behaviour of respondents as reported in the household survey and to facilitate further analysis, the following elements in the process will be examined more closely:

1. *Patients:*
   Respondents in the survey who reported themselves ill in the preceding twelve months as opposed to those who had not been ill.
2. *Perceived morbidity:*
   The illnesses which respondents who had been ill during the previous twelve months believed they had been suffering from, together with the duration of such illnesses.
3. *Alternative sources of health care:*
   Which of the three medical systems in the area people as a consequence had consulted for treatment. Three main categories of patients are used.
4. *Illness steps taken by patients:*
   The number of times the above patients visited one or more institutions in order to discover a remedy for their reported illness.

These elements in the complex health care seeking process will now be examined in more detail.

Table 6.1: *Reported illness episodes of respondents over the preceding twelve months, according to sex*

| illness reporting | sex | | | | total | |
|---|---|---|---|---|---|---|
| | male | | female | | | |
| | N | % | N | % | N | % |
| number of reported illness episodes | 243 | 36.2 | 258 | 37.9 | 501 | 37.1 |
| no reported cases of illness episodes | 428 | 63.8 | 422 | 62.1 | 850 | 62.9 |
| Total | 671 | 100.0 | 680 | 100.0 | 1351 | 100.0 |

## Patients

Of the total sample population of 1351 persons in the survey, 501 (37.1%) reported themselves ill in the preceding twelve months as opposed to 850 (62.9%) who said they had not been ill to any extent.

Table 6.1 shows the reported occurrence of illness episodes among respondents in the twelve preceding months according to sex. There is little difference between the sexes as regards the reported incidence of illness (36.8% and 37.9%). Table 6.2 shows that within the sample, the incidence of reported illness rises with age from 35.4% among children via 36.8% among middle-aged people to 49.0% among the elderly. The fact that the majority of the population of Babile tend to regard diseases such as chicken pox, whooping cough and measles – often referred to as 'children's diseases' – as an inescapable part of childhood rather than as illness probably accounts for the relatively small number of cases of illness reported for children. Of course, the illness of an adult has a much greater effect on the economic life of the family and is therefore more likely to be remembered and reported.

Of the reported cases of illness within the context of the main ethnic groups, it is evident that the largest number of patients come from the Oromo (45%), followed by Somali (36.4%), with the Amhara forming the smallest group (26.8%). Comparison of the figures in Table 6.3 with the socio-economic status of households in the survey according to ethnic group (Table 4.12), shows that 38.1% of the Oromo patients belong to the poorest socio-economic class whereas only 13.8% of the Amhara patients came from this category.

Table 6.2: *Reported illness episodes of respondents over the preceding twelve months according to age*

| illness reporting | 0–15 | | 16–25 | | 26–45 | | 46–45 | | 66+ | | Total | |
|---|---|---|---|---|---|---|---|---|---|---|---|---|
| | N | % | N | % | N | % | N | % | N | % | N | % |
| number of reported illness episodes | 240 | 35.4 | 53 | 35.8 | 152 | 36.8 | 50 | 49.0 | 6 | – | 501 | 37.1 |
| no reported illness episodes | 438 | 64.6 | 95 | 64.2 | 261 | 63.2 | 52 | 51.0 | 4 | – | 850 | 62.9 |
| Total | 678 | 100.0 | 148 | 100.0 | 413 | 100.0 | 102 | 100.0 | 10 | – | 1351 | 100.0 |

Table 6.3: *Reported illness episodes of respondents over the preceding twelve months according to ethnic group*

| illness reporting | ethnic groups | | | | | | | | Total | |
|---|---|---|---|---|---|---|---|---|---|---|
| | Oromo | | Amhara | | Somali | | Other | | | |
| | N | % | N | % | N | % | N | % | N | % |
| number of reported illness episodes | 322 | 45.0 | 139 | 26.8 | 32 | 36.4 | 8 | 28.6 | 501 | 37.1 |
| no reported illness episodes | 493 | 55.0 | 381 | 73.2 | 56 | 63.6 | 20 | 71.4 | 850 | 62.9 |
| Total | 715 | 100.0 | 520 | 100.0 | 88 | 100.0 | 28 | 100.0 | 1351 | 100.0 |

Table 6.4: *Categories of the most frequent cases of illness reported by respondents over the preceding twelve months*

| *categories of frequently reported illnesses* | N | % |
|---|---|---|
| infectious and parasitic diseases | 156 | 31.1 |
| respiratory diseases | 57 | 11.4 |
| stomach and intestinal diseases | 54 | 10.8 |
| skin diseases | 48 | 9.5 |
| allergies, etc. | 47 | 9.4 |
| nervous complaints and mental disorders | 22 | 4.4 |
| other non-specific illnesses | 117 | 23.4 |
| Total | 501 | 100.0 |

## Perceived morbidity

As was indicated in the theoretical orientation of the study in Chapter 2, perceived morbidity of respondents is to be regarded as a significant determinant of utilisation of the plural medical system. It has already been pointed out that the 'subjective' perceived illness need not correspond exactly to the 'objective' status of the psycho-biological system of the patient. For the analytical purpose of the study – which is to obtain insight into illness behaviour without attempting to evaluate the medical services consulted by patients – the individual's interpretation and experience of his state of health are more important determinants of the related process of seeking and obtaining medical care than his state of health established by standardised, clinical criteria. As the illness behaviour of respondents is 'triggered off' by the individuals' perception of his morbidity, a wide variety of action (or non-action) is initiated which leads to relief of the complaint or recovery from a disease. With a view to achieve minimal under-reporting of cases during the health interview survey over the rather long recall period of time, the main reported illness episodes have been recorded in order to examine the processual nature of response to illness in Babile.[2] This implies that attention can focus on the individual as a patient suffering from a disease rather than as a carrier of a disease, given the fact that in the tropics patients often suffer from several diseases simultaneously (cf. Vervoorn 1974: 1, 2). In this context, the analysis of morbidity data will additionally discriminate both between 'severe' and 'mild' illnesses and between 'acute and 'chronic' diseases.

Table 6.4 shows the most common categories of illnesses reported by respondents in the survey. Infectious and parasitic diseases, mainly amoebiasis, tuberculosis, venereal diseases, lint worm, etc., are the diseases most widely reported (31.1%), corresponding to the general pattern of morbidity in the tropics. Similar figures for respiratory diseases (11.4%), the most common being pneumonia, bronchitis and influenza, and for stomach and intestinal complaints (10.8%), chiefly gastritis, stomach ulcers and liver complaints, indicate the severity of these illnesses generally perceived by the local population as second and third in the list of severe diseases which present a real threat to health. Parasitic diseases of the skin which achieved relatively high scores in 'objective' medical surveys described in Chapter 3, were experienced as 'mild' illnesses by respondents and accordingly reported to a much smaller extent (9.5%). Nevertheless, on the basis of medical studies conducted earlier in the region, it is fair to assume that a number of diseases with negative social sanctions, including 'shameful diseases' such as syphilis, gonorrhoea, leprosy and vitiligo and 'magic diseases' such as the 'evil eye' and epilepsy were relatively under-reported in the household interview surveys.

With a view to the earlier mentioned discrimination in the classification of perceived morbidity, an important distinction can additionally be made in the reported cases of illness between 'acute' illnesses (from 1 day to 4 weeks) and 'chronic' illnesses (from 1 to 12 months). These categories are based largely on the local population's own experience and interpretation of the duration of symptoms and are not indicative of chronic illnesses determined on medical grounds such as rheumatism, high blood pressure, cardiac and vascular diseases, lumbar complaints, diabetes, epilepsy, etc. For analytic purposes it is also necessary to classify a number of reported illness episodes as either 'naturalistic' or 'personalistic' illnesses. This indigenous classification of perceived morbidity established partly on the basis of qualitative research is explained in detail in Chapter 4.

Tables 6.5 and 6.6 show reported cases of illness according to perceived duration and indigenous classification of illness.

Evidently, these figures indicate that less than one-third of the reported cases of illness are perceived as chronic (28.9%). More than one-third of the cases of illness in the survey are regarded by the population as naturalistic (35.3%) while one-fifth (20.2%) are attributed to personalistic causes. Since the local population tends

Table 6.5: *Illness episodes reported by respondents over the preceding twelve months, according to acute and chronic diseases*

| categories of reported illnesses | N | % |
|---|---|---|
| acute | 356 | 71.1 |
| chronic | 145 | 28.9 |
| Total | 501 | 100.0 |

Table 6.6: *Illness episodes reported by respondents over the preceding twelve months according to naturalistic, personalistic and non-specified diseases*

| categories of reported illnesses | N | % |
|---|---|---|
| naturalistic | 177 | 35.3 |
| personalistic | 101 | 20.2 |
| non-specified | 223 | 44.5 |
| Total | 501 | 100.0 |

to be dubious about the posibility of treating some acute diseases and personalistic illnesses successfully in the modern medical system, the above categories will be introduced as separate variables of perceived morbidity into the analysis later in this chapter.

## Alternative sources of health care

During the qualitative research, it became clear that members of the community have a choice from a wide range of medical facilities in the event of illness. The successive stages in the illness process vary from not taking any action after symptoms have been observed to making use, to a certain extent, of the latest developments in modern medicine. The following section examines the distribution of the various choices of action aimed at recovery or non-action among respondents in the survey.

Previous research has shown that in the event of illness, individuals may choose between five different types of action, including non-action, or a combination of these:

1. the patient does not take action of any kind;
2. the patient uses self-care;
3. the patient consults the traditional medical system;
4. the patient consults the transitional medical system;
5. the patient consults the modern medical system.

Table 6.7: *Categories of patients from the survey distributed according to the reported type of action or non-action taken to obtain treatment during the preceding twelve months*

| category of patients | N | % |
|---|---|---|
| non-action patients | 15 | 2.9 |
| internal action patients | 30 | 5.9 |
| external action patients | 456 | 91.2 |
| Total | 501 | 100.0 |

As indicated above, 501 people of the sample covering 1351 respondents reported that they had been ill or unwell during the previous twelve months. Further, 15 of the 501 did not take any action to seek treatment. Of the remaining 486, 30 reported self-care and 456 consulted one or more medical systems.

By analogy with the preceding Rural Health in Ethiopia Project, the patients in the health interview survey can be divided into three main categories:

- non-action patients: patients who do not take any action to obtain treatment;
- internal action patients: patients who make exclusive use of internal help or self-care which includes the use of home remedies;
- external action patients: patients who seek medical care on one or more occasions from an official or institution of a traditional, transitional and/or modern medical system

Table 6.7 shows the totals for the three categories of patients in the survey.

The table shows that the majority of patients (91.2%) reported the use of medical treatment from an external source, i.e. had consulted a functionary from one of the three major health care systems on one or more occasions. Each of these three categories will now be examined separately in greater detail.

## The non-action patients

This category of 15 patients (2.9% of the total) who had refrained from any action after symptom experience, was composed of 12 women and 3 men. Despite the small numbers, this could illustrate the weak position of women in the event of illness. Of the women, 8 were over 41 years of age and 9 of the 12 patients were Oromo. There were 3 children among non-action patients aged 0–15 suffering from 'childhood diseases' for which no medical treatment was considered necessary. Likewise, 4 people were in the 16–25 age group and more than half of the non-action patients were over the age of 46.

It was revealed that 5 of the patients did not wish to seek any medical treatment in order to allow 'nature to take its own course to healing'. All of them were Oromo, who regard Allah as responsible for illness and therefore believe that supernatural forces determine the patient's recovery. In keeping with their faith, a number of Oromo included the strict observance of religious practices in the course of the recovery process. Two of the 9 Oromo patients gave 'lack of money' as the main reason for not taking any action to obtain treatment.

Finally, 3 of the non-action patients were Amhara and they too gave 'lack of money' as the reason for not seeking any treatment. The remaining 2 patients, who were Somali, both said that their perceived illnesses (respiratory complaints) were not sufficiently serious to merit medical treatment. Generally speaking, the non-action patients suffered from non-chronic illnesses such as muscular cramps, 'children's diseases' and abdominal complaints.

## The internal action patients

This category covers patients in the survey who used the various forms of self-care such as traditional home remedies described in Chapter 5 to treat their illnesses. It consists of 30 patients (5.9%) who reported that they made exclusive use of local home remedies, in the majority of cases successfully. They comprised 12 male patients and 18 female patients, 17 of whom were in the 0–15 age group and 8 in the 46–65 age group. The symptoms of infants and young children were treated in the first instance by their mothers and grandmothers within the family with traditional remedies. As far as ethnic groups are concerned, the Oromo accounted for the largest number of patients (21) who used this type of curative medicine. Also, 3 Amhara and 3 Somali made use of this type of remedy.

Among traditional home remedies, a particularly important method of treatment consists of eating the flesh and drinking the blood of a sheep or goat after its ritual slaughter. For example, a patient suffering from amoebiasis or an intestinal complaint, will eat the contents of the stomach of the slaughtered animal. Someone suffering from muscular or back pains will have the animal's blood and fat rubbed on the affected part of the body. Another common technique of treatment is to employ butter, to which strong healing powers are attributed. Often it is rubbed on the head of the patient or massaged into aching joints of the body.

Local medicinal plants, sometimes in combination with honey, are also used in specific cases to prepare medicinal drinks, tablets and powders. In a number of cases it was reported that headaches were treated by patients inhaling the smoke of the burning leaves of certain plants. Roots and tubers of specific plants are also attributed with considerable healing properties and are used mainly during the practise of self-care to prepare extracts and medicinal pastes. During the qualitative research it became clear that the use of medicinal plants, roots and tubers forms an important part of daily life in Oromo culture.

Although the survey indicates that all of the ethnic groups make substantial use of animal ingredients in relation to health and healing, the use of medicinal plants was most frequently reported among the Oromo as a form of self-care. Finally, 40 patients reported that they had attempted self-care as a means of internal action prior to a visit to one of the medical systems.

## The external action patients

The number of patients of this category who actually left their homes and sought some form of external medical care in one of the available medical systems during the preceding twelve months consisted of 456 individuals or 91.2% of the total number of respondents who reported some form of illness (N = 501). While all 456 external action patients reported contacts with the traditional, transitional or modern medical systems, in various ways, 40 of them had first attempted to use home remedies without success, after which they had decided to take external action. As described in Chapter 5, the traditional medical system includes the local Cushitic medical sub-system and the regional Arabic and Amhara sub-systems, while the transitional system consists largely of

Table 6.8: *First-step utilisation of the three medical systems in Babile by the external action patients during the preceding twelve months*

| number of external action patients | | type of medical system | | | | | |
|---|---|---|---|---|---|---|---|
| | | traditional medical system | | transitional medical system | | modern medical system | |
| N | % | N | % | N | % | N | % |
| 456 | (100.0) | 197 | 43.2 | 87 | 19.1 | 172 | 37.7 |

pharmaceutical services of drug vendors, 'needlemen' and 'injectors'. The modern medical system is made up of the official health care organisations in the area, the main ones being the health station in Babile, the health centre in Gursum and the hospitals in Bisidimo, Harar and Dire Dawa.

Table 6.8 shows the external action patients classified according to the type of medical system they first consulted in the event of illness.

Almost half of the external action patients (43.2%) consulted the traditional medical system as a first step while more than one-third (37.7%) consulted the modern medical system first. Less than one-fifth (19.1%) initially referred to the transitional medical system. However, the picture is complicated by the fact that a number of patients often seek treatment from several systems for the same illness rather than confining themselves to one system of health care delivery. Despite the tendency among patients to consult one type of system for a particular kind of illness, in practice patients use different systems in certain cases. Such multiple utilisation or 'healer shopping' may be simultaneous or successive and may involve different medical systems or be within the same system. The complex behaviour of external action patients in relation to the plural medical system forms the basis for the subsequent calculation of utilisation scores as emerged from the health interview survey.

### *6.1.2 External action: the choice of treatment*

As noted above, some patients make use of the opportunities available to them to obtain medical care by taking one step whilst other patients consult several different systems in succession or simultaneously.

Table 6.9: *Number of reported steps taken by the 456 external action patients during the preceding twelve months*

| number of reported illness steps | number of patients | |
|---|---|---|
| | N | % |
| 1 illness step | 395 | 86.6 |
| 2 illness steps | 53 | 11.6 |
| 3 illness steps | 8 | 1.8 |
| Total | 456 | 100.0 |

The latter group who take several steps for one illness may conveniently be described as 'flow-through cases' (cf. Buschkens and Slikkerveer 1982: 101–103). Multiple utilisation within medical systems where, for example, patients consult both a *kabira* (Oromo) and a *tanqway* (Amhara), has been recorded in quantitative terms but has not been worked out in detail in the analysis of the patterns of utilisation because of its complexity. During the research it became apparent that highly selective utilisation within medical systems is less than that between medical systems. As far as 'healer shopping' is concerned, the present study emphasises the multiple contacts between patients and representatives of the traditional, transitional and/or modern medical systems, by means of which inter-relationships between the systems can be explained.

The survey shows that 47 of the 546 external action patients reported that they had consulted several representatives of the same system for one particular illness. These were mainly Oromo who had used various forms of traditional health care. Section 6.2.1 deals with multiple utilisation of the three systems.

Table 6.9 shows the 456 external action patients according to the number of steps they took to obtain medical treatment for one reported illness. These findings confirm that the majority of patients take one step and that a much smaller number take either two steps (11.6%) or three steps (1.8%). In other words, the majority of external action patients discontinue their medical treatment after having consulted their first choice of 'external' health care.

If Tables 6.8 and 6.9 are combined with the reported number of non-patients and patients in the survey and the three categories of non-action patients, internal action patients and external action patients mentioned above, it becomes possible to construct a

Figure 6.1: *Decision tree showing the movement of patients in the survey through the plural medical system in Babile*

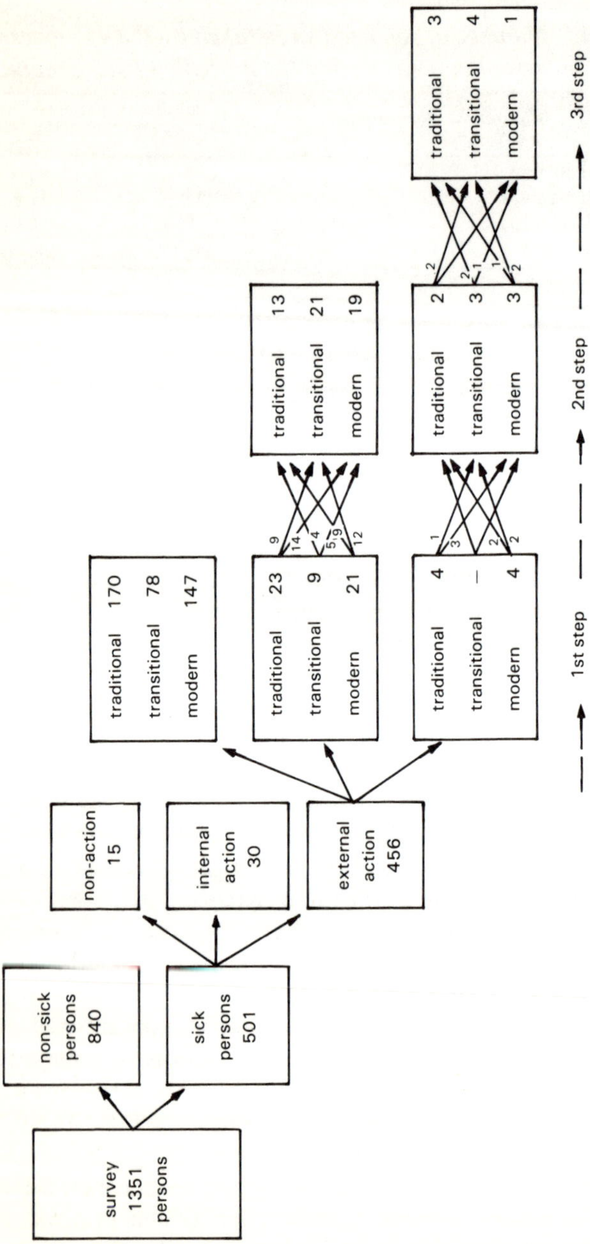

'decision-tree' to chart the illness episodes and the progress of patients through the plural medical systems. This shows both the distribution of the 456 external action patients over the systems and the number of steps taken by them (cf. Figure 6.1). Here, it should again be emphasised that multiple utilisation covers both simultaneous and successive visits to different medical systems.

From Figure 6.1 it can now clearly be seen that of the 1351 people in the survey, 501 (37.1%) reported that they had been ill, unwell or injured during the preceding twelve months. Of these people, 15 (1.1%) did not take action of any kind while 30 (2.2%) only used traditional home remedies. In addition, the action taken by the largest group – the 456 external action patients (33.8%) – to consult the traditional, the transitional or the modern system can easily be followed through the course of the health care seeking process. While 395 patients took only one step, of which almost half (43%) consulted the traditional medical system, more than one-third of the 395 (37.2%) made use of the services of the transitional medical system.

Further examination of the category of patients who took two illness steps reveals that 21 and 3 patients respectively from the traditional and modern systems consulted the transitional system, making a total of 24 patients who consulted the transitional system as a second step. Similarly, 14 patients consulted the traditional medical system as a second step, and 22 consulted the modern system. Finally, there were 8 'flow-through cases' who took three steps, almost all of whom consulted all three systems in search of treatment.

## 6.2 Patterns of Health Care Utilisation

As Chapter 2 explained, the present study employs an analytical model at systems level in order to describe and explain the factors which seem to play a role in the process of utilisation of the different medical systems. The research into health care utilisation concentrates on the number of contacts which the population have had with components of the plural medical system over a period of twelve months expressed in the form of scores, referred to as attendance or utilisation rates.

### *6.2.1 Overall patterns of utilisation rates for the plural medical system*

The reported contacts of patients with one or more components of the plural medical system have been entered as independent variables in the analytical model. Generally speaking, the best way of establishing these independent variables would be by just recording them in the field, but since no such facilities exist within the systems, health interview surveys have been used to provide a workable method for the analysis of utilisation. The shortcomings of this technique have already been pointed out in Chapter 2. Since the external action patients of all illness-reporting persons in the survey indicated that they had consulted a representative or service of one of the available medical systems in the previous twelve months, this category of patients will determine the overall pattern of utilisation in the analysis. In this way it will be possible to relate the total pattern of utilisation resulting from the action taken by illness-reporting respondents to the various categories of independent variables: predisposing, enabling and morbidity factors.

The overall pattern of utilisation resulting from the reported illness behaviour of the 456 external action patients should now be compiled on the basis of the individual action reported and the number of steps taken per illness episode. This involves the calculation of the total number of visits or 'scores' by patients who consulted one or more medical systems during the research period of twelve months. Such utilisation rates at system level can rather simply be obtained by combining the data on the type of action taken with the number of illness steps taken by patients. Consequently, the combination of the figures in Table 6.9 with those in Figure 6.1, produces the totals shown in Table 6.10 for the number of visits to the three medical systems.

Table 6.10 shows that the 456 patients in the survey, who consulted an external health care facility, paid a total of 525 visits to the various medical systems, establishing the overall utilisation pattern in Babile. Of these 525 visits, 215 (40.9%) were to the traditional medical system, 115 (21.9%) to the transitional medical system and 195 (37.2%) to the modern medical system. The total picture of action undertaken by the external action patients (n = 456) and the resulting pattern of health care utilisation expressed in the total number of contacts with the traditional, transitional and modern

Table 6.10: *Total number of visits by the 456 external action patients in the survey to the three medical systems in Babile*

| number of external action patients | number of steps | number of visits to the plural medical system: traditional medical system n | % | transitional medical system n | % | modern medical system n | % | total number of visits n | % |
|---|---|---|---|---|---|---|---|---|---|
| 395 | 1 | 170 | 43.0 | 78 | 19.7 | 147 | 37.3 | 395 | 100.0 |
| 53 | 2 | 36 | 33.9 | 30 | 28.3 | 40 | 37.8 | 106 | 100.0 |
| 8 | 3 | 9 | 37.5 | 7 | 29.2 | 8 | 33.3 | 24 | 100.0 |
| 456 | – | 215 | 40.9 | 115 | 21.9 | 195 | 37.2 | 525 | 100.0 |

medical system (N = 525) is presented in Table 6.11. It is clear, that the shift in utilisation rates is caused by multiple utilisation and referral of patients between the systems for the treatment of the same illness episode.[3]

Roughly half of the external action patients (43.2%) consulted the traditional medical system as a first step in the health seeking process. In this group, 27 respondents reported that they had consulted another medical system for the same illness. Of these 27 'multiple users' of the traditional system, 10 patients applied to the transitional system while 17 consulted the modern system. Table 6.11 also shows that almost one-fifth of external action patients (19.1%) consulted the transitional medical system in the first instance. Of the 9 'multiple users' in this category, 4 patients sought treatment in the traditional system and 5 patients consulted the modern system. Finally, more than one-third (37.7%) of respondents reported that their first visit was paid to the modern medical system. Of this last category of patients, 25 reported multiple utilisation resulting in: 11 attendances at the traditional system and 14 visits to the transitional medical system. The overall pattern reveals that from the total number of 456 external action patients, who initially sought treatment in one of the existing medical systems, 61 patients also contacted a second system and 8 of the 61 even took a third step: 3 consulted the traditional, 4 consulted the transitional and 1 consulted the modern medical system. Multiple utilisation of all three systems is roughly the same, averaging 15% of the 456 external action patients in the survey.

In order to make the above analysis of the health care seeking process as clear as possible, Table 6.11 also attempts to express the illness behaviour of respondents in the survey and the subsequent pattern of utilisation in the form of a combined flow-through chart.

### *6.2.2 Differential- and under-utilisation of health care*

The previous section described the variety and dynamics in the illness behaviour of respondents in the survey. In the first place, 15 respondents did not take any form of action. This phenomenon, known as the 'symptom iceberg' indicates the limited number of illness episodes referred to doctors, nurses and other health care personnel (cf. Nuysens 1973: 35; Kroeger 1983: 157). Self-care, the use of home remedies and consulting the family, neighbours and villagers often leads to the use of medical practices by laymen which Freidson (1973: 107–211) has called the *lay referral system*. Moreover, this type of care and lay referral sometimes precedes the use of professional health care services. As noted above, 30 of the 501 respondents in the survey made exclusive use of this kind of medical treatment while 40 respondents reported such internal 'experimentation' before consulting one or more medical systems in Babile. Finally, 456 external action patients consulted professional medical systems in the research area. The analysis in the following sections concentrates mainly on the pattern of utilisation exhibited by this latter category of respondents. As indeed these patients, who generally reported perception of serious illness episodes causing social dysfunction, undertook one or more steps seeking external aid, here the dynamics in the illness process find expression in the transition to successive stages of alternative behaviour. It is in the context of such transitions that not only bio-medical, but economic and socio-cultural determinants seem to play a crucial role.

As Table 6.11 clearly shows there is differential utilisation of health care in Babile: the local population tend to use the three medical systems to varying degrees. The variation in the extent to which patients use the plural medical system indicates also that illness behaviour cannot solely be explained by an analysis of perceived morbidity and that other factors play a key role in addition to the nature and perception of illness. As, for example, ethnic affiliation of the patients of the sample is discriminated in the aforementioned Table 6.11, comparison of the utilisation rates of

Table 6.11: *Flow-through chart of patients: illness behaviour of the 501 patients of the sample and the resulting total number of 525 utilisation rates, distributed over the three medical systems in Babile*

| patients | | | | | | | | | | | | medical system | visits | |
|---|---|---|---|---|---|---|---|---|---|---|---|---|---|---|
| total number of patients | non-action patients | internal action patients | external action patients | | | | | | | | | | utilisation rates | |
| | | | | first step | | flow-through cases | second step | | flow-through cases | third step | | | | |
| N | N | N | N | N | (%) | N | N | (%) | N | N | | | N | (%) |
| 501 | 15 | 30 | | | | | | | | | | | | |
| | | | | 197 | (43.2) | 27 | 15 | (24.6) | 2 | 3 | | Trad. m.s. | 215 | (41.0) |
| | | | 456 | 87 | (19.1) | 9 | 24 | (39.3) | 3 | 4 | | Trans. m.s. | 115 | (21.9) |
| | | | | 172 | (37.7) | 25 | 22 | (36.1) | 3 | 1 | | Mod. m.s. | 195 | (37.1) |
| 501 | 15 | 30 | 456 | 456 | (100.0) | 61 | 61 | (100.0) | 8 | 8 | | | 525 | (100.0) |

Table 6.12: *Illness behaviour of the 501 patients of the sample and the resulting pattern of differential utilisation of the three medical systems, distributed according to the main ethnic groups in Babile*

| | patients | | | | | | | | | | visits | | | | | | | |
|---|---|---|---|---|---|---|---|---|---|---|---|---|---|---|---|---|---|---|
| ethnic group | non-action patients | internal action patients | external action patients | | | | | | total | | utilisation rates | | | | | | total | |
| | | | trad. m.s. | | trans. m.s. | | mod. m.s. | | plural m.s. | | trad. m.s. | | trans. m.s. | | mod. m.s. | | plural m.s. | |
| | N | N | N | % | N | % | N | % | N | % | N | % | N | % | N | % | N | % |
| Oromo | 9 | 21 | 173 | 59.5 | 55 | 18.9 | 63 | 21.6 | 291 | 100.0 | 192 | 56.5 | 67 | 19.7 | 81 | 23.8 | 340 | 100.0 |
| Amhara | 4 | 3 | 11 | 8.2 | 25 | 18.8 | 97 | 73.0 | 133 | 100.0 | 11 | 7.3 | 38 | 25.3 | 101 | 67.4 | 150 | 100.0 |
| Somali | 2 | 6 | 10 | 41.7 | 5 | 20.8 | 9 | 37.5 | 24 | 100.0 | 9 | 33.3 | 9 | 33.3 | 9 | 33.3 | 27 | 100.0 |
| Other | – | – | 3 | – | 2 | – | 3 | – | 8 | 100.0 | 3 | – | 1 | – | 4 | – | 8 | – |
| Total | 15 | 30 | 197 | 43.2 | 87 | 19.1 | 172 | 37.7 | 456 | 100.0 | 215 | 41.0 | 115 | 21.9 | 195 | 37.1 | 525 | 100.0 |

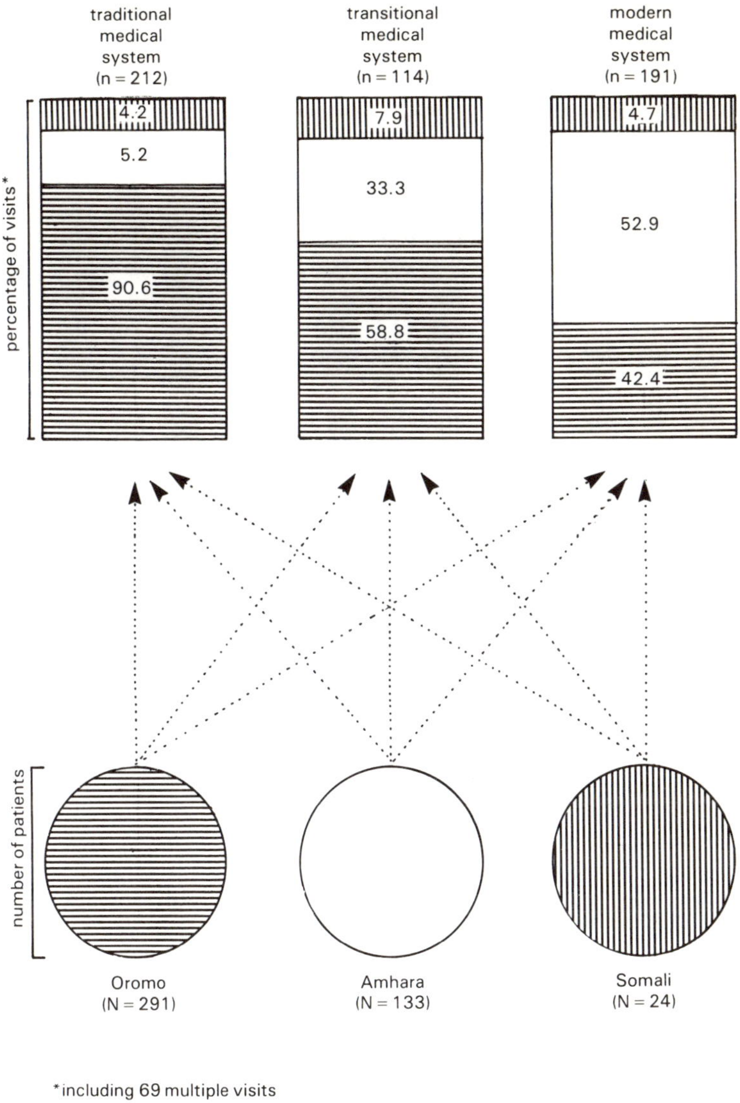


Figure 6.2: *Differential pattern of health care utilisation of the three medical systems by patients from the three major ethnic groups of the sample (N = 448; n = 517)*

the three medical systems by patients from the three major ethnic groups displays a highly differential pattern of utilisation.

By consequence table 6.12 shows the illness behaviour of the 501 patients, resulting in a differentiated pattern of utilisation of the plural medical system, distributed according to the Oromo, Amhara, Somali, and other ethnic groups in the sample. It is evident that more than half of the Oromo patients who account for 192 visits (56.5%) refer to the traditional system, compared with 11 visits (7.3%) by the Amhara and 9 visits (33.3%) by Somali. Utilisation of the modern medical system by the three ethnic groups is completely different: the Amhara account for the largest number of visits, 101 (67.4%) compared with 81 (23.8%) by the Oromo. Somali patients consult the three systems to more or less the same extent. The transitional system occupies a middle position in terms of utilisation by both the Oromo: 67 visits (19.7%) and the Amhara: 38 visits (25.3%). The differences between these two ethnic groups are considerably less in relation to the transitional system than in relation to the traditional and modern systems (19.7–25.3% versus 56.5–7.3% and 23.8–67.4%). Thus, while Oromo and Somali patients tend to show a clear preference in case of illness to engage in transactions with the traditional medical systems, Amhara patients prefer to seek treatment at the modern medical services. This differential pattern among patients is less obvious within the transitional medical system, in which only a slightly increased preference among Somali patients exists.

In order to assess this highly complicated pattern from the medical system's point of view, Figure 6.2 attempts to clarify schematically the differential pattern of utilisation of the three medical systems, as it emerges from the transactions with Oromo, Somali and Amhara groups in Babile. In this figure the increasing utilisation rates of the Oromo of the traditional system contrasting with the increasing rates of the Amhara of the modern system – together with the rather equal distribution of the Somali throughout the plural medical system – are further substantiated.

Previous studies in health services use have shown that factors other than perceived morbidity and ethnic affiliation have a significant influence on differential utilisation. However, before looking at these and other determinants or groups of determinants which are likely to be involved in this process, it is useful first to consider a specific form of utilisation in the research area, namely under-utilisation of modern health care facilities.

Health care utilisation is usually expressed as the number of contacts or scores between patients and a particular medical institution or service, calculated, for example, by recording the number of visits made over a certain period of time. The total number of scores obtained in this way indicates a certain level of utilisation and can be converted into a ratio in order to enable different results to be compared with one another. Ratios can also provide insight into utilisation of doctors, nurses or specific hospital services and enable comparison between levels of utilisation by different populations.

As Chapter 2 explained, the utilisation ratio is usually obtained by dividing the total number of visits paid to a medical facility by consumers/patients belonging to a population or specific group over a period of one year, by the total number of people in the population or group concerned:

$$\text{utilisation ratio} = \frac{\text{number of visits by patients}}{\text{number of individuals in population}}$$

As was noted in Chapter 2, King (1966: 2, 5) estimates that a realistic norm in relation to health care planning in Africa is two visits per adult and three visits per child per year resulting in an average of 2.5 visits per person per year to a modern health care facility.

It becomes quite evident that the modern system of health care delivery in Babile is highly under-utilised by patients if the results of the health interview surveys are compared with this norm. The sample population of 1351 persons paid a total of 195 visits to the modern medical system during a period of twelve months, producing the following ratio:

$$\frac{\text{number of visits to the modern medical system}}{\text{number of respondents in the sample}} = \frac{195}{1351} = 0.14 \text{ visits per person per year}$$

According to King's norm of 2.5 visits per person per year, the above ratio should be $1351 \times 2.5 = 3377.5$ visits to a modern health care institution in the research area. However, the reported scores which produce a utilisation ratio of 0.14 visits per person in the previous year reaches only 5.7% of the ideal standard.

Government figures, though scarce, confirm this picture of extremely low utilisation of the modern medical system by the local populaton in this part of Ethiopia. The *Comprehensive Health Service Directory* (1976: 114) gives a total of 800 out-patient visits to the health station in Babile in the year in question. If visits to the health centre outside the research area at Gursum and visits to the various hospitals at Bisidimo and Harar are excluded, then this total number amounts to the following utilisation ratio:

$$\frac{80}{4000} = 0.20 \text{ visits per person per year}$$

It is clear that this ratio together with that of 0.14 emerging from the health interview survey is extremely low in comparison to King's norm of 2.5 visits per person per year.

The picture of under-utilisation of the modern medical system in Eastern Ethiopia ties in with the results of research earlier conducted in the rural part of the Hararghe Highlands. Using official figures from the *Comprehensive Health Service Directory* (1976) supplemented with field studies in five villages, Buschkens and Slikkerveer (1982: 105–107) arrive at the following general utilisation ratio by the total population of the highlands, which applies to both rural and urban areas:

$$\frac{285{,}653}{2{,}000{,}000} = 0.142 \text{ visits per person per year}$$

Using the norm devised by King (1962: 2, 5) this would be:

$$\frac{5{,}000{,}000}{2{,}000{,}000} = 2.5 \text{ visits per person per year}$$

In other words, utilisation should be 17.6 times higher than that actually established during the research among the *Kottu* Oromo. Schneider (1975: 46) suggests that only 0 to 1% of the population of the Highlands of Hararghe make use of the modern medical services available to them. In view of the limited number of government services operating in rural areas it might be expected that they would be functioning just above capacity but this is not always the case in practice.

It is therefore clear that in Ethiopia, with its current pattern of morbidity and mortality and given the present situation of the official health care infrastrucutre, there is a high degree of under-utilisation of modern services. Under-utilisation of the modern medical system in the Eastern Highlands with ratios of 0.14 and 0.16 is also extremely high compared, for example, with urban areas such as Addis Ababa where a ratio of 0.25 visits per person per year has been recorded (cf. Freij *et al.* 1973).

## Notes

1. Following Johns Hopkins University's (1976: 42) definition, this study regards an 'illness episode' as a: '... *reported period of uninterrupted illness or injury irrespective of the number of symptoms or conditions simultaneously present'.*
2. As Kroeger (1985: 18) notes: '*Little is known about the optimal recall period in developing countries.*' Short recall periods in health interview surveys have the advantage of rather accurate description of current illnesses, while longer recall periods enable matching of seasonability and chronicity of diseases. In order to attempt avoidance of both under- and over-reporting, the study in Babile has compared quantitative results of the twelve months health interview survey with qualitative data of longitudinal case-studies following the patient's course in the health care seeking process for particular illness episodes.
3. Quantification of multiple health care utilisation reported for the cure of the same illness period requires accurate memory of respondents of different actions taken. In view of the relative long recall period of the health interview survey, several longitudinal case studies were included in the research to complement the household data and to ascertain the 'shift' in utilisation rates from traditional via transitional to modern medicine and vice versa.

# 7

# Choice of Therapy: Analysis and Interpretation

## 7.1 Bivariate Analysis of Determinants of Utilisation

The previous sections have shown that in the Eastern Highlands illness behaviour and the accompanying pattern of health care utilisation which together form the central theme of this study, encompass a complex process of seeking and obtaining medical care expressed in terms of multiple and differential utilisation of the plural medical system. According to the results of the health interview survey, the Oromo substantially utilise the traditional system while the Amhara make more use of the modern system with the transitional system occupying a middle position for both groups. In addition, a comparison between utilisation ratios of the modern medical system and the planning-norm devised by King (1966) for the whole of Africa has shown that the modern medical system is under utilised by the population in the research area to a very great extent.

In this stage of the study it now becomes a challenge to consider which factors play an important role in influencing the evident variation in utilisation of health care services in the area. In order to find an answer to this question, utilisation of the three systems will be examined in relation with the various groups of factors selected in advance for the study: predisposing factors, enabling factors, and perceived morbidity factors. Bivariate analysis will then be used to determine the relative influence of these factors on utilisation. As was stated in Chapter 2, the systems factors will be retained as a constant variable in the analysis. The role of system factors in the health care seeking process will be examined in qualitative terms in relation to geographical and financial accessibility when the analytical model is being considered.

### *7.1.1. Predisposing factors*

Predisposing factors comprise a group of variables which are postulated to influence illness behaviour at the individual level and in which context personal characteristics and the background of respondents can be related to utilisation of health care services. This category includes situational, socio-cultural, cognitive and attitudinal variables such as sex, age, level of education, medical knowledge, ethnic affiliation, religion, occupation, household size, marital status and opinions on quality of medical services. Table 7.1 shows the successive distribution of multiple utilisation of 525 visits reported by the 456 external action patients in the sample, according to the predisposing factors of the model.

#### Sex and age

Table 7.1 shows that although women seem to make greater use of traditional medicine than men, generally speaking there is no specific pattern of utilisation according to sex. However, if the composition of the group of women patients is examined more closely, it becomes clear that Oromo and Somali women score relatively higher in relation to the traditional system than Amhara women. This can be explained by the fact that the roles of the sexes are more clearly defined in the Muslim communities of the Oromo and Somali. As regards the age of the patients, it is noticeable that children are treated to a large extent by traditional practitioners (45.5%) whereas older age groups score higher in relation to the modern medical system (54.1%). Older people, particularly older Amhara, increasingly make use of the 'poverty certificate' officially issued after the revolution, which entitles them to free treatment at the clinic in Babile.[1] In the transitional medical system the treatment of children dominates the pattern of utilisation (25.1%). During the household interviews it was discovered that cheaper medicines in particular were bought from traditional and transitional practitioners for the treatment of children. In such situations,

Table 7.1: *Multiple health care utilisation in 525 cases of illness reported by 456 external action patients*

| variable | | plural medical system | | | | | | total | |
|---|---|---|---|---|---|---|---|---|---|
| | | trad. | m.s. | trans. | m.s. | modern | m.s. | | |
| | | N | % | N | % | N | % | N | % |
| *sex* | | | | | | | | | |
| male | (1) | 105 | 39.3 | 59 | 22.1 | 103 | 38.6 | 267 | 100.0 |
| female | (2) | 110 | 42.6 | 56 | 21.7 | 92 | 35.7 | 258 | 100.0 |
| *age* | | | | | | | | | |
| 0–15 | (1) | 116 | 45.5 | 64 | 25.1 | 75 | 29.4 | 255 | 100.0 |
| 16–25 | (2) | 23 | 43.4 | 9 | 17.0 | 21 | 39.6 | 53 | 100.0 |
| 26–45 | (3) | 57 | 35.2 | 33 | 20.4 | 72 | 44.4 | 162 | 100.0 |
| 46–65 | (4) | 14 | 29.2 | 8 | 16.7 | 26 | 54.1 | 48 | 100.0 |
| 65 + | (5) | 4 | – | – | – | 3 | – | 7 | – |
| *education* | | | | | | | | | |
| none | (1) | 189 | 45.1 | 88 | 21.0 | 142 | 33.9 | 419 | 100.0 |
| primary | (2) | 23 | 23.0 | 26 | 26.0 | 51 | 51.0 | 100 | 100.0 |
| secondary | (3) | 3 | – | 1 | – | 2 | – | 6 | – |
| *medical knowledge* | | | | | | | | | |
| below average | (1) | 145 | 39.1 | 83 | 22.4 | 143 | 38.5 | 371 | 100.0 |
| above average | (2) | 70 | 45.4 | 32 | 20.7 | 52 | 33.9 | 154 | 100.0 |
| *ethnic group* | | | | | | | | | |
| Oromo | (1) | 192 | 56.5 | 67 | 19.7 | 81 | 23.8 | 340 | 100.0 |
| Amhara | (2) | 11 | 7.3 | 38 | 25.3 | 101 | 67.4 | 150 | 100.0 |
| Somali | (3) | 9 | 33.3 | 9 | 33.3 | 9 | 33.3 | 27 | 100.0 |
| other | (4) | 3 | – | 1 | – | 4 | – | 8 | – |
| *religion* | | | | | | | | | |
| Muslim | (1) | 186 | 58.3 | 63 | 19.7 | 70 | 22.0 | 319 | 100.0 |
| Christian | (2) | 29 | 14.1 | 52 | 25.2 | 125 | 60.7 | 206 | 100.0 |

| | | | | | | | | | |
|---|---|---|---|---|---|---|---|---|---|
| farmer | (1) | 92 | 48.5 | 43 | 22.6 | 55 | 28.9 | 190 | 100.0 |
| trader | (2) | 32 | 39.1 | 23 | 28.0 | 27 | 32.9 | 82 | 100.0 |
| public servant | (3) | 65 | 29.9 | 44 | 20.3 | 108 | 49.8 | 217 | 100.0 |
| other | (4) | 26 | 72.2 | 5 | 13.9 | 5 | 13.9 | 26 | 100.0 |
| *size of household* | | | | | | | | | |
| 1–3 members | (1) | 211 | 49.5 | 93 | 21.8 | 122 | 28.6 | 426 | 100.0 |
| 4–6 members | (2) | 4 | – | 18 | 21.9 | 60 | 73.1 | 82 | 100.0 |
| 7+ members | (3) | – | – | 4 | – | 13 | – | 17 | – |
| *marital status* | | | | | | | | | |
| married | (1) | 67 | 34.0 | 38 | 19.3 | 92 | 46.7 | 197 | 100.0 |
| unmarried | (2) | 127 | 45.2 | 68 | 24.2 | 86 | 30.6 | 281 | 100.0 |
| prev. married | (3) | 21 | 44.7 | 9 | 19.1 | 17 | 36.2 | 47 | 100.0 |
| *opinion on quality of transitional medical system* | | | | | | | | | |
| no opinion | (1) | 9 | – | 1 | – | 8 | – | 18 | – |
| poor | (2) | 8 | – | 4 | – | 7 | – | 19 | – |
| average | (3) | 153 | 45.8 | 62 | 18.6 | 119 | 35.6 | 334 | 100.0 |
| good | (4) | 45 | 29.2 | 48 | 31.2 | 61 | 39.7 | 154 | 100.0 |
| *opinion on attitude of transitional staff* | | | | | | | | | |
| no opinion | (1) | 9 | – | 1 | – | 8 | – | 18 | – |
| poor | (2) | 48 | 35.0 | 30 | 21.9 | 59 | 43.1 | 137 | 100.0 |
| average | (3) | 115 | 52.7 | 44 | 30.2 | 59 | 27.1 | 218 | 100.0 |
| good | (4) | 43 | 28.3 | 40 | 26.3 | 69 | 45.5 | 152 | 100.0 |
| *opinion on quality of modern medical system* | | | | | | | | | |
| no opinion | (1) | 9 | – | 5 | – | 4 | – | 18 | – |
| poor | (2) | 17 | 42.5 | 9 | 22.5 | 14 | 35.0 | 40 | 100.0 |
| average | (3) | 101 | 40.7 | 54 | 21.8 | 93 | 37.5 | 248 | 100.0 |
| good | (4) | 88 | 40.2 | 47 | 21.5 | 84 | 38.5 | 219 | 100.0 |
| *opinion on attitude of modern medical staff* | | | | | | | | | |
| no opinion | (1) | 9 | – | 5 | – | 4 | – | 18 | – |
| poor | (2) | 37 | 54.5 | 13 | 19.1 | 18 | 26.5 | 68 | 100.0 |
| average | (3) | 102 | 43.2 | 57 | 19.1 | 77 | 32.6 | 236 | 100.0 |
| good | (4) | 67 | 33.0 | 40 | 19.7 | 96 | 47.3 | 203 | 100.0 |

perceived morbidity also plays a role. As noted in Chapter 4, a number of children's diseases are usually not regarded as serious and in many cases the head of the household considers local home remedies or cheap pharmaceutical products to be sufficient treatment for these so-called 'children's diseases'.

## Education and medical knowledge

Table 7.1 affirms that respondents with some form of education tend to use the modern system rather than the traditional one (51% to 23%). It is worth asking here whether this is in any way connected with the *zemecha* campaign described in Chapter 3 which was carried out in the Highlands of Hararghe during the survey. This is part of a programme of national awakening of consciousness, including a new approach to health promotion in the form of intensive health care information programmes. Since the 1974 revolution, schools have attempted to include in their programmes a general attention on the principles of modern medicine. In addition, formal training and education usually involve a first contact with western culture, of which modern medicine is an important expression. There is little difference in utilisation of modern and traditional health care among patients with below average medical knowledge, measured on a 10-points scale. Respondents with above average knowledge are not necessarily more likely to use the modern medical system; in fact the reverse is true. There is also little variation in utilisation of the transitional system, which is lower than that of the other two, in relation to below average or above average medical knowledge (22.4% as against 20.7%).

## Ethnic affiliation and religion

The pattern of health care utilisation in Babile varies considerably according to the ethnic and religious background of patients. The Oromo make virtually twice as much use of traditional medicine as they do of modern health care (56.5% against 23.8%). By way of sharp contrast, Amhara patients make almost ten times more use of the modern medical system than they do of the traditional medical system (67.4% against 7.3%). They also consult the transitional system relatively more frequently. It is noticeable here that the religion of respondents produces an almost diametrically opposite picture of utilisation as far as the traditional and modern systems are concerned. During the household survey it became clear that there are two main religious groupings in the community, the Christian Amhara and the Muslin Oromo and Somali. In the light of the ethno-cultural pluralism of the community, there are clearly patterns of utilisation in Babile which relate specifically to ethnic and religious background. The bivariate analysis confirms the qualitative survey indicating the crucial role of group treatment of *beteseb, ollaa* and *reer* respectively.

## Occupation of household head

Farmers who had consulted one of the three medical systems in the year preceding the health interview survey expressed a preference for traditional medicine. The same was true to a lesser extent of traders, but civil servants and other heads of households preferred the use of cosmopolitan medicine. This clearly ties in with the fact that most farmers are Oromo while most civil servants and soldiers belong to the Amhara group in Babile.

## Household size and marital status

It might be expected that larger families would tend to make relatively less use of the modern medical system because of their extended social pattern of action. This, however, is not the case. Respondents in this category actually make more use of modern medicine, whereas respondents belonging to the 'nuclear family' prefer traditional medicine.

Utilisation of the transitional medical system shows little variation in this respect (49.5% and 21.8% respectively). It is interesting to note that married household heads reported more contact with the modern medical system whereas unmarried household heads and those who had previously been married reported the opposite. In the qualitative household survey, household heads sometimes reported a different pattern of utilisation from that of the other members of their households. For example, particularly among the Oromo, in a number of cases when the head of the household became ill, medicines were provided through collective efforts of the *gosa* to raise the necessary funds for expensive treatment at the clinic. In the case of a major threat to the economic future of a complete household, the traditional community spirit and group responsibility – the *gadaa* system of the Oromo – seem to take over, proving that the group still has an important social function when serious illness affects one of its members. When a marriage ends, the household in question usually breaks up. The illness behaviour of respondents who had previously been married showed marked similarities with that of the unmarried members of the community.

## Opinions on quality and attitudes in the transitional system

Table 7.1 also contains figures showing the relationship between utilisation behaviour on the one hand and respondents' opinions of the quality of treatment provided by the three medical systems and the attitude of medical staff to patients on the other. As far as the transitional system is concerned, a positive rating of the treatment it provides is reflected in a relatively high utilisation score (31.2%). The opinions of users of the two other systems regarding the quality of the service provided by the transitional system do not show any marked variation, but users of the modern system scored the attitude of transitional staff markedly higher than users of the traditional system (45.5% against 28.3%).

## Opinions on quality and attitude in the modern medical system

The relation between a general positive evaluation of the modern medical system and illness behaviour is less marked. The increase in utilisation rates by respondents who thought the knowledge and skills of modern staff were good as opposed to poor was only slight (from 35% to 38.3%) and variation in utilisation of the two other systems was also minimal. However, the attitude of modern medical staff to patients in Babile would appear to be extremely important. The *higher* respondents scored the attitude of official health care staff, the greater the use they made of the modern system with the result that the percentages almost doubled from 26.5% to 47.3%. The reverse was also true. The *lower* respondents scored communication between patients and modern trained staff, the more likely they were to consult the traditional medical system, utilisation of which then went up from 33% to 54.4%. By contrast with opinions concerning the transitional medical system, a certain relationship can therefore be established between utilisation of traditional medicine and opinions concerning the attitude of modern medical personnel. Utilisation of the transitional system does not, however, show any variation to speak of in relation to this factor.

Table 7.2: *Distribution of multiple health care utilisation in 525 cases of illness reported by 456 external action patients in the survey according to enabling factors*

| variable | | plural medical system | | | | | | total | |
|---|---|---|---|---|---|---|---|---|---|
| | | trad. | m.s. | trans. | m.s. | modern | m.s. | | |
| | | N | % | N | % | N | % | N | % |
| *socio-economic status* | | | | | | | | | |
| poor | (1) | 85 | 53.4 | 37 | 23.3 | 37 | 23.2 | 159 | 100.0 |
| average | (2) | 116 | 35.9 | 66 | 20.4 | 141 | 43.7 | 323 | 100.0 |
| well-to-do | (3) | 14 | 32.6 | 12 | 27.9 | 17 | 39.5 | 43 | 100.0 |
| *cost of treatment* | | | | | | | | | |
| free | (1) | 45 | 41.3 | 1 | – | 63 | 57.8 | 109 | 100.0 |
| 0–1 bir | (2) | 93 | 53.1 | 55 | 31.4 | 27 | 15.5 | 175 | 100.0 |
| 2–5 bir | (3) | 61 | 35.3 | 54 | 31.2 | 58 | 33.5 | 173 | 100.0 |
| 6–10 bir | (4) | 3 | – | 3 | – | 4 | – | 10 | 100.0 |
| 10+ bir | (5) | 13 | 22.8 | 1 | 1.8 | 43 | 75.4 | 57 | 100.0 |

## *7.1.2 Enabling factors*

Enabling factors, as Chapter 2 explained, include parameters which in principle cannot be changed by the individual but rather depend on the social and economic sub-systems of the society. These are independent variables which enable the individual to pay for medical treatment in the event of illness such as financial resources, socio-economic status, fees for treatment and cost of transport. For this study, factor analysis was used to determine the socio-economic status (SES) of respondents who were then divided into three classes: poor, average and well-to-do.[2] The amounts paid by patients for treatment were also recorded and divided into four categories. Table 7.2 presents a detailed picture of the pattern of multiple utilisation in 525 cases of illness reported by the 456 external action patients in the sample according to enabling factors.

### Socio-economic status (SES) and fees for treatment

The table shows that respondents in the lowest socio-economic class make most use of the traditional medical system (53.4%) and that the higher the socio-economic status of respondents, the more use they make of the modern medical system (39.5% against 23.2%). In the transitional system, the increase in utilisation in relation to socio-economic status is less marked (from 23.3%, via 20.4% to 27.9%). It is fair to conclude that as the socio-economic status of patients rises, the use they make of the traditional system decreases while utilisation of the modern system increases in proportion.

Turning now to treatment fees paid by respondents in the preceding year, it is remarkable that 41.3% of cases in the traditional system and 57.8% of cases in the modern system were treated free of charge. There were hardly any such cases reported in the transitional system. As far as the traditional system is concerned, this can be explained by the fact that many traditional practitioners in both local and regional sub-systems work 'to the greater glory of God' and in some cases are paid in kind either by the community, by the patient or, more commonly, by his or her lineage group. A relatively high number of cases are treated free of charge in the modern system because patients had been able to obtain poverty certificates via the *kebele* entitling them to free treatment at the clinic.

Table 7.2 further shows that fees for treatment in the modern system ranged from 15.5% below 1 bir to 75.4% which were 10 bir or more; in the traditional system, on the other hand, the percentage went down from 35.3% costing more than 2 bir to 22.8% costing over 10 bir. With the exception of free treatment and therapy costing 10 bir or more, a number of variations can be seen between the distribution of the cost of treatment and utilisation. Although traditional practitioners charged more than 10 bir in almost one-quarter of the cases they treated (22.8%), approximately three-quarters of all cases in this price category were carried out by the modern medical system (75.4%). Since the geographical distribution of both the traditional and modern as well as the transitional health care resources in the highlands roughly overlapped, there emerged no significant variation in the cost of transport – if paid at all – to reach one of the available medical institutions in the research area. By consequence, this variable has not been included in the bivariate analysis of the enabling factors, but will be looked into later on in the context of the factors of the plural medical system.

Table 7.3: *Distribution of multiple health care utilisation in 525 cases of illness reported by 456 external action patients in the survey according to perceived morbidity*

| variable | | plural medical system | | | | | | | |
|---|---|---|---|---|---|---|---|---|---|
| | | trad. | m.s. | trans. | m.s. | modern | m.s. | total | |
| | | N | % | N | % | N | % | N | % |
| *duration of perceived illness* | | | | | | | | | |
| acute | (1) | 145 | 43.1 | 80 | 23.3 | 115 | 33.6 | 355 | 100.0 |
| chronic | (2) | 66 | 36.3 | 34 | 18.7 | 82 | 45.0 | 145 | 100.0 |
| *traditional classification of perceived illness* | | | | | | | | | |
| naturalistic | (1) | 54 | 28.3 | 45 | 24.1 | 89 | 47.6 | 187 | 100.0 |
| personalistic | (2) | 48 | 54.5 | 25 | 28.4 | 15 | 17.1 | 88 | 100.0 |
| unspecified | (3) | 114 | 45.6 | 45 | 18.0 | 91 | 36.4 | 250 | 100.0 |

## *7.1.3 Perceived morbidity factors*

As noted in Chapter 2, the majority of medical anthropological studies have confirmed that the individual's perception of the type of illness is an important determinant of illness behaviour which can be related to differentiation in utilisation of health care services. In the explanatory model for the present study, perceived morbidity is used as an independent variable by means of which the need to utilise health care is initiated. Table 7.3 sets out the pattern of utilisation as revealed by the survey according to perceived morbidity. Here, perceived morbidity is regarded both in terms of acute versus chronic and personalistic versus naturalistic illness episodes.

### Acute and chronic morbidity

The table shows that patients with acute illnesses consult the traditional medical system relatively more frequently than the modern system (43.1% against 33.6%), while those with chronic illnesses tend to use the modern system. It also shows that more acute than chronic illnesses are treated by the transitional medical system. It should be noted that respondents reported that they had consulted the traditional system first in a number of cases of acute illness and had then consulted the modern system later when they needed more time for effective treatment.

### Traditional disease classification

Chapter 2 stressed the importance of classifying perceived illnesses according to the respective etiological concepts of Foster (1983) as naturalistic or personalistic in relation to the health care seeking process in developing countries. Using these categories in the analysis it becomes clear that more reported cases of naturalistic illnesses were treated by the modern system than by the traditional system (47.6% to 28.3%) and that variation in utilisation of traditional and transitional systems to treat illnesses in this category was very slight. Even more striking is the fact that more than half of the perceived cases of personalistic illnesses were treated by traditional practitioners (54.5%) with less than one-fifth (17.1%) being presented to modern medicine. The differentiation between the modern and traditional systems as regards non-specified illnesses is not particularly marked. It is evident that this analysis also confirms a direct relationship between utilisation of a particular system and the local classification of diseases into the two categories described above. This is particularly evident in the choice between modern and traditional health care. The extent of the explanatory value of perceived morbidity for the choice of treatment as compared with other factors will be assessed in the following multivariate analysis in section 7.2.

### *7.1.4 Factors of the plural medical system*

The account in Chapter 2 of the theoretical approach to the process of illness behaviour and health care utilisation used in the present study points to the important role played by the geographical and financial accessibility of medical services. As both factors are equally important to the local population, they could have been retained as constant in the analytical model. Although there are considerable variations between the individual systems as regards, for example, organisation, education of personnel, medical knowledge and practices, etc., the analysis is restricted to the relationship between geographical and financial accessibility and variation in health care utilisation.

First, the geographical accessibility of the various medical systems in the research area would appear to be roughly the same. As noted before, representatives of the various systems live in and around Babile on a permanent basis and various practitioners visit the community, particularly the local market, at fixed times. The household survey found that geographical distance to the three systems in Babile was reported the same for almost all respondents. If, however, particular treatment meant travelling to a health centre or hospital outside the highland area of the community it then became an important factor in illness behaviour.

As the section on the cost of treatment in relation to utilisation explained (Table 7.2), the modern medical system was consistently described by respondents as the most expensive form of health care. If the five categories of reported fees for treatment paid by patients are averaged out and then divided up among the three medical systems, the average financial threshold per system can be calculated and expressed as follows:

| | |
|---|---|
| traditional medical system: | 2.00 bir |
| transitional medical system: | 2.25 bir |
| modern medical system: | 3.50 bir |

The average financial threshold to obtain health care in Babile from the traditional via the transitional to the modern medical system obviously rises from 2.00 bir to 3.50 bir despite the fact that the modern medical system officially includes provision of free treatment for members of the lowest socio-economic class. The possible link between the cost of treatment and variation in utilisation of the systems is reflected in the ways available to individuals of paying for treatment. This has already been described in the analysis of enabling factors. Clearly the cost of modern health care could be reduced by changes in government policy. On the other hand, barring government intervention, treatment fees in the traditional and transitional systems will tend to respond to the free market forces of supply and demand for medical services.

To conclude the bivariate analysis of the research, it can be stated that a relationship exists between a series of separate, pre-selected factors and variation in health care utilisation. As far as predisposing factors are concerned, it is noticeable that the predominantly Muslim women make more use of the traditional medical system than do children, while older men make greater use of the modern system. The level of education of patients also plays a role both in relation to contacts with the transitional system and with the modern medical system, while the possession of medical knowledge is linked with variation in utilisation of the traditional and modern systems. Ethnic affiliation and religion have a most marked effect on utilisation of traditional and modern health care: the Muslim Oromo in particular prefer the traditional system, whereas the Christian Amhara have a strong preference for modern medicine. The similar differentiation in relation to religion justifies the conclusion that there is a specific pattern of utilisation based on the ethnic and religious backgrounds of patients. As far as occupation goes, farmers in the survey make more use of traditional medicine and less of the modern system but the reverse was true for civil servants. Utilisation of the transitional system showed some variation in this connection. The relationship between size of household and utilisation of the medical systems shows that the nuclear family prefers traditional medicine, as do unmarried people and people who have previously been married. With regard to the role of socio-psychological factors in the utilisation of health care, a high rating of both the quality of service and the attitude of staff in the transitional system towards patients is linked with a preference for using this system. There is a less consistent relationship between these factors and utilisation of the modern medical system.

Respondents with a low socio-economic status make greater use of the traditional system whereas the well-to-do prefer modern health care. Respondents able to obtain free treatment from the modern system prefer the modern system but if the cost of treatment is the same up to 10 bir, they make relatively greater use of the traditional system. The modern system accounts for the largest number of cases of treatment costing more than 10 bir. Utilisation of the transitional system shows little variation in relation to financial cost.

As far as perceived morbidity is concerned, patients suffering from chronic diseases consult the modern system more often but those with personalistic and non-specified illnesses make greater use of the traditional system. Finally, despite the recent introduction by the government of the poverty certificate to impecunious patients, the analysis shows that the modern medical system is the most expensive form of health care in the area. This makes it difficult, particularly for members of the lower socio-economic class, to pay for modern health care without financial support from relatives or members of their own ethnic group.

This analysis confirms that the patients within major ethnic groups in Babile show a high degree of similar variation in their utilisation of traditional, transitional and modern health care primarily based on differences in perceived morbidity, sex, age, ethnic background, religion, education, occupation, opinion on the various medical systems and socio-economic status. An interesting point in the context of religion and illness and illness behaviour is the fact that differences exist between the Muslim Oromo and Somali on the one hand and the Christian Amhara and a few Oromo converts on the other, but that there are at the same time strong similarities within these groups with regard to utilisation of health care.

The next section examines how variations in utilisation of the plural medical system in Babile can be explained in terms of the correlation and interaction among variables.

## 7.2 Multivariate Analysis of the Factors in the Model

The results of the aforegoing bivariate analysis of the quantitative data suggest a certain coherence between predisposing factors, enabling factors and perceived morbidity factors on the one hand and factors of utilisation of the plural medical system on the other. Within the first three selected groups of variables, cross-tabulations have also revealed variations in the separate coherence between preselected factors and utilisation. How then do the factors relate to one another with regard to utilisation of the plural medical system?

Once this question is answered, an explanatory model of health care utilisation in this part of Africa can be developed, based on the descriptive analysis of the above section. Such a model examining the relative effects of a number of variables on health care utilisation has already been developed in Chapter 2, by incorporating the various factors into four blocks of independent and dependent variables (cf. Figure 2.3). In this context, however, the structure and inter-relationship of selected variables cannot be explained by mere analysis of cross-tabulations. Indeed, roughly 300 tables would at least be needed to analyse 20 variables and this would be both unwieldy while the identification of significant relationships would be extremely arbitrary.

Following the most widely known efforts to develop a multivariate model of utilisation by Suchman (1965), Anderson (1968), Greenlick *et al.* (1973) and Kohn and White (1976) as noted in Chapter 2, the present explanatory model is based on an advanced type of multivariate analysis: the *non-linear canonical correlation analysis*. The reasons for choosing this particular type of analysis which attempts to prove insight into the relationship between two sets of variables are set out in Appendix 1. It comprises a specific form of multivariate analysis which has been developed by the 'Vakgroep Datatheorie' of the University of Leiden, together with a model and computer programme based on the technique known as CANALS. For a more detailed account see, *i. a.*, De Leeuw (1973), Stoop (1980), Gifi (1981), Van den Burg (1983) and Van den Burg and De Leeuw (1983).

### *7.2.1 Canonical correlation analysis of health care utilisation*

Non-linear canonical correlation analysis of the research data renders it possible for this study to establish the coherence between various background variables and the utilisation of health care in Babile and subsequently to interpret such coherence and incorporate it into an explanatory model. The method can be seen as factor analysis of two sets of variables whereby the factor from the first set should have maximum correlation with the factor from the second set. The correlation between the two factors is called *canonical correlation (r)*. There is a second way in which the canonical correlation can be interpreted. If the number of variables from the second set consists of one single variable, then a weighted combination of variables from the first set is chosen which has maximum correlation with one variable from the second set. In such cases, canonical correlation is similar to multiple regression.

In order to apply the CANALS-programme on the quantitative data of the household survey, a canonical correlation model of utilisation for the total number of variables in the blocs in the analytical model must first be produced schematically. This is done by subjecting the individual variables of the 'external action' patients in the sample and reported utilisation of health care to a non-linear canonical correlation analysis. Beforehand, however,

14 individuals were removed from the file as 'outliers' tending to dominate the solution[3]. In addition, a limited reduction of the number of categories of variables was introduced to facilitate processing.

In this way, the block of predisposing variables comprises: SEX: *sex* (1), (1 = male, 2 = female); ETHN: *ethnic* affiliation (2) (1 = Oromo, 2 = Amhara); EDUC: *education* (3), (1 = none, 2 = some); RELIG: *religion* (4), (1 = Muslim, 2 = Christian); OPTRA: *opinion on the quality of the transitional system*(5), (1 = poor, 2 = average, 3 = good); ATTRA: *opinion on the attitude of transitional staff* (6), (1 = poor, 2 = average, 3 = good); OPMOD: *opinion on the quality of the modern system* (7), (1 = poor, 2 = average, 3 = good); ATMOD = *opinion on the attitude of modern health care staff* (8), (1 = poor, 2 = average, 3 = good); HUW: *marital status* (9), (1 = married, 2 = unmarried); HHOMV: *size of household* (10), (1 = 1–3, 2 = 4+); PROF: *occupation* (11), (1 = farmer, 2 = civil servant, 3 = other); AGE: *age* (12), 1 = 0–15, 2 = 16–25, 3 = 26–45, 4 = 46–65, 5 = 65+); MEDK; *medical knowledge* (13): (1 = none, 2 = some).

The perceived morbidity block includes the following variables: CHRON: *duration of the illness episode* (14), 1=0–1 month, 2=1+ month) and PMCL: *traditional disease classification* (15), (1 = naturalistic, 2 = personalistic, 3 = non-specified). The block of enabling factors consists of SES: *socio-economic status* (16), (1 = poor, 2 = average, 3 = well-to-do). Finally, the block of dependent variables includes TRAD: *the traditional medical system* (17), TRAN: *the transitional medical system* (18) and MOD: *the modern medical system* (19).

Fig. 7.1 shows that if no distinction is made between predisposing variables, enabling variables and variables of perceived morbidity and if they are put in a single block of predictor-variables opposite 'utilisation', relatively high canonical correlations between both sets in the first and second dimension are produced of respectively $r_1 = 0.703$ and $r_2 = 0.471$. In addition, the figure shows that *ethnic affiliation* (ETHN), *religion* (RELIG), *traditional medicine* (TRAD) and *modern medicine* (MOD) play the most important role in the first dimension as does *traditional disease classification* (PMCL) to a smaller extent. The most important variables in the second dimension are *duration of the illness episode* (CHRON), *opinion on the attitude of transitional medical staff* (ATTRA),

| correlations 1. dim. | correlations 2. dim. | variables | values 1. dim. | values 2. dim. |
|---|---|---|---|---|
| −0.045 | 0.007 | SEX | −0.063 | 0.065 |
| 0.525 | 0.051 | ETHN | 0.416 | 0.013 |
| 0.185 | 0.068 | EDUC | 0.052 | 0.214 |
| 0.514 | 0.072 | RELIG | 0.420 | 0.076 |
| 0.198 | 0.091 | OPTRA | 0.301 | 0.322 |
| −0.013 | −0.222 | ATTRA | 0.030 | −0.526 |
| −0.070 | 0.052 | OPMOD | −0.127 | 0.167 |
| −0.040 | −0.167 | ATMOD | −0.080 | −0.329 |
| 0.145 | 0.075 | HUW | 0.194 | −0.199 |
| −0.001 | −0.001 | HHOMV | 0.047 | −0.073 |
| −0.091 | 0.167 | PROF | −0.253 | 0.354 |
| 0.116 | −0.028 | AGE | 0.010 | 0.167 |
| 0.137 | −0.042 | MEDK | 0.033 | −0.285 |
| 0.099 | −0.254 | CHRON | 0.091 | −0.621 |
| −0.239 | 0.016 | PMCL | −0.357 | 0.057 |
| 0.212 | 0.033 | SES | 0.158 | 0.003 |

predictor variables

(r1 = 0.703)

(r2 = 0.471)

'utilisation'

| correlations 1. dim. | correlations 2. dim. | variables | values 1. dim. | values 2. dim. |
|---|---|---|---|---|
| −0.922 | −0.290 | TRAD | −0.666 | −1.543 |
| 0.105 | 0.105 | TRANS | −0.016 | −0.943 |
| 0.843 | −0.416 | MOD | 0.460 | −1.568 |

Figure 7.1: *Schematic representation of canonical correlation for both dimensions ($r_1 = 0.703$; $r_2 = 0.471$) between the first set and the second set of the total number of variables in the survey*

*occupation* (PROF), *opinion on the attitude of modern medical staff* (ATMOD) and on the *quality of the transitional medical system* (OPTRA).

On the basis of the calculated correlations in Figure 7.1, the first dimension confirms the conclusions from the bivariate analysis reflecting the importance of ethnic affiliation, religion and to a smaller extent, traditional and modern medicine. In the second dimension, attention is focussed on the role played by the duration of perceived morbidity and opinions on the attitude of transitional staff by users of the transitional system.

### *7.2.2 Projections of variables and objects in the canonical space*

A further understanding of the complex coherence between variables and their accompanying observations or categories can be obtained by projecting the correlations as points onto the space of the canonical variates known as *canonical space*. If the variable points are geographically connected with zero, a vector diagram is created illustrating the links between the variables and the canonical variates. In addition, the length of the vectors will indicate the relative importance of the variables. In such a diagram the vectors point in the direction of a high score, measured from zero on the plot.

Figure 7.2 shows the plot of the 19 optimally scaled variables from the survey data in the canonical space of the second solution. The utilisation variables have been projected onto the space of the 16 predictor variables. From the plot it is clear that the traditional and modern system form the first dimension. From all background variables *ethnic affiliation* (ETHN) and *religion* (RELIG) express the strongest coherence with the first dimension. This is not surprising in view of the fact that *ethnic affiliation* (ETHN) and *religion* (RELIG) are closely related to the contrast between utilisation of the *traditional* (TRAD) and the *modern medical system* (MOD) which was also indicated in the bivariate analysis.

It is noticeable that background variables such as sex (SEX), *age* (AGE) and *size of household* (HHOMV) do not really play any role in the interaction analysis; the vectors are relatively short and the directions in question are extremely divergent. Other important variables in the first dimension are *opinion on the quality of the*

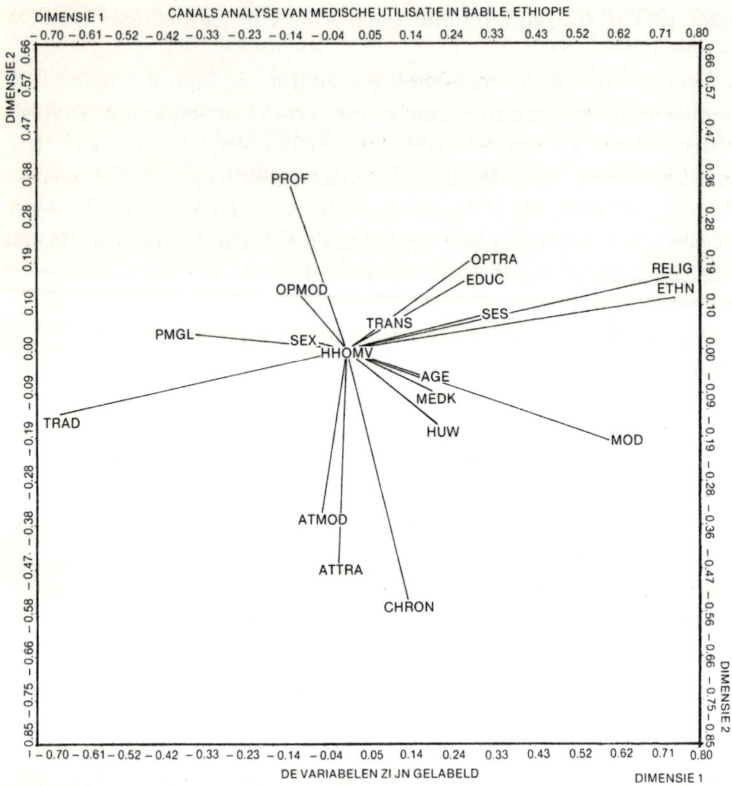


Figure 7.2: *CANALS analysis of health care utilisation in Babile: Projection of the optimally scaled variables onto the canonical space of the second solution (variables are labelled)*

*transitional system* (OPTRA), *traditional disease classification* (PMLC), *education* (EDUC) and *socio-economic status* (SES). The variable *traditional disease classification* (PMLC) strongly points in the direction of the *tradition medical system* (TRAD), which can be explained from the category quantifications of traditional disease classification. This variable is categorised: 1 = naturalistic; 2 = personalistic and 3 = non-specified. The quantification of CANALS proves to ascribe the following corresponding values to the categories: naturalistic = −1.26, non-specified = 0.4 and personalistic = 1.4. This means that in the plot the category personalistic diseases is projected on the outer end of the vector indicating that patients suffering from personalistic diseases are most likely to use the traditional medical system.

Although variables such as *sex* (SEX), *size of household* (HHOMV) and *age* (AGE) play a relatively limited role in the first dimension in relation to traditional and modern medicine, the categories concerned point in the direction of utilisation of the *modern medical system* (MOD). For example, men make relatively more use than women of modern medicine and, as people get older, they tend to make more use of the modern system. The category quantifications of *age* (AGE) show that only the youngest age group (0–15) has a quantification different from the rest, indicating that when children fall ill they initially tend to use the traditional medical system. The same applies to *marital status* (HUW): married people are more likely to use the *modern medical system* (MOD) than unmarried people. Another group of background variables which expresses interaction with utilisation of the traditional as opposed to the modern medical system in the first dimension is made up of *education* (EDUC), *socio-economic status* (SES) and *opinion on the quality of the transitional medical system* (OPTRA). As *opinion on the transitional medical system* (OPTRA) becomes more positive, *education* (EDUC) increases and *socio-economic status* (SES) is higher, utilisation of the *transitional medical system* (TRANS) tends to increase proportionally.

Figure 7.2 also shows a certain correlation between *opinion on attitude of transitional staff* (ATTRA) and *opinion on the attitude of modern staff* (ATMOD). However, since these variables are at right angles to the variables from the first dimension, it must be concluded that they do not have predictive value for utilisation of traditional and modern health care. Some users of traditional and modern health care would appear to have changing opinions about the quality and attitude of the staff in both systems. The category quantifications seem to have undergone changes here too.

The second dimension of Figure 7.2 is characterised by utilisation of the *transitional medical system* (TRANS). Two groups of variables show a strong coherence with this type of utilisation: *duration of illness episode* (CHRON), *opinion on the attitude of transitional staff* (ATTRA) and *opinion on the attitude of modern staff* (ATMOD) on the one hand and *occupation* (PROF), *opinion on the quality of the transitional system* (OPTRA) and *opinion on the quality of the modern system* (OPMOD) on the other. As *duration of illness episode* (CHRON) increases, so utilisation of transitional medicine declines. *Occupation* (PROF) also plays an important role in relation to utilisation of the transitional medical system; patients are more likely to use this system if they are members of the armed forces or civil servants rather than if they are farmers.

As the bivariate analysis has already shown, *opinion on the quality of the modern system* (OPMOD) does not show substantial interaction with utilisation of modern as opposed to traditional medicine. *Opinion on the attitude to the transitional system* (OPTRA), on the other hand, does have a correlation with utilisation of the actual system.

As has been indicated above, the vectors of socio-psychological variables from the second dimension (OPTRA, ATTRA, OPMOD and ATMOD) are being projected at right angles to the first dimension, suggesting that they play hardly any role in the prediction of utilisation of the modern medical system. In this connection similar projections of the vectors of *occupation* (PROF) and *duration of illness episodes* (CHRON) from the second dimension indicate that they similarly cannot optimally predict utilisation of the traditional or modern medical systems.

The results from the plot of the canonical correlation analysis in Figure 7.2 for both dimensions can be summarised as follows. First of all, as far as the first dimension is concerned, a very strong correlation emerges between ethnic affiliation and religion versus utilisation of the traditional as opposed to the modern medical system. Then, the plot shows for the second dimension a significant interaction between socio-economic status, education and opinion on the quality of the transitional system and the utilisation of transitional medicine. In other words, ethnic groups, religion and classification of perceived morbidity are the most important *predictors* of utilisation of traditional and modern medicine while the level of education and socio-economic status of patients constitute the best *predictors* of utilisation of transitional medicine.

Since the variables of ethnic affiliation and religion as well as the traditional classification of disease with regard to the process of health care utilisation clearly relate to the two major ethno-cultural groups in the highlands, the Muslim Oromo and the Christian

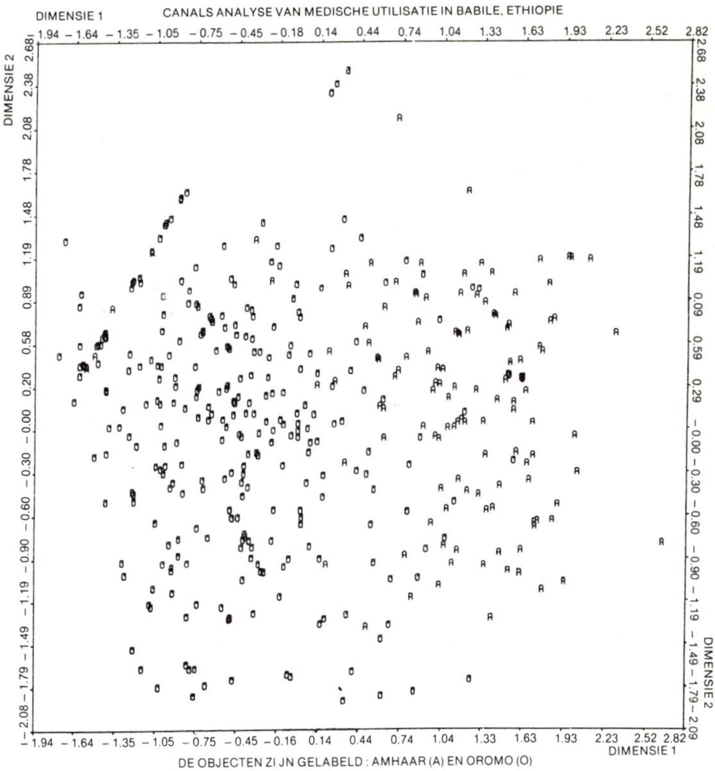


Figure 7.3: *Projection of patients onto the canonical space, specified according to the two major ethnic groups in Babile. Objects are labelled: Oromo (O) and Amhara (A)*

Amhara, it is illustrative here to itemise and amplify the projection of individual patients from both groups onto the canonical space as plotted O's and A's in Figure 7.3. Here the position of each patient is a function of his scores on all variables. This figure clearly shows that the Oromo are projected mainly in the left segment of the canonical space in which the traditional medical system is plotted (cf.

Figure 7.2) whereas the Amhara are mainly projected in the right segment in which the modern medical system is located. In the central area of the canonical space where the transitional system is operational, Amhara as well as Oromo have been plotted, indicating an overlap of the two ethnic groups in utilisation of this system. The existence of a strong interaction and prediction in the first dimension between the two groups vis à vis the traditional and modern system is confirmed in a convenient fashion by this projected configuration of the patients concerned.

### *7.2.3 The analytical model: stepwise non-linear multiple regression analysis*

In the preceding sections, multivariate analysis has covered all the variables in the survey without discriminating between variables or blocks of variables. Certain conclusions have been drawn on correlation, interaction and predictability using canonical correlation analysis of the total number of 19 variables.

Since the objective of the study includes the development of an explanatory model of health care utilisation, multivariate analysis should now be used to examine the correlation among the blocks of predisposing factors, factors of perceived morbidity and enabling factors and determine the interaction with the factors of utilisation of the plural medical system in the model. The obvious way to do this would be to develop a pathway model using non-linear partial canonical correlation analysis (PARTHALS, cf. Van den Burg and De Leeuw 1983). However, since this programme is still being developed, another way needs to be found of determining the relative importance of each of the three blocks of variables vis à vis utilisation. As was mentioned in Section 7.2 on the introduction of the CANALS programme, with a single variable in the second set, CANALS can be regarded as a multiple regression analysis. An additional complication as far as the present research is concerned is the fact that 3 (instead of 1 dichotome) dependent variables have been incorporated into the model. However, as will be demonstrated below, the correlations and values are not affected to any appreciable extent, which indicates the existence of a rather stable block of utilisation. This stability justifies the introduction of a stepwise multiple regression analysis using the CANALS programme. Moreover, as regards content, this block from the model

Table 7.4: *Stepwise CANALS analysis, with utilisation of the plural medical system (TRAD; TRANS; MOD) in the second set*

| variables | blocks | correlation of 1st dimension | | | regression values of 1st dimension | | | correlations of 2nd dimension | | | regression values of 2nd dimension | | |
|---|---|---|---|---|---|---|---|---|---|---|---|---|---|
| TRAD | health | 0.941 | 0.926 | 0.922 | 0.759 | 0.661 | 0.666 | 0.276 | 0.293 | 0.290 | 1.417 | 1.540 | 1.543 |
| TRANS | care | 0.125 | 0.123 | 0.105 | 0.060 | 0.005 | 0.016 | 0.297 | 0.117 | 0.105 | 0.694 | 0.930 | 0.943 |
| MOD | util. | 0.811 | 0.837 | 0.843 | 0.362 | 0.463 | 0.460 | 0.530 | 0.420 | 0.416 | 1.538 | 1.566 | 1.568 |
| SEX | pre- | 0.044 | 0.044 | 0.045 | 0.092 | 0.056 | 0.063 | 0.014 | 0.007 | 0.007 | 0.135 | 0.068 | 0.065 |
| ETHN | disposing | 0.527 | 0.525 | 0.525 | 0.483 | 0.415 | 0.416 | 0.016 | 0.051 | 0.051 | 0.091 | 0.011 | 0.013 |
| EDUC | variables | 0.189 | 0.186 | 0.185 | 0.090 | 0.083 | 0.052 | 0.057 | 0.068 | 0.068 | 0.210 | 0.211 | 0.214 |
| RELIG | | 0.517 | 0.514 | 0.514 | 0.440 | 0.470 | 0.420 | 0.040 | 0.073 | 0.072 | 0.179 | 0.070 | 0.076 |
| OPTRA | | 0.203 | 0.197 | 0.198 | 0.327 | 0.285 | 0.301 | 0.093 | 0.092 | 0.091 | 0.442 | 0.341 | 0.322 |
| ATTRA | | 0.006 | 0.008 | 0.013 | 0.007 | 0.033 | 0.030 | 0.212 | 0.221 | 0.222 | 0.633 | 0.544 | 0.526 |
| OPMOD | | 0.103 | 0.091 | 0.070 | 0.197 | 0.163 | 0.127 | 0.005 | 0.015 | 0.052 | 0.294 | 0.150 | 0.167 |
| ATMOD | | 0.023 | 0.096 | 0.040 | 0.010 | 0.049 | 0.080 | 0.169 | 0.166 | 0.167 | 0.526 | 0.354 | 0.329 |
| HUW | | 0.139 | 0.144 | 0.145 | 0.005 | 0.211 | 0.194 | 0.094 | 0.076 | 0.075 | 0.213 | 0.144 | 0.199 |
| HHOMV | | 0.000 | 0.000 | 0.001 | 0.050 | 0.045 | 0.047 | 0.001 | 0.001 | 0.001 | 0.129 | 0.076 | 0.073 |
| PROF | | 0.136 | 0.093 | 0.091 | 0.306 | 0.298 | 0.253 | 0.128 | 0.153 | 0.167 | 0.355 | 0.305 | 0.354 |
| AGE | | 0.143 | 0.073 | 0.116 | 0.203 | 0.054 | 0.010 | 0.092 | 0.005 | 0.028 | 0.080 | 0.136 | 0.167 |
| MEDK | | 0.134 | 0.137 | 0.137 | 0.039 | 0.057 | 0.033 | 0.053 | 0.042 | 0.042 | 0.302 | 0.274 | 0.285 |
| CHRON | perc. | | 0.099 | 0.099 | | 0.063 | 0.091 | | 0.254 | 0.254 | | 0.629 | 0.621 |
| PMCL | morb. var. | | 0.238 | 0.239 | | 0.354 | 0.357 | | 0.014 | 0.016 | | 0.056 | 0.057 |
| SES | enabl. var. | | | 0.212 | | | 0.158 | | | 0.033 | | | 0.033 |
| MC | | 0.667 | 0.703 | 0.703 | | | | 0.371 | 0.463 | 0.471 | | | |

refers to utilisation of the overall plural medical system which includes traditional, transitional and modern health care. Accordingly, such stepwise multiple regression analysis with CANALS enables the assessment of the contribution of the three blocks of variables in predicting utilisation patterns of health care.

The following multiple regression analyses have been carried out. Per step, the block of health care utilisation is predicted first from an increasing group of successively predisposing variables, then from predisposing variables enlarged with variables of perceived morbidity, and finally from predisposing variables and variables of perceived morbidity enlarged with the variable socio-economic status.

The implementation of this type of stepwise analysis should pay attention to the appearance of *multi-collinearity*; by adding new variables to the predicting variables, sharp changes in regression values can occur rendering certain instability in these values. Stoop (1980: 101–103) points to the difficulty of interpreting results in such cases.

Table 7.4 contains the results of the analysis on predicting utilisation by the patients in the survey from an increasing number of background variables. It shows from left to right respectively the variables, the correlations and the regression values from the first and second dimensions while the bottom line states the multiple regression-coefficients. The values and correlations are otherwise given without signs. Each column is the result of a separate analysis. The first column refers to the first block of background variables, the second column to two blocks with a total of 15 variables and finally the third column refers to three blocks with a total of 16 background variables. Analogously to the secondary analysis of the data from the '*Van Jaar tot Jaar*' study by De Leeuw and Stoop (1979) and the stepwise CANALS analysis by Stoop (1980), the following inferences can be made with regard to the different blocks from the analytical model for this study.

First, the three variables of health care utilisation are again predicted to a large extent by the three blocks of variables. The multiple correlation-coefficient goes steadily up with a stepwise increase in the number of variables per block from 0.667 via 0.703 to 0.703 in the first dimension and from 0.371 via 0.463 to 0.471 in the second dimension. The contribution is therefore most substantial in the second dimension. Subsequently, it is evident that intro-

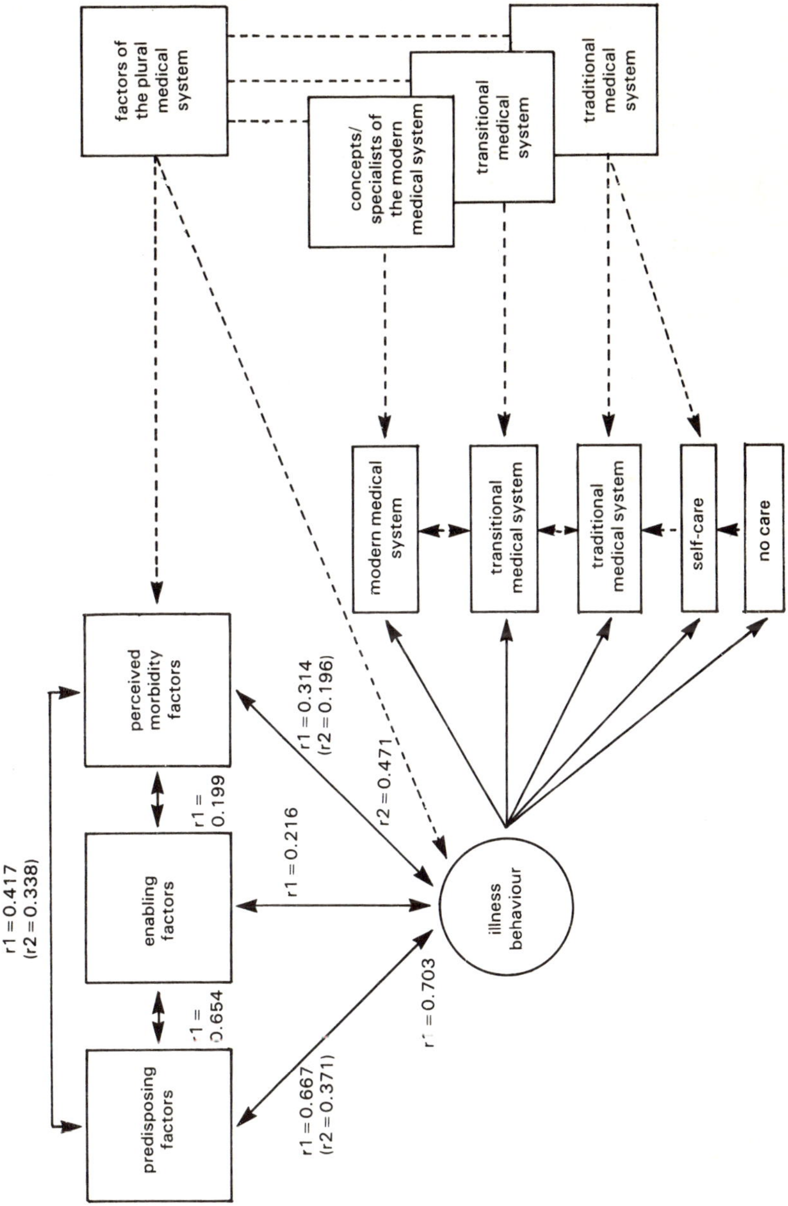


*calculated correlation coefficients are indicated separately*

duction of new groups of variables to the analysis has virtually the same effect on correlations and values, which indicates a relatively stable result.

However, this stepwise multiple regression analysis has not as yet made it clear whether perceived morbidity has a large *overlap* with predisposing factors, as a result of which the multiple correlation-coefficient is barely raised. To establish whether there is overlapping, a separate CANALS analysis was carried out between perceived morbidity and utilisation of the plural medical system. The multiple correlation-coefficient here is $r_1 = 0.314$, $r_2 = 0.196$ which most remarkably confirms that predisposing factors make a direct contribution to health care utilisation independent of perceived morbidity. These and the remaining calculated canonical correlations between the four blocks of factors from the explanatory model are presented in Figure 7.4. This figure establishes the ultimate model of transcultural health care utilisation as completed on the base of successive analyses of quantitative data from the sample survey in Babile.

*Ethnic affiliation* (ETHN), *religion* (RELIG) and *traditional disease classification* (PMCL) emerge from the analyses as the variables in the first dimension which contribute most towards prediction of health care utilisation from the second set. The highest correlations were found in utilisation of the traditional and modern medical systems in the final analysis: 0.992 and 0.843. In the second set of variables, *opinion on the attitude of transitional staff* (ATTRA) and *size of household* (HHOMV), however, make virtually no contribution to predicting utilisation. Closer examination of the regression values of the predictors *ethnic affiliation* (ETHN), *religion* (RELIG) and *traditional disease classification* (PMCL) from the first dimension shows that despite a strong coherence among these variables, there is no multi-collinearity. Values remain stable after addition of variables from the various blocks, which actually strengthens the interpretation.

Although the variables *occupation* (PROF) and *age* (AGE) have not been included in the interpretation of the analyses because of their relatively low correlations, it should be pointed out that multi-collinearity does occur here. These two variables have a high correlation with *traditional disease classification* (PMCL) as a result of which, after addition of the other variables, the regression value of *age* (AGE) decreases considerably from 0.203 to 0.010. Such instability in the regression values of these two variables could therefore jeopardise any possible interpretation of this solution.

As regards the second dimension, which largely reflects utilisation patterns of the transitional medical system, Table 7.4 shows that *duration of illness episode* (CHRON) makes the greatest contribution towards prediction of this type of utilisation.

As the previous analyses have shown, the possible contributions to the prediction of utilisation by the variables *opinion on the attitude of transitional staff* (ATTRA) and *opinion on the attitude of modern staff* (ATMOD) cannot be interpreted because of the occurrence of multi-collinearity. Both variables correlate strongly with utilisation. After addition of the other variables, the value of the variable *opinion on the attitude of modern staff* (ATMOD) goes down more sharply than the value of *opinion on the attitude of transitional staff* (ATTRA). In view of the possibility of misleading or erroneous inferences, efforts to further interpretation of the importance of the first of these variables should be abandoned.

Finally, the stepwise multiple regression analyses confirm that prediction of utilisation of traditional and modern medicine in the first dimension is strongly dominated by ethnic affiliation and religion from the block of predisposing factors. After addition of the block of perceived morbidity variables, the predictability of utilisation increases slightly in which the traditional disease classification plays a particularly important role. The inference therefore is that in itself, the block of perceived morbidity has a low predictive value in relation to utilisation, from which it may be concluded that predisposing factors exercise a rather independent influence on health care utilisation in Babile. It is also striking that addition of the block of enabling factors does not make any contribution towards utilisation in the first dimension, while in the second dimension the contribution is also small, from 0.463 to 0.471.

The result of the corresponding analyses for the second dimension, which reflects utilisation of the transitional medical system in particular, shows that the block of predisposing variables similarly makes a strong contribution to the prediction of health care utilisation of this system. Within this block, *opinion on the attitude of transitional staff* (ATTRA) is particularly dominant. When the block of perceived morbidity variables is subsequently added, the predictability of transitional utilisation rises. By contrast with health care utilisation for the first dimension, in this latter block of variables, *duration of illness episode* (CHRON) is particularly dominant. Addition of the block of enabling factors, as has previously been noted, increases slightly the predictability for the second dimension.

## 7.3 Interpretation of the Results of the Analyses

In the first part of the chapter, bivariate analysis of data confirmed the description of the significance of the socio-cultural background of patients as a determinant of illness and utilisation behaviours. Multivariate analyses then considerably increased the prospect of developing a model to explain and predict patterns of health care utilisation in the plural community of Babile. In addition to such insight into the overall coherence between background variables and utilisation of the available health care systems, subsequent canonical correlation analysis established a relatively high correlation between the two (cf. Figure 7.1). A two-dimensional configuration of both sets of variables from the model could then be projected onto the canonical space. This technique made it not only possible to identify the most important background variables, but it also enabled specification of interaction among certain groups of variables in relation to utilisation of the three medical systems as well as the direction in which the category quantifications of the variables concerned increase (cf. Figure 7.2).

The results of the canonical correlation analysis strongly indicate that two of the predisposing factors, ethnic affiliation and religion are accurate predictors of utilisaton of both the traditional and modern systems, followed by perceived illness. The qualitative research shows that the Oromo who refer to the traditional system mainly use the local Cushitic and regional Arabic sub-systems, although this has not been further examined in quantitative terms. The Somali tend to follow the same pattern. The Amhara, on the other hand, reported only sporadic utilisation of the regional Amhara system. The majority of patients from the latter ethnic group reported a high level of utilisation of the modern system in Babile.

A number of techniques can be used to interpret these differences in utilisation according to ethnic group and religion more closely. The relevance of socio-cultural factors as major determinants of illness and utilisation behaviours was noted already in Chapter 2, based on the great number of relevant studies. As perception of illness is culturally defined, differences in perception tend to affect utilisation of health care in a differential way as well. These differences emerging from previous studies have been abundantly confirmed by the present research; they concern primarily traditional disease classification, etiology and the manner in which symptoms are being experienced. Again, the socio-cultural context is in evidence here. Yet, multiple regression analysis showed ethnicity and religion to explain differences in utilisation directly. These results admit of an alternative interpretation, inasmuch as tolerance levels towards utilisation of traditional cures may very well differ among Muslim Oromo and Somali on the one hand and Christian Amhara on the other, within their respective cultural identities. Indeed, qualitative research yielded some evidence in this direction. Ecclesiastical precept of Ethiopean Christianity for instance, is far less tolerant of superstition, amulets and magic than Islam's 'Great-Tradition', which to a certain extent allows incorporation of culture traits of the 'Little-Tradition', including such elements of the local medical (sub) system.

Furthermore, the concept of the plural society discussed earlier on, which is applicable to the research area, permits the interpretation that diverse sub-groups are not only socio-culturally differentiated, but that such plural characteristics also refer to the differential way in which means of production and political power have been incorporated. Such means include also the formal health care resources in Ethiopia predominantly in the hands of the Amhara groups who in Babile tend to use them most.

The picture of ethno-cultural contrasts, mentioned in the previous discussion of post-revolutionary Ethiopian society, obviously seems to occur again in the field of health and healing. For instance, Figure 7.3, which clearly confirms the importance of the socio-cultural predictors, ethnic affiliation and religion for health care utilisation, has visualised a strong differentiation in the projection of the rather opposite configuration of dots onto the canonical space depicting Oromo and Amhara patients in the survey.

Canonical correlation analysis disclosed duration of illness episode, opinion on the attitude of transitional staff as well as the occupation of household heads to be the most important predictors for utilisation of that system. The household survey yielded information on transitional healers reputedly offering potent medicines for several acute diseases, which is most probably connected with the commercial use of transitional and modern medicine such as drugs and antibiotics. Mutual trust would seem to mark relationships observed between these transitional healers and the local population as they meet in shops and in the marketplace. The role of profession of household head in the choice of utilisation of transitional medicine evidently shows a strong coherence with the fact that those who are not employed in agriculture, are less inclined to turn to the traditional medical system; they would sooner avail themselves of the transitional or modern systems.

Finally, the stepwise, non-linear multiple regression analysis has rendered feasible the development of an explanatory model of health care utilisation showing, incidentally, the stepwise approach in the analysis and the choice of the model in terms of components or blocs of variables to have been warranted for the present research. Within these blocs, moreover, dominant predictors for utilisation could be further identified.

Among the major conclusions corroborated by these analyses of the quantitative field data is the confirmation that the health care seeking process first and foremost is dominated by socio-cultural background characteristics such as ethnicity and religion and subsequently by perceived morbidity factors, comprising duration of illness episode and traditional disease classification. The current approach in most medical-anthropological studies on illness and utilisation behaviours to consider the type of perceived morbidity as '*the principal determinant of use*' (Kohn and White) (1976: 13) in usually homogeneous societies has evidently to be readjusted for the health care seeking process in a plural society such as Babile.

The differential use of the traditional versus the modern medical system in the region studied is dominated by ethnic-religious dissimilarity between the Christian Amhara and the Muslim Oromo and their kindred Somali. Although it is true that variation in utilisation in Babile can be explained by evoking varied perception of illness and the respective etiological conception, the ethnic-religious factor prevails in the whole process rather independently. In this context, the analysis further showed the enabling factor socio-economic status to be a more minor predictor for health care utilisation than expected for the situation in the highlands.

Since, in the multi-ethnic society studied, the perception of illness episode does not emerge as the most important determinant of health care utilisation, one might expect perceived morbidity to gain influence as the predictors ethnicity and religion are held constant. Such experiment in actually 'neutralising' the heterogeneous character of the household survey in Babile in a multivariate analysis of each single ethno-cultural group has indeed increased substantially the predictive value of the type of illness, thus confirming the argument that such groups play a crucial role in the choice of therapy.

Kroeger (1983) in his review of contemporary literature on illness behaviour and utilisation in developing countries, observes that there seem to be two schools of thought, followed by medical anthropologists and non-western sociologists respectively. Some researchers stress predisposing factors and traditional concepts of illness, whereas others mainly focus on enabling factors in the explanation of health care utilisation.

As the present study shows the plural character of a society to be a prime condition for predisposing factors to determine the health care seeking process, as against perceived morbidity, it would be interesting to investigate elsewhere in Africa, and for that matter, in the Third World whether, and to what extent, the conclusions arrived at in the Horn of Africa hold for plural societies in general.

## Notes

1. Since the 1974 revolution the Central Government introduced free health care for the poor. Members of households earning less than 30 bir annually qualify for a poverty certificate.
2. Factor analysis was undertaken in order to determine 'socio-economic status' of respondents by using the following variables: type and state of housing; income of head of household; size of land owned; number of sheep and goats owned; heads of cattle, donkeys owned. Subjective impressions of the interviewers were taken into account. The categorisation chosen was: 'well-to-do', 'average' and 'poor' (cf. Van de Geer 1971; Rademaker 1978).
3. Analysis of the data showed fourteen persons on the random sample to report significantly erratic behaviour. Further research proved them to be non-systematic 'outliers', not representing any sort of specific groups (cf. Cook and Weisberg 1982: 2).

8

# Conclusions and Implications

## 8.1 Conclusions

Since the end of the Second World War a great many strategies aiming at amelioration of health care have been introduced and implemented in the Third World. Yet, after more than forty years, the objective of optimal physical, mental and social well-being for the population at large has not been achieved. Even in the West, despite spectacular developments in medicine and biology, achievements fall short of the ideal, but in a number of developing countries, especially in the rural areas, health conditions are downright critical. In the Sahel region of Africa, and particularly in Ethiopia and The Horn, this serious situation has recently led to a recrudescence of poverty, hunger and mass starvation as a result of subsequent, extreme drought conditions, prompting world-wide action programmes of emergency food and medicine supplies.

Previous attempts to solve the complex problems associated with health care delivery in Africa, Asia and Latin America have shown social and cultural factors to be pivotal and social scientists have increasingly become involved in the health field. Nor have their efforts been confined to the realms of theoretical interest in the socio-cultural context of health and disease: even since the fifties and sixties applied anthropologists and development sociologists have engaged in efforts to find alternative solutions for health problems in the Third World. In the course of the seventies out of the general field of epidemiology, social scientists developed several areas in socio-cultural epidemiological study, in which particular health problems were related to processes of urbanisation, modernisation and – most promising – health care utilisation.

However, the inadequacy of research methodology and analysis of data, peculiar to the situation in the West is evident whenever instead of 'mainstream' medicine, plural medical systems co-exist, such as is the case in many developing countries. The study of illness and utilisation behaviours here focusses on the sequential steps taken by those seeking treatment. Hence, in the course of the eighties the analysis of health care utilisation has emerged as a core theme in policy-oriented studies. Accordingly, the complex utilisation of traditional, transitional and modern health care systems has engendered a specifically designed and analytical model guiding the research of multiple use of plural medical systems by different ethnic groups.

This ethnomedical study in highland Babile in the centre of the Horn has examined the delicate health care situation among different ethnic groups in a plural community, using both existing historical documents and statistical resources as well as empirical data, gathered in the field over a four years' period. Fieldwork encompassed longitudinal, qualitative research on health and healing, supplemented with an extensive household interview survey. The study was carried out as a first follow-up research in the medical social sciences to the joint 'Rural Health in Ethiopia' project between the University of Addis Ababa and the University of Leiden under the auspices of the Netherlands University Foundation for International Cooperation (NUFFIC).

The study has sought to link up on a rather revised ethnomedical perspective to the study of indigenous patterns of medical traditions and behaviour aimed at generating alternative strategies of 'development from the bottom' in rural health care improvement, yielding the results described below.

The general objective was to gain insight into the health care seeking behaviour of members of a plural society and to develop an explanatory model of health care utilisation in a transcultural perspective. Indeed, such a mulitvariate model should not only provide a more profound understanding of the interaction among discrete factors and their relative effects on health care utilisation but would also have predictive value for planning purposes. Factors were to be identified which either impede or, alternatively, encourage patients to avail themselves of services offered. In addition to the theoretical implication of the study, results may provide a base for future policy formulation in terms of facilitating optimal use of appropriate health care services for specific population groups.

Moreover, such a model offers the possibility of complementarity of local, regional and cosmopolitan medical systems, bridging the 'classical gap between ethno-and biomedicine'. Thus, the incorporation of alternative forms of health care in the formal medical system by, for instance, employing traditional and transitional healers would lead to predictable changes in the illness behaviour and eventually more groups of the population could be provided with more relevant care. From this general perspective, a household health survey has been carried out in the multi-ethnic community of Babile in the Eastern Highlands of Ethiopia. In addition to several qualitative studies, a random sample of 1351 respondents provided background information on the health care seeking process of patients from different ethnic groups. To complement the major findings of this study, a number of derived objectives have been cited in the introduction.

*First of all*, an inventory and analytical scheme has been made of various traditional medical practices and perceptions prevailing among different ethnic groups in the area. Also, a typology of healers was conceived in order to describe and classify the diverse health care systems in the research area following Dunn's (1977) classification of local, regional and cosmopolitan medical systems. The peculiar phenomenon of the transcultural process of different medical systems and sub-systems was shown in the outcome of historical events and mutual contacts over centuries between border groups inhabiting the major culture areas of Africa and the Mediterranean. Successive processes of internal differentiation and external interaction among these cultures in the course of history were shown to have evolved into a plural society in Ethiopia and the Horn of Africa. The most remarkable expression of the transculturation process in medicine in the highlands has been the recorded invocation of Muslim healers or 'sheikhs' on genealogical descent of their 'ancestral' preceptor 'Sheikh' Hippocrates. The knowledge and practice of Arabic medicine of such healers or sheikhs and the residual concepts of classical Graeco-Arabic medicine among representatives of the literate, regional Arabic medical system confirm the: '*centuries-old influence of Graeco-Arabic medical culture*' (Young 1982: 23) in the Horn of Africa to this day.

*Secondly*, an indigenous disease classification has been constructed for the two major ethnic groups in the research area: the Amhara and the Oromo. The categorisation *personalistic, naturalistic* and *non-specific diseases* yielded a comprehensive list of names for various diseases, in use with both groups, giving the names with which they are locally called, as well as their etiology as traditionally perceived (cf. Table 4.13). The relevance of this traditional disease classification for illness behaviour has been shown later on in this study.

*Thirdly*, the sequence of stages in the illness and utilisation behaviour has been described over a one year's period of time as reported by patients from a sample survey of 1351 respondents. Here, the rather typical phenomenon of simultaneous or successive use of various medical systems for the same illness episode – 'healer shopping' – became manifest. A total of 525 cases of such multiple utilisation was registered for 456 patients in the sample. Often these patients tend to turn primarily to their 'own' medical (sub) system for treatment, before trying an alternative system. In specific cases, however, such a sequence is upset when circumstances call for deviance: certain diseases prompt patients to consult the alternative system first as, for instance, is the case with acute infections and 'shameful' diseases. The pattern of multiple use appeared to be very complex and some methodological problems had to be solved. Within the traditional system, where professional healers and part-time practitioners were active, a total of 47 'internal' referrals among diverse local and regional medical sub-systems were recorded. The overall pattern of utilisation of the plural medical system varied strongly among diverse ethnic-religious groups. Muslim Oromo and their kindred Somali mostly use the traditional system, whereas the Christian Amhara reported a predilection for the modern system. The phenomenon of a high rate of under-utilisation of modern health care in the highlands was given special attention. Futher analysis showed women and children of Oromo-Somali background to under-utilise the modern medical system most significantly. The same is true in general for those who suffer from diseases considered to be of a personalistic nature. In order to examine and analyse differentiation in reported use of health care, a number of appropriate data analysis techniques have been introduced to specify the interaction and coherence among significant factors vis à vis patterns of utilisation.

Initially, bivariate cross-tabulation analysis yielded identification and description of significant relationships here. Muslim women, for instance, used traditional medicine more often, whereas men preferred the modern medical system. Ethnic and religious factors clearly differentiate the overall utilisation pattern in Babile. Psychosocial factors, such as medical knowledge, opinion on proficiency and attitude of medical personnel were shown to be less decisive than the socio-demographic factors mentioned above. Remarkably, socio-economic status hardly correlated with variation in usage of the plural medical system. Finally, bivariate analysis revealed chronic illness episodes to be presented to the modern medical system more often, whereas personalistic diseases were treated more frequently by traditional healers.

*Fourthly*, in addition to bivariate analysis, it was attempted on the strength of quantitative data of the household survey to initiate a multivariate model of health care utilisation. A non-linear, canonical correlation analysis (CANALS), developed at the University of Leiden rendered practicable the exposition of the interaction and total coherence of all background variables among themselves vis à vis the utilisation of the plural medical system. It then became evident that relatively high correlations were achieved ($r_1 = 0.703$ and $r_2 = 0.471$) so long as the various predictor variables in their mutual relationship vis à vis health care utilisation were left undifferentiated. This result, incidentally, showed the model chosen for the research to be suitable for such transcultural situation of different groups and systems. The sixteen predictor variables and three utilisation variables were later on presented in the form of a spatial projection onto the canonical space, which further enhanced predictive power.

The results of the canonical correlation analysis enabled the explanation of differential utilisation in more detail; also, a number of factors such as ethnicity, religion and traditional disease classification were identified as strong predictive variables. Here the ethnoreligious contrasts which distinguish modern Ethiopian society are also observed as reflecting in the pattern of health care utilisation; a projected cloud of points representing patients in the sample reveals a strongly dichotomous picture of Muslim Oromo and Somali on the one hand, who use the traditional medical system primarily, and the Christian Amhara on the other hand, who present their illness to the modern medical system for treatment (cf. Figure 7.3).

Following certain interpretations of coherence and interaction revealed between a number of factors and differential use based on qualitative data, implementation of a stepwise multiple regression analysis has finally led to refinement of the multivariate utilisation model. Further differentiation was undertaken of the various contributing effects of blocs comprising predisposing factors, enabling factors and factors of perceived morbidity vis à vis utilisation of the plural medical system.

One of the most important conclusions of the multivariate analysis is that, in the plural society of the area, utilisation of transitional and modern health care strongly correlates with ethno-religious differences among patients. Contrary to the often held notion that perceived illness is the major determinant of health care utilisation of one 'mainstream' system or in homogeneous settings, socio-cultural factors of ethnicity and religion in this multi-ethnic society dominate illness behaviour rather independently from perceived morbidity factors (Figure 7.4).

*Finally*, a fifth, derived objective includes the indication of a number of implications for applied medical-anthropological and sociological research in the Horn of Africa, and perhaps in other areas of the Third World. The next paragraph will describe such policy implications both for Ethiopia and The Horn as well as for other developing nations in addition to an overview of the theoretical implications of the study in Babile.

## 8.2 Implications

In addition to the above-mentioned key findings of the study, some implications on both theoretical and policy level will now be presented.

### *8.2.1 Theoretical implications*

As to both continuities and shifts in theoretical orientation in medical anthropology and sociology over the past half-century, the general approach of this study is derived from the ecological model in which health and disease are viewed as relationships between population groups, their cultures and their environments. In order to contribute to the development of a theoretical framework for the comparative study of ethnomedical systems, distinct from the biomedical paradigm, a primarily behavioural basis for cross-cultural comparison has been chosen which concentrates on management of illness episodes within the socio-cultural context of the community. In contrast with previous, rather normative views focussing on either traditional or modern medicine in developing countries, the study links up with the new, more realistic perspective of medical pluralism, in which various medical systems can be conceptualised as pluralistic medical configurations (Leslie 1977, 1980). Such research interest in the plural character of medical systems accommodating a wider variety of traditional, transitional and modern knowledge, perceptions, practices and behaviour related to health and disease has called for a more holistic approach, recently referred to as the 'new' ethnomedical approach. Expanding Hughes' (1968) original but limited definition of the discipline of ethnomedicine in terms of a research interest in predominant indigenous beliefs and practices, more and more scholars tend to include different forms of biomedicine as part of the new ethnomedical approach (Press 1980, Yoder 1982).

As one of the first comparative studies of ethnomedical systems undertaken in Ethiopia, the main contribution of the present study includes establishing that several local and regional medical systems persist alongside pharmaceutical and cosmopolitan medicine, confirming Ethiopia's present pluralistic medical configuration. Based on geo-historical data on successive processes of acculturation, an analytical scheme has been presented on the composition of such medical pluralism in the Horn of Africa in terms of a classification of perceptions, practices and types of healer. Most remarkable in the acculturation process between the 'Great' and 'Little' traditions in medicine, in which local Cushitic, regional Amhara and regional Arabic medicine have constituted the present configuration of the traditional medical system, is the revelation that Muslim 'sheikhs' practice 'prophetic medicine' in their treatment of patients following ancient prescripts of their Arabic medical textbooks, often based on early Syriac translations of classical Greek medical works of Hippocrates, Galen and Paul of Aegina. Sporadic references in such medical books in Babile to the principle of 'Hot-Cold' opposites in food, illness and therapy, the concept of 'life-breath' and alphabetical lists of Graeco-derived names of illnesses and medicaments can be attributed with modest certainty to a process of 'simplification' or 'degeneration' of the Hippocratic system in Africa as a result of culture trait selection, similarly observed in Latin America and South Asia (Logan 1977, Foster 1978).

Indeed, with the influx of Arabic sciences and their religious Muslim overtones during the process of Islamisation of East Africa for centuries, it is not surprising that 'prophetic medicine' has dominated acculturation, emphasising the use of natural products in the treatment of disease according to the revelations of the Prophet. However, 'Sheikh' Hippocrates 'legacy' in the Horn of Africa can be conceived of as the early introduction and adaption of classical Graeco-Arabic perceptions, therapies and medical products to indigenous African medical systems, based on naturalistic principles of humoral medicine. Although within the present ethnomedical configuration in this part of Africa only evidence of a 'stripped down' system has been recorded, research findings strongly support extension of the 'diffusion model' of the humoral theory beyond the cultural areas of Greece, India and China into the coastal plains and highlands of the Horn of Africa. General tolerance of the 'Great Tradition' towards incorporation of the indigenous practices and herbal medicines of the 'Little Tradition' of local Cushitic medicine into the regional Arabic system has reinforced the crucial role that ethno-religious affiliation plays in the choice of therapy among Muslim Oromo and Somali. For the study of health and disease in Africa, a focus on the origin and use of such naturalistic components of ethnomedical systems in a transcultural setting opens new ways to enter a field of study in which medicine becomes increasingly disengaged from the personalistic context of myth, ritual and religion. The study not only confirms O'Leary's (1964) statement on the careful observation and clinical practice of Arab physicians, inherited from the Greeks, but strongly supports Young's (1982) delimitation of the prolonged influence of the Graeco-Arabic medical culture on Ethiopia's practice of medicine, especially operational in the highlands bordering on Somalia.

Research data from the regional Arabic system indicate an important and wide-spread component in the contemporary ethnomedical systems of the Horn of Africa. They certainly invite further ethnohistorical and ethnomedical study of the interactions between contrasting humoral traditions and prophetic medicine of ancient Graeco-Arabic systems on the one hand, and the indigenous systems of Africa on the other hand, in particular in the coastal regions of the Red Sea and the Indian Ocean.

Furthermore, the traditional disease classification, in which folk taxonomies of disease of the two major Oromo and Amhara ethnic groups have been constructed on the base of reported indigenous etiological concepts, lexemes and local names of diseases (Table 4.13) is presented according to Foster's (1983) criteria of 'personalistic' versus 'naturalistic' diseases. The quantitative data confirm the conclusion of Yoder (1982: 15) on the present study of ethnomedicine in Africa as: *'emerging as a domain of research separate from ritual and religion'*. While 35.3% of all patients reported symptom experience of naturalistic diseases, only 20.2% explained 'personalistic' causes of illness during the 12 months' period of the research (Table 6.6).

The classification of medical ideas and practices in Babile has been undertaken from a rather holistic point of view following the ethnomedical approach of Bibeau (1979), Janzen (1978), Warren (1974) and Young (1976) to substantiate the insight into the cognitive aspects of the health care seeking process. In contrast to the cosmopolitan disease classification serving a transcultural reference for diagnosis, both indigenous Oromo and Amhara classifications seem to be confined within the boundaries of the culture area of the Horn of Africa. Although evidence indicates the importance of classification of medical ideas and perceptions for the use of services, considerable allowance should be made for a wider interpretation of such perceptions in terms of worldview, socio-cultural environments and solidarity groups.

Accordingly, the study has examined perceived illness episodes in relation to all actions (or non-action) patients undertake in case of illness, thereby classifying non-action patients, self-care patients and external-action patients in the sample survey. In the analysis of utilisation behaviour the external action patients in particular have subsequently been followed in their course through the different components of the plural medical system. Despite some methodological problems, the approach has enabled the calculation of patterns of differential health care utilisation on systems level resulting from recorded visits of patients. Moreover, the relevant socio-cultural context of both patients and systems has been recorded for the purpose of later analysis of relationships and interactions among pre-selected variables. In this way, the overall pattern of health care utilisation showed a highly differentiated picture, in which typical phenomena such as multiple or concurrent utilisation of various systems ('healer shopping') and under-utilisation of the modern system of health care delivery came to full expression.

The development of the explanatory model for this study was faced with several methodological problems. First of all, it should accommodate the whole range of traditional, transitional and modern medical systems of health care delivery in order to obtain a non-normative, balanced view on utilisation of all available resources on an empirical, in this case 'equal' basis. Thus, a model of transcultural health care utilisation of different medical traditions was designed, based on previous utilisation models of 'mainsteam' medicine of Suchman (1965), Anderson (1968), Greenlick *et al.* (1973) and Kohn and White (1976). The factors of the plural medical system of the model therefore included the concepts of geographical and financial accessibility, labelled with relevant variables, indicators and categories, as shown in Table 2.4. Equally, factors of utilisation of the plural medical system, introduced as dependent variables in the model, were recorded as contacts of patients at system level (Table 2.5).

Secondly, it became clear that the model should not confine itself to descriptive properties of the health care seeking process on a bivariate base, limiting an understanding of differential usage: what is needed is a type of multivariate model explaining the relationships and interactions among relevant variables and their relative importance in utilisation in order to increase the predictive value of the model. To this end, the analytical model includes several categories or 'blocks' of predisposing, enabling and perceived morbidity factors, as worked out in Tables 2.1, 2.2 and 2.3. The eventual model of transcultural health care utilisation, in which the resulting correlation-coefficients have been indicated, is shown in Figure 7.4.

Thirdly, in order to examine the relative effects of a number of determinants of transcultural health care utilisation, a refined multiple regression analysis has been introduced, known as non-linear canonical correlation analysis (CANALS). Subsequent projection of variables onto the canonical space and plotting of patients from different ethnic groups, followed by a further step-wise, non-linear multiple regression analysis has led to a significant conclusion. In contrast with most medical anthropological and sociological studies on utilisation of usually *one type* of 'mainstream' medicine in which perceived morbidity is often shown to be the most important explanatory variable for the patient's choice of treatment, this study strongly supports research stressing the crucial role of the socio-cultural environment of patients in the health care seeking process, such as ethnic or religious groups, lineage groups, residential groups or household groups. As noted above, the ethnographic findings of this study clearly indicate the predominant factor of the residential grouping *ollaa* (Or.) of the Muslim Oromo whose members involve themselves in often cooperative efforts to seek medical treatment for patients from among their groups. Similarly, their fellow Muslim brothers and sisters of the Somali groups primarily activate their clan *reer* (Som.), to find appropriate therapy for their patients. Also Amhara patients tend to consult their household group *beteseb* (Am.), initially to choose and obtain treatment, in which utilisation patterns the type of illness is often secondary to the choice between alternative forms of therapy. Eventually, as the findings of the research strongly indicate that patients from among the different ethno-religious groups in the highlands of Babile tend to turn to specific types of available medical systems or healers to find suitable remedy, explanation for such particular illness behaviour should complete this study.

Several studies have provided general explanations for preference among sub-groups to turn to specific types of treatment which are often universally applicable across such groupings. In Chapter 2 explanations were mentioned, such as the difference and availability of certain types of services, variation in cost of treatment, contrasting 'cultures' between patients and healers, the onset of culture-specific syndromes often caused by 'personalistic' disease agents, applications of special religious practices in healing and contrasting language use in clinical settings.

In the African context of the Horn, in-depth health interview surveys conducted among respondents of the main ethnic groups in Babile have resulted in findings clarifying the transcultural pattern of utilisation, observed within these groups. These explanations for sub-group-specific behaviour seem to be limited to the members of the ethno-cultural groups in the research area, although wider application is often indicated. Within the Oromo residential groupings based on lineage (Or. *ollaa*), the response to illness is largely determined by collective interpretation of symptoms and cooperative action after the complaint has been diagnosed. Although Oromo households rarely comprise members who are not immediate kin, consultation and illness management usually happens within the wider corporate body of the *ollaa*. This lineage system limits itself not only to diagnosis and choice of treatment but in some cases raises money for fees and medicines. Similar practice is used among the settled Somali groups in Babile, where *reer* performs collective duties such as the care of their patients.

Unlike the Oromo household, the Amhara *beteseb* usually form larger homesteads containing several related families and retainers. As these groupings are actually politico-economic units whose members perform specific tasks according to sex, age, etc., authority is executed by a senior male. In addition to daily tasks such as ploughing, harvesting, herding, carrying water, cutting wood, etc., the type of illness and choice of therapy is usually determined by the household authority. As the households of the Amhara group in Babile have been connected through their ethno-religious and socio-political relationships since their arrival from the turn of the century onwards, it is clear, that consultation and treatment of patients similarly take place within these groups.

In sum, while the Oromo and their related Somali ethnic groups in the highlands functionalise their *ollaa* and *reer* as 'collective associations' (Levine 1974) for the predominant traditional treatment of their patients, the Christian Amhara tend to refer to their *beteseb* in case of illness, in which a rather 'individualistic association' (Levine 1974) determines the appropriate kind of action towards recovery.

The effects of socio-cultural relationships within groups on patterns of illness behaviour have earlier been found in class and caste differences affecting access and utilisation of health services (Simmons 1958, Foster 1958, Erasmus 1961, Lieban 1967). Also, factionalism, family, kinship and similar solidarity factors among individuals have shown a differentiating effect in disease management in several settings (Foster 1958, Kunstadter 1960 and Weaver 1970). This result has been supported by research undertaken by, *inter alia*, Ludwig and Gibson (1969: 125 – 133) who arrived at similar conclusions for the role of illness perception among two diverse groups in the U.S. Later on, several comparative studies have indicated such variation among ethnic sub-groups in their health and illness behaviours (Bullough 1972; Spicer 1977; Weidman 1978). Also, differences in health care practices among various ethnic groups have been examined by Hill (1973) and Hand (1976). In addition to Lieberson's (1963), Kantrowitz's (1973) and Kain's (1975) coherent research findings on the indirect influence of ethnic residential segregation on health care utilisation, Harwood (1981) notes a similar preference among different ethnic sub-groups for 'social' treatment by usually 'non-mainstream' healers. As for the African context, Janzen (1978) found equally strong ethno-cultural factors in the healing process among the Bakongo in Lower Zaire indicating similar types of collectiveness in the group-specific approach to illness, employing his useful concept of 'therapy management group'.

The general conclusion, that the predominant significance of the type of illness and the related etiological concepts in the health care seeking process would seem to be thwarted by strong ethno-religious factors of sub-groups in Africa appears to warrant further study of transcultural health care utilisation in comparable situations elsewhere.

### *8.2.2 Policy Implications*

Although major changes have taken place over the past decade guided by international organisations such as WHO, UNICEF and UNFPA, the global situation in 1985 indicated that half the world's population was still living and dying without regular access to some form of adequate services. In spite of the introduction of the PHC-strategy in 1978 aimed at 'Health for All by the year 2000' and its incorporation into national health policies in most developing nations, access by all to an acceptable level of health care before the turn of the century seems, especially in Africa, to remain an uncertain gamble.

This study has analysed the complex problems of health care delivery among different groups in a central area in the Horn of Africa, where in addition to 'common' problems of overpopulation, high morbidity and mortality rates for communicable diseases, unequal social and geographic distribution of services, lack of financial resources, shortage of personnel and inadequate infrastructure, a critical situation of poverty, hunger and starvation has emerged from opposition, violence, war and severe drought in this part of Africa.

In Ethiopia, where, since the revolution of 1974, the central government has been confronted with a wide variety of socio-economic and political problems ranging from a decline in economic growth to political instability and armed struggle with several liberation movements, discussions on the main health question have been dominated by the issue of health care coverage of the total population. In view of such upheavals on top of the generally slender means and inadequate resources, efforts towards successful health care development have so far failed to reach ethnic groups and 'nationalities' in the rural areas, which as the majority of the population continue to rely on their 'own' cultural traditions of medicine.

Based on accumulation of in-depth knowledge of the complex health situation among such groups in the border region of Ethiopia and Somalia, the policy implications of the study in Babile should eventually pertain to a more detailed plan of action, identifying and devoting appropriate services to individuals and groups who have emerged from the analysis as being at special risk of having inadequate health care.

Following previous recommendations for improvement of health care utilisation of modern health services by the Eastern Oromo in Ethiopia and the suggestion for initiation of a medical-sociological project on 'Distance Reduction in Rural Health Care' in Hararghe based on the extension of services and manpower outwards into the villages (Buschkens and Slikkerveer 1982), this study seeks to contribute to a rather ethonomedical approach to the problem of health care coverage of different population groups on the periphery. Indeed, as the afore-going chapters provide detailed information on the different medical perceptions, practices and patterns of behaviour among disinct ethno-religious groups, certain key-findings can be distinguished which could directly bear on the development of guidelines for future policy.

The comparative study of local, regional and cosmopolitan medicine, based on the management of illness episodes, has shown that among the Muslim Oromo and their kindred Somali groups, as well as among the Christian Amhara, the choice of treatment correlates closely with residential lineage and household groups, respectively *ollaa, reer* and *beteseb*, allowing for specific health action geared towards these groupings.

Here, the development of a general risk approach focussed on high-risk groups such as mothers, infants, young children, school children and the elderly (WHO 1978) should be extended into special programmes for specific ethno-religious groups as mentioned above. Beside the necessary expansion and improvement of existing staff and services, national and local planning authorities and policy-makers should seriously take into their consideration the indigenous, socio-cultural context of target communities in terms of design and implementation of *culturally appropriate and integrative health care programmes.* Only such, more relevant programmes are likely to contribute to the delivery of proper care to specific groups, in this way redressing existing inequalities in health and consequently increasing community involvement and the participation of individuals and their families within and between ethno-religious boundaries.

The complex problem of under-utilisation of the modern health care system, in particular, can be addressed effectively once patterns of illness behaviour established in the present study are recognised. Health planners generally try to identify factors whose change can positively influence patterns of utilisation and the results here set forth indicate the feasibility of socio-cultural and political integration of major ethnic groups.

Hence, future national plans of action should adopt a more *pluralistic strategy* for health care improvement in which at the same time room for expanded access will be left to 'alternative' forms of traditional and transitional therapy, as has successfully been the case elsewhere in Africa: the ARO-programme in Nigeria (Lambo 1978), the TMP-programme in Swaziland (Green and Makhubu 1984) and the meanwhile world-famous PRHETIH-programme among the Bono in Techiman, Ghana (Warren 1982). In Ethiopia, initial steps towards recognition and possible collaboration between traditional medicine and biomedicine has been reported by Slikkerveer (1982) and Akerele (1984). In this context, a dynamic policy aimed at *culturally appropriate health care* should also include the rehabilitation and integration of certain aspects and functionaries of indigenous, local and regional traditional health care systems often closely related to health beliefs and behaviours of ethno-religious groups in the area.

However, since the services of specific types of traditional healer, such as 'witch doctors' and 'diviners', are officially disapproved of and discouraged by the central government since the revolution of 1974, it seems necessary to convince political decision-makers that certain forms of *indigenous medical knowledge and practise* in

Ethiopia, as elsewhere, not only implies great potential, but in fact forms a prerequisite for genuinely improving the health care development process. This situation supports the need to link-up the study of medical pluralism with the examination of the socio-political processes in which the phenomenon is embedded. Although WHO and its Regional Committee for Africa issued several resolutions on the priority of traditional medicine and its role in health care development in Africa, and international collaboration between WHO and UNDP, OAU, CAMES and EDNA has given strong impetus to establishing traditional medicine programmes in a number of countries of the African region, Ethiopia so far has adopted a rather distant attitude towards collaboration between traditional and conventional systems. Despite pioneering work on the identification of medicinal plants and other substances used in local drugs and therapies, carried out at the Department of Pharmacology at the Black Lion Hospital in Addis Ababa, a latent conflict between political ideology of the state and indigenous healing practices seem to create hesitation in the development and implementation of collaborative efforts between modern and traditional medicine. In this respect, the study in Babile aims to support efforts to bring about recognition, official and legal status and collaboration, based on the local population's point of view, where patterns of illness behaviour indicate the socio-cultural identity among ethnic groups and 'nationalities' as an inalienable part of their cultural heritage. The Institute of Nationalities established in 1985 in Addis Ababa could also serve here as a vehicle to bring this heritage back into official favour and function.

In sum, this study has focussed on cross-cultural comparison of patterns of illness behaviour of different groups in a pluralistic medical configuration in the Horn of Africa, examining the way in which members of distinct ethno-religious groupings respond to illness and express intracultural variation in the health care utilisation process. As regards policy implications of the understanding of this highly complex process, the inclusion of culturally appropriate health care programmes for specific, ethno-religious target groups in national, pluralistic plans of action is proposed, in which certain indigenous medical perceptions, practices and healers are integrated in order to achieve optimal use of all available resources by the entire population.

# Bibliography

Aall-Jilek, L.M. and W.G. Jilek
1970 The Problem of Epilepsy in a Rural Tanzanian Tribe, in: *African Journal Medical Science*, 1: 305–307.
Abdul Hafiz
1976 *Introduction to the Local History of Babile*. Unpublished manuscript.
Abdullahi
1976 Unpublished Year Report, Babile.
Abrahams, R.G.
1959 'African Concepts of Health and Disease', in: *Symposium on Attitudes to Health and Disease among some East African Tribes*. Makarere Institute for Social Research, Kampala.
Ackerknecht, E.
1955 *A Short History of Medicine*. Ronald Press Company, New York.
Adams, P.L. and N.F. MacDonald
1968 'The Clinical Cooling Out of Poor People', in: *American Journal of Orthopsychiatry*, 38 (April): 457–463.
Aday, L.A. and R. Andersen
1975 *Development of Indices of Access to Medical Care*. Health Administration Press, Ann Arbor, Michigan.
Akerele, O.
1984 'WHO's traditional medicine programme: progress and perspectives', in: *WHO Chronicle* 38: 76–81.
Aklilu Lemma
1973 'Schistosomiasis: the Social Challenge of Controlling a Man-Made Disease', in: *Impact of Science on Society*, Vol. 23.
Alula Abate
1969 *Studien zur jüngeren Entwicklung der Kulturlandschaft im Hochland von Harar*. Doctoral dissertation, Rheinischen Friedrich-Wilhelms Universität.
Alula Abate and Tesfaye Teklu
1980 'Land Reform and Peasant Associations in Ethiopia – Case studies of two widely differing regions', in: *Northeast African Studies*, 2, 2: 1–51.

Amelsvoort, V.F.P.M. van
1964 *Culture, Stone Age and Modern Medicine. The early introduction of integrated rural health in a non-literate society. A New Guinea case study in medical anthropology*. Van Gorcum, Assen.
1979 *Basisklapper 'Gezondheidszorg Ontwikkelingslanden'*. Stafleu, Leiden.
Andargatchew Tiruneh
1981 'Eritrea, Ethiopia and Federation (1941–1952)', in: *Northeast African Studies*, 3, 1: 99–119.
Andersen, R.
1968 *A behavioral Model of Families' Use of Health Services*. Center for Health Administration Studies, Research Series 25, University of Chicago.
Anderson, James G. and David E. Bartkus
1973 'Choice of Medical Care: a Behavior Model of Health and Illness Behavior', in: *Journal of Health and Social Behavior*, 14 (December): 348–362.
Antonovsky, Aaron
1967 'Social Class and Illness: a Reconsideration', in: *Sociological Inquiry* (Spring): 311–322.
1972 'A Model to Explain Visits to the Doctor: With Specific Reference to the Case of Israel', in: *Journal of Health and Social Behavior*, 13 (December): 446–454.
Armelagos, G.J. (*et al.*)
1976 Disease and the Ecological perspective, in: *Ecologist* 6, 2.
Asfaw Desta
1971 *National Health Planning in Ethiopia*. Doctoral dissertation, The Johns Hopkins University, Baltimore.
Asmarom Legesse
1973 *Gada: Three Approaches to the Study of African Society*. Free Press, New York.
Azais, R.P. and F. Chambard
1931 *Cinq Années de Recherches Archéologiques*. Paris.
Baker, T.D. and M. Perlman
1967 'Health Manpower in a Developing Economy. Taiwan, a case study on planning', in: *The Johns Hopkins Monographs in International Health*. The Johns Hopkins Press, Baltimore.
Banerji, D.
1979 'Place of Indigenous and Western Systems of Medicine in the Health Services of India', in: *International Journal of Health Services*, 9: 511–520.
Bank, B. (*et al.*)
1973 *Readings in Health Care*. University of Columbia Medical Center, Columbia.

Bannerman, R.H.
1977 'WHO Programme for the Study of Traditional Medicine', in: *WHO Chronicle*, 31, no. 11.
Bannerman, R.H., J. Burton and Ch'en Wen-Chiehn (Eds.)
1983 *Traditional Medicine and Health Care Coverage; a reader for health administrators and practitioners.* World Health Organization, Geneva.
Baxter, P.T.W. and Hector Blackhurst
1978 'Vercingetorix in Ethiopia: Some Problems Arising from Levine's Inclusion of the Oromo in his Delineation of Ethiopia as a Culture Area', in: Jean Chavallion (Ed.), *Abbay. Documents pour servir à l'histoire de la civilisation Ethiopienne*. Cahier no. 9: 159–166. Centre National de la Recherche Scientifique. Meudon, France.
Beck, R.G.
1973 'Economic Class and Access to Physician Services under Public Medical Care Insurance', in: *Journal of Health Services*, 3 (Summer): 341–355.
Becker, Marshall H. (Ed.)
1974 *The Health Belief Model and Personal Health Behavior*. Society for Public Health Education, San Francisco.
Becker, Marshall H. and Lois A. Maiman
1975 'Sociobehavioral Determinants of Compliance with Health and Medical Care Recommendations', in: *Medical Care*, 13 (January): 10–24.
Becker, Marshall H., Lois A. Maiman and John P. Kirscht
1977 'The Health Belief Model and Prediction of Dietary Compliance: a Field Experiment', in: *Journal of Health and Social Behavior*, Vol. 18 (December): 348–366.
Behets, L. and L. Vermost
1972 *Socio-Kulturele determinanten in het Ziekte- en Gezondheidsgedrag. Een literatuuranalyse*. S.O. I, Leuven.
Bellin, Seymour S. and H. Jack Geiger
1972 'The Impact of a Neighborhood Health Center on a Patient's Behavior and Attitudes Relating to Health Care: a Study of Low Income Housing', in: *Medical Care*, 10 (May-June): 224–239.
Benyoussef, A. and A.F. Wessen
1974 'Utilization of Health Services in Developing Countries – Tunisia', in: *Social Science and Medicine*, 8: 287–305.
Berkanovic, Emil and Leo G. Reeder
1974 'Can Money Buy the Appropriate Use of Services? Some notes on the meaning of utilization data', in: *Journal of Health and Social Behavior*, 15 (June): 93–99.

Berki, S.E. and Marie L. Ashcraft
1979 'On the Analysis of Ambulatory Utilization. An investigation of the roles of need, access and price and predictors of illness and preventive visits', in: *Medical Care*, Vol. XVII, 12 (December): 1163–1181.
Bhardwaj, S.M.
1975 'Attitude toward Different Systems of Medicine: a Survey of Four Villages in the Punjab – India', in: *Social Science and Medicine*, 9: 603–612.
1980 'Medical Pluralism and Homoeopathy: a Geographic Perspective', in: *Social Science and Medicine*, Vol. 14B, 4: 209–216.
Bibeau, Gilles
1979 *De la Maladie à la Guérison; essai d'analyse systématique de la médicine des Agbandi du Zaire*. Doctoral Dissertation, Laval University.
1981 'Current and Future Issues for Medical Social Scientists in Less Developed Countries', in: *Social Science and Medicine*, Vol. 15A: 357–370.
1982 'New Legal Rules for an Old Art of Healing. The case of Zairian healers associations', in: *Social Science and Medicine*, Vol. 16, 21: 1843–1849.
Bice, T.W. and K.L. White
1969 'Factors related to the Use of Health Services – an International Comparative Study', in: *Medical Care*, 7: 124–133.
Bice, Thomas W., Robert Eichhorn and Peter D. Fox
1972 'Socioeconomic Status and Use of Physician Services: a Reconsideration', in: *Medical Care*, 10 (May-June): 261–271.
Blum, R. and E. Blum
1965 *Health and Healing in Rural Greece. A study of three communities*. Stanford University Press, Stanford.
Boer, Leen
1981 'A Typology of Local Rural Development Situations: Problems and Prospects'. *ICA Working Paper* 11, University of Leiden.
Branch, M.F. and P.P. Paxton
1976 *Providing Safe Nursing Care for Ethnic People of Color*. Appleton-Century-Crofts, New York.
Brink, P.J.
1976 'Introduction', in: *Transcultural Nursing: A Book of Readings*. Prentice Hall, Englewood Cliffs, New Jersey.
1982 'Traditional Birth Attendants among the Annang of Nigeria. Current Practices and Proposed Programs', in: *Social Science and Medicine*, Vol. 16, 21: 1883–1893.

Broekhuizen, A.
1935 *Abessynië. Het land, het volk en zijn geschiedenis*. Thieme, Zuthpen.

Brokensha, D., D.M. Warren and O. Werner (Eds.)
1980 *Indigenous Knowledge Systems and Development*. University Press of America, Lanham, New York, London.

Brooke, Clarke Harding
1956 *Settlements of the Eastern Galla, Hararghe Province, Ethiopia*. Unpublished doctoral dissertation, University of Nebraska.

Bruce, J.
1790 *Travels to Discover the Source of the Nile*. Edinburgh.

Brummelkamp
1956 *Ethiopië's Ontwikkeling in de Twintigste Eeuw van Middeleeuwse tot Moderne Staat*. Meppel.

Brunswick, Ann F., John M. Boyle and Carol Tarica
1979 'Who Sees the Doctor? A Study of Urban Black Adolescents', in: *Social Science and Medicine*, 13A: 45–56.

Bryant, John
1971 *Health & the Developing World*. Cornell University Press, Ithaca.

Buck, Alfred A. (*et al.*)
1968 *Health and Disease in Four Peruvian Villages. Contrasts in Epidemiology*. The Johns Hopkins Press, Baltimore.

Buck, Alfred A., Robert I. Anderson, Tom T. Sasaki and Kazuyoshi Kawata
1970 *Health and Disease in Chad. Epidemiology, culture, and environment in five villages*. The Johns Hopkins Press, Baltimore.

Bullough, B.
1972 'Poverty, Ethnic Identity and Preventive Health Care', in: *Journal of Health and Social Behavior* 13: 347–359.

Burg, Eeke van der
1983 *Canals User's Guide*. Department of Datatheory, University of Leiden.

Burg, Eeke van der and Jan de Leeuw
1983 'Non linear Canonical Correlation', in: *British Journal of Mathematical and Statistical Psychology*, 36: 54–80.

Burton, Sir Richard F.
1856/1894 *First Footsteps in East Africa, or an Exploration of Harar*. J.M. Dent & Sons, London.

Buschkens, W.F.L.
1979 'De Houding van de Bevolking van de Derde Wereld tegenover Verschillende Geneeswijzen', in: *Geneesmiddelen Voorziening in de Ontwikkelingslanden*. Rijksuniversiteit te Leiden.

Buschkens, W.F.L. and L.J. Slikkerveer
1976 *Project RUL/22* Addis Ababa/Leiden [Questionnaire].
1980 *Illness Behavior of the Eastern Oromo in Hararghe. Recommendations for rural health planning in Ethiopia*. Institute of Cultural and Social Studes, Leiden.
1982 *Health Care in East Africa. Illness behaviour of the Eastern Oromo in Hararghe (Ethiopia)*. Van Gorcum, Assen.
Bush, Patricia J. and Marian Osterweis
1978 'Pathways to Medicine Use', in: *Journal of Health and Social Behavior*, Vol. 19, 2 (June): 179–189.
Buijs, H.Y.
1979 *Access and Participation: on the Access Problems of the Poor People and Participation as a Solution*. ICA Publication No. 33, University of Leiden.
Bwibo, N.O.
1971 'Whooping Cough in Uganda', in: *Scandinavian Journal of Infant Diseases*, 3, 41.
Cassel, J.
1970 'Physical Illness in Response to Stress', in: S. Levine and N.A. Scotch (Eds.) *Social Stress*, Aldine, Chicago: 189–209.
1974 'Psychosocial Processes and Stress: Theoretical Formulation', in: *Journal of Health Services* 4: 471–482.
Caulk, Richard
1971 'The Occupation of Harar: January 1877', in: *Journal of Ethiopian Studies*, Vol. IX, 2.
Cecchi, A.
1886 *Da Zeila alle Frontiere del Caffa*. Roma.
Cerulli, Enrico
1922 *The Folk-Literature of the Galla*. Cambridge, Mass.
1936 *La Lingua e la Storia di Harar*. Studie Ethiopia, Roma
Cerulli, Ernesta
1957 *Peoples of South-West Ethiopia and its Borderland*. London.
Chabot, H.T.J.
1973 *A Comparison Between Four Health Centres in Indonesia. With a general description of the peripheral health service*. Erasmus University, Rotterdam.
Chen, P.C.Y.
1975 'Medical Systems in Malaysia', in: *Social Science and Medicine*, 9: 171–180.
Chrisman, N.J.
1977 'The Health Seeking Process. An approach to the natural history of illness', in: *Culture Medicine Psychiatry* 1, 4.

Chrisman, N.J. and T.W. Maretzki (Eds.)
1984 *Clinically Applied Anthropology; Anthropologists in Health Science Settings*. Reidel Publishing Company, Dordrecht.
Clapham, Christopher
1969 *Haile-Selassie's Government*. Praeger, New York.
Cobb, S.
1976 'Social Support as a Moderator of Life Stress', in: *Psychosomatic Medicine* 38: 300–314.
Cockerham, William C.
1978 *Medical Sociology*. Prentice-Hall, Inc., New Jersey.
Coe, R.
1970 *Sociology of Medicine*. McGraw-Hill, New York.
Coleman, J.S., E. Katz and H. Menzel
1966 *Medical Innovation: A Diffusion Study*. Bobbs-Merrill, New York.
Colson, A.C.
1971 'The Differential Use of Medical Resources in Developing Countries', in: *Journal of Health and Social Behavior*, 12: 226–237.
Colson, A.C. and K.E. Selby
1974 'Medical Anthropology', in: B.J. Siegel *et al.* (Eds.) *Annual Review of Anthropology*, Vol. 3, Annual Review Inc., Palo Alto, California.
*Comprehensive Health Service Directory 1968 E.C. (1976 G.C.)*
1977 Planning and Programming Bureau, Addis Ababa.
Conti-Rossini, Carlo
1928 *Storia d'Etiopia*. Milan.
1937 *Etiopia e genti di Etiopia*. Firenze.
Cook, R. Dennis and Sanford Weisberg
1982 *Residuals and Influence in Regression*. Chapman and Hall, New York.
Croizier, Ralph C.
1977 'The Ideology of Medical Revivalism in Modern China', in: Charles Leslie (Ed.), *Asian Medical Systems: a Comparative Study*. University of California Press, Berkeley: 341–355.
Cunningham, C.E.
1970 'Thai Injection Doctors, Antibiotic Mediators', in: *Social Science and Medicine*, 4: 1–21.
Dechering, W.
1977 *Inleiding tot de Data-Theorie. Voor Cultureel Antropologen en Niet Westerse Sociologen*. ICA, University of Leiden.
1981 'Het Bepalen van Doelgroepen voor Accesbeleid met Behulp van Loglineaire Analyse? *Paper ICA-Festival 1981*. University of Leiden.

Demissie Gebre Michael
1974 *The Kottu of Harerge, an Introduction to the Eastern Oromo.* (Experiment Station Bulletin no. 68). College of Agriculture, Dire Dawa (Alemaya).
Demoz, Abraham
1968 *Ethiopia Today*, Stanford University Press.
Denton, John A.
1978 *Medical Sociology*. Houghton Mifflin Company, Boston.
Djukanovic, V. and E.P. Mach
1975 *Alternative Approaches to Meeting Basic Health Needs in Developing Countries*. World Health Organization, Geneva.
Djurfeld, G. and S. Lindberg
1975 'Pills against Poverty. A study of the introduction of Western medicine in a Tamil town', in: *Indien Studenti Litteratur*, Scandinavian Institute of Asian Studies. Monograph Series No. 23. Curzon Press, New York.
Douglass, C.W.
1971 A Social-Psychological View of Health Behavior for Health Services Research, *Health Services Research*, Spring 1971: 6–14.
Drewes, A.J.
1962 *Inscriptions de l'Ethiopie Antique*. Doctoral dissertation, University of Leiden.
1970 'Bilingualism in Ethiopia', in: *Proceedings of the Third International Conference of Ethiopian Studies, Addis Ababa.*
1976 *Classical Arabic in Central Ethiopia*. Publ. nr. 7, Oosters Genootschap in Nederland, Leiden.
Dubos, R
1965 *Man Adapting*. Yale University Press, New Haven.
Dunn, Frederick L.
1977 'Traditional Asian Medicine and Cosmopolitan Medicine as Adaptive Systems', in: Charles Leslie (Ed.), *Asian Medical Systems. A comparative study*. University of California Press, Berkeley: 133–158.
Dutton, Diana B.
1978 'Explaining the Low Use of Health Services by the Poor: Costs, Attitudes, or Delivery Systems?', in: *American Sociological Review*, Vol. 43 (June): 348–368.
Ehrenreich, B. and J. Ehrenreich
1971 *The American Health Empire: a Report from the Health Policy Advisory Center*. Random House, New York.
Eisenberg L. and A. Kleinman (Eds.)
1980 *The Relevance of Social Sciences for Medicine*. Reidel, Dordrecht.

Elliott, K. (Ed.)
1979 *Auxiliaries in Primary Health Care*. Intermediate Technology Group, London.
Engel, G.L.
1962 *Psychological Development in Health and Disease*. Saunders, Philadelphia.
Erasmus, Charles J.
1961 *Man Takes Control*. University of Minnesota Press, Minneapolis.
Etten, G.M. van and J.G.F. Anten
1972 'Evaluation of Health Education in a Tanzanian Leprosy Scheme', in: *International Journal of Leprosy*, 40: 402–409.
1976 *Rural Health Development in Tanzania*. Van Gorcum, Assen.
Evans-Pritchard, E.E.
1937 *Witchcraft, Oracles and Magic Among the Azande*. Clarendon Press, Oxford.
Fabrega, H.
1972 'The Study of Disease in Relation to Culture', in: *Behavioral Science*, 17: 183–203.
1973 'Toward a Model of Illness Behavior', in: *Medical Care*, 11 (Nov.-Dec.): 470–484.
Fabrega, H.
1974 *Disease and Social Behavior*. MIT Press, Cambridge, Mass.
1977 'The Scope of Ethnomedical Science', in: *Cultural Medical Psychiatry*, 1: 210.
Fabrega, H. and P.K. Manning
1979 'Illness Episodes, Illness Severity and Treatment Options in a Pluralistic Setting', in: *Social Science and Medicine*, 13B:
Feacham, R.
1973 *Environment and Health in a New Guinea Highlands Community*. Doctoral dissertation, University of New South Wales.
Fink, Raymond
1969 'The Measurement of Medical Care Utilization', in: Merwyn R. Greenlick (Ed.), *Proceedings of a Conference on Conceptual Issues in the Analysis of Medical Care Utilization Behavior*. Portland: 5–32.
Fink, R., S. Shapiro and J. Lewis
1968 'The Reluctant Participant in a Breast Cancer Screening Program', in: *Public Health Reports*, 83 (June): 479–490.
Foster, George M.
1952 'Relationships between Theoretical and Applied Anthropology: a Public Health Program Analysis', in: *Human Organization*, Vol. 11, 3: 5–16.

1958 *Problems of Intercultural Health Programs.* Social Science Research Council, Pamphlet 12, New York.
1983 'An introduction to ethnomedicine', in: R.H. Bannerman, J. Burton and Ch'en Wen-Chieh (Eds.) *Traditional Medicine and Health Care Coverage. A reader for health administrators and practitioners.* World Health Organization, Geneva: 17–25.
Foster, George M. and Barbara Gallatin Anderson
1978 *Medical Anthropology.* Wiley, New York.
Fowler, H.W. and F.G. Fowler
1975 *The Concise Oxford Dictionary.* Clarendon Press, Oxford.
Frankenberg, R.
1968 'The Beginning of Anthropology: the Challenge of the New Africa to the Sociological Study of Small-Scale Social Processes, in: *Proceedings of the VIIth International Congress of Anthropological and Ethnological Sciences,*' Tokyo, Vol. 2.
Frankenberg, R. and J. Leeson
1976 'Disease, Illness and Sickness: Social Aspects of the Choice of Healer in a Lusaka Suburb', in: J.B. Loudon (Ed.), *Social Anthropology and Medicine.* Academic Press, New York: 223–258.
Freidson, Eliot
1973 'Client Control and Medical Practice', in: Gartly Jaco, E., *Patients and Illness. A sourcebook in behavioral science and health.* The Free Press, New York: 204–211.
Freij, Lennart (*et al*)
1973 *Exploring Child Health and its Ecology.* Journal of Development Research, Supplement to Vol II, no 2. Institute of Development Research, Addis Ababa University.
Fromm, E. and M. Maccoby
1970 *Social Character in a Mexican Village.* Prentice-Hall, Englewood Cliffs, New Jersey.
Furnivall, J.S.
1939 *Netherlands India, A Study of Plural Economy.* Cambridge University Press, London.
Gaag, Jacques van der and Wijnand van de Ven
1978 'The Demand for Primary Health Care', in: *Medical Care,* Vol. XVI, 4 (April): 299–312.
Gabre Emanuel Teka
1975 *The Public Health College & Training Centre Gondar. Review of its origin and development in twenty years of national service.* Haile Selassie I University, Public Health College Gondar.

Galjart, Benno F.
1978 'Ontwikkeling: Processen en Strukturen. Een analytisch model voor de Ontwikkelingssociologie'. (mimeo)
Galjart, Benno F. (*et al*)
1982 'Participatie, Toegang tot Ontwikkeling. verslag van een onderzoek naar de mogelijkheden van participatie in ontwikkelingsprojekten', *Leiden Development Studies* 1, Institute of Cultural and Social Studies, University of Leiden.
Galjart Benno F. and D. Buijs (Eds.)
1982 'Participation of the Poor in Development; contribution to a seminar', *Leiden Development Studies* 2, Institute of Cultural and Social Studies, University of Leiden.
Galvin, Michael L. and Margaret Fan
1975 'The Utilization of Physician's Services in Los Angeles County, 1973', in: *Journal of Health and Social Behavior*, 16 (March): 75–94.
Geer, John. P. van de
1971 *Introduction to Multivariate Analysis for the Social Sciences* Freeman, San Francisco.
Geertsen, R. (*et al.*)
1975 'A Re-examination of Suchman's Views on Social Factors in Health Care Utilization', in: *Journal of Health and Social Behavior*, 16: 226–237.
Gelfand, M.
1964 *Medicine and Custom in Africa*. Livingstone, Edinburgh.
Gerlach, L.P.
1959 'Some Basic Digo Conceptions of Health and Disease', in: *Symposium on Attitudes to Health and Diseases among some East African Tribes*. Makarere Institute for Social Research, Kampala.
Gesler, W.M.
1979 'Morbidity Measurement in Household Surveys in Developing Areas', in: *Social Science and Medicine*, 13D: 223–226.
Gifi, A.
1981 *Non Lineur Multivariate Analysis*. Datatheory, University of Leiden.
Ginneken, J.K. van and A.S. Muller (Eds.)
1984 *Maternal and Child Health in Rural Kenya, an epidemiological study*. Croom Helm, London.
Ginzberg, Eli and Herbert A. Smith
1967 *A Manpower Strategy for Developing Countries: Lessons from Ethiopia*. Columbia University Press, New York.

Gish, O.
1973 'Resource Allocation, Equality of Access, and Health', in: *International Journal of Health Services*, 3: 399–412.
Gish, O. (Ed.)
1971 *Health Manpower and the Medical Auxiliary*. Intermediate Technology Group, London.
Glick, L.
1967 'Medicine as Ethnographic Category: the Gimi of the New Guinea Highlands', in: *Ethnology*, 6: 31–56.
Gonzalez, N.S.
1966 'Health Behaviour in Cross-cultural Perspective: A Guatemalan Example', in: *Human Organization*, 25: 122–125.
Good, C.M. and M.J. DelVecchio Good
1980 'The Meaning of Symptoms: a Cultural Hermeneutic Model for Clinical Practice', in: L. Eisenberg and A. Kleinman (Eds.), *The Relevance of Social Sciences for Medicine*. Reidel, Boston.
Good, C.M., J.M. Hunter, S.H. Katz and S.S. Katz
1979 'The Interface of Dual Systems of Health Care in the Developing World: toward Health Policy Initiatives in Africa', in: *Social Science and Medicine*, 13D: 141–154.
Gould, G.C. (Ed.)
1971 *Health and Disease in East Africa; the community approach*. East African Literature Bureau, Nairobi.
Gould, H.A.
1957 'The Implications of Technological Change for Folk and Scientific Medicine', in: *American Anthropology*, 59: 507–516.
1965 'Modern Medicine and Folk Cognition in Rural India', in: *Human Organization* 24: 201–208.
Gragg, G.B. (Ed.)
1982 *Oromo Dictionary*. African Studies Center, MSU, East Lansing.
Green, E.C. and L. Makhubu
1984 'Traditional Healers in Swaziland: Toward improved cooperation between the traditional and modern health sectors', in: *Social Science and Medicine* 18: 1071–1079.
Greene, S.B. (*et al*)
1979 'Who Shops for Medical Care in a Southern Rural Community – how much and why', in: *Inquiry*, 16: 62–72.
Greenlick, Merwyn R., Arnold V. Hurtado, Clyde R. Pope, Ernest W. Saward and Samuel S. Yoshioka
1968 'Determinants of Medical Care Utilization', in: *Health Services Research*, (Winter 1968): 296–315.

Greenlick, Merwyn R. (*et al*)
1969 *Proceedings of a Conference on Conceptual Issues in the Analysis of Medical Care Utilization Behavior*. Kaiser Health Services Research Centre. Portland, Oregon.
Greenlick, Merwyn R., Donald K. Freeborn, Theodore J. Colombo, Jeffery A. Prussin and Ernest W. Saward
1972 'Comparing the Use of Medical Care Services by a Medically Indigent and a General Membership Population in Comprehensive Prepaid Group Practice Program', in: *Medical Care*, 10 (May-June): 187–200.
Greenlick, Merwyn, R., Donald K. Freeborn, Gary L. Gambill and Clyde R. Pope
1973 'Determinants of Medical Care Utilization: the Role of the Telephone in Total Medical Care', in: *Medical Care*, II (March): 121–134.
Griaule, M.
1930 *Le Livre de Recettes d'un Dabtara Abyssin*. Paris.
Grunebaum, Gustave E. von
1955 *Kritik und Dichtkunst, Studien zur Arabischen Literaturgeschichte*. Wiesbaden.
Gunawan, L.A. (*et al*)
1972 'Research into the Health Service Delivery System'. *LKN Papers*. (The National Research Institute for Community Health) Surabaya.
Haberland, Eike
1963 *Galla Süd-Athiopiens*. W. Kohlhammer Verlag, Stuttgart.
Hand, Vayland D. (Ed.)
1976 *American Folk Medicine: A Symposium*. University of California Press, Berkeley.
Harrison Church, R.J. (*et al*)
1977 *Africa and the Islands*. Wiley, New York.
Harwood, A.
1981 *Ethnicity and Medical Care*. Harvard University Press, Cambridge, Mass.
Hatfield, C.
1968 *The Nfumu in Tradition and Change. A study of the position of religious practitioners among the Sukuma of Tanzania, East Africa*. Ph.D. Dissertion, The Catholic University of America.
Heggenhougen, J.K.
1978 'Hospital Assistants in Malaysian Rural Health Care', in: *Medical Journal of Malaysia*, 33: 165–177.
Heller, P.S.
1982 'A Model of the Demand for Medicals and Health Services in

Peninsular Malaysia', in: *Social Science and Medicine*, 16: 267–284.

Heller, P.L., H.P. Chalvant, G.M. Queseda and C. Rivera-Worley
1981 'Class, Familism and Utilization of Health Services in Durango, Mexico: a Replication', in: *Social Science and Medicine*, 15A.

Hershey, John C., Harold S. Luft and Joan M. Gianaris
1975 'Making Sense Out of Utilization Data', in: *Medical Care*, Vol. XIII, 10 (October): 838–854.

Hightower, William L.
1978 'Development of an Index of Health Utilizing Factor Analysis', in: *Medical Care*, Vol. XVI, 3 (March): 245–254.

Hill, Carole E.
1973 'Black Healing Practices in the Rural South', in: *Journal of Popular Culture* 6: 829–853.

Hinderling, P.
1973 *Communication between Doctor and Patients in Thailand. Interview with traditional doctors*. Part III. Socio-Psychological Research Centre on Development Planning. University of the Saar.

Hoben, Allan
1972 'Social Anthropology and Development Planning: a Case Study in Ethiopian Land Reform Policy', in: *Journal of Modern African Studies* 10, 4: 561–582.

Hoefnagel, A.H.J.M.
1978 'Systeemtheorie / Systeemtheoretische Sociologie', in: L. Rademaker (Ed.), *Sociologische Encyclopedie* 3. Het Spectrum, Utrecht: 717–722.

Hoorweg, J.C. and I. McDowell
1969 'Nutrition Education in Uganda', in: *Kroniek van Afrika*, 2: 185–197.

Horton, R.
1973 'African Traditional Thought and Western Science, Part I and II,' in: *Africa* 37:71; 155–187.

Hughes, C.C.
1968 'Ethnomedicine', in: *International Encyclopedia of the Social Sciences*, Macmillan, New York: 87–93.

Hulka, B. (*et al.*)
1972 'Determinants of Physician Utilization', in: *Medical Care*, 10: 300–309.

Hunt, E.E. Jr.
1978 'Ecological Frameworks and Hypothesis Testing in Medical Anthropology', in: M.H. Logan and E.E. Hunt (Eds.), *Health and the Human Condition. Perspectives on Medical Anthropology*. Duxbury Press, North Scituate.

Hunter, David E. and P. Whitten
1975 *Encyclopedia of Anthropology*. Harper & Row, New York.
Huntingford, G.W.B.
1955 *The Galla of Ethiopia*. International African Institute, London.
Igun, U.A.
1979 'Stages in Health-Seeking: a Descriptive Model', in: *Social Science and Medicine*, 13A: 445–456.
Imperato, P.J.
1966 'Witchcraft and Traditional Medicine among the Luo of Tanzania', in: *Tanganyika Notes and Records*, 66: 193–201.
Janzen, J.M.
1978 *The Quest for Therapy in Lower Zaire*. University of California Press, Berkeley.
Janzen, J.M.
1982 'Lubanzi: The History of a Kongo Disease', in: Yoder, Stanley P. (Ed.), *African Health and Healing Systems: Proceedings of a Symposium*. Crossroads Press, University of California, Los Angeles: 107–121.
Jeffery, Roger
1982 'Policies towards Indigenous Healers in Independent India', in: *Social Science and Medicine*, Vol. 16, 21: 1835–1841.
Johanson, D. and M. Edey
1981 *Lucy: The Beginnings of Humankind*. Simon & Shuster, New York.
Jolly, Richard and Maurice King
1966 The Organization of Health Services', in Maurice King (Ed.) *Medical Care in Developing Countries*. Oxford University Press, Nairobi: 2.1–2.15.
Jong, Gaspard A. de (Ed.)
1980 *Ongelijkheid in Gezondheid en Gezondheidszorg*. Verslag van het congres ter gelegenheid van het 50–jarig bestaan van de Algemene Nederlandse Vereniging voor Sociale Geneeskunde, 24 en 25 April 1980 te Arnhem. Supplement bij het Tijdschrift voor Sociale Geneeskunde, jaargange 58, 28 Oktober 1980.
Josselin de Jong, J. P. B. de
1935 'The Malay Archipelago as a Field of Ethnological Study', in: P. E. de Josselin de Jong (Ed.), *Structural Anthropology in the Netherlands. A reader*. Martinus Nijhoff, 1977. The Hague: 164–182
Josselin de Jong, P. E. de
1977 *Structural Anthropology in the Netherlands. A reader*. Martinus Nijhoff, The Hague.

1980 'The Concept of the Field of Ethnological Study', in: James Fox (Ed.), *The Flow of Life.* Harvard University Press, Cambridge, Mass.

Kadushin, C.

1967 'Social Class and Ill Health: the Need for Further Research. A reply to Antonovsky', in: *Sociological Inquiry*, 37 (Spring): 323–332.

Kain, John F.

1975 'Race, Ethnicity, and Residential Location,' in: *Urban Planning: Policy Analysis and Administration.* Paper D75–3, Harvard University.

Kantrowitz, Nathan

1973 *Ethnic and Racial Segregation in the New York Metropolis: Residential Patterns among White Ethnic Groups, Blacks and Puerto Ricans.* Praeger, New York.

Kaplan, B., J. Cassel, and S. Gore

1977 'Social Support and Health, in: *Medical Care* 15 (May, suppl.): 47–58.

Kapur, R. L.

1979 'The Role of Traditional Healers in Mental Health Care in Rural India', in: *Social Science and Medicine*, 13B: 27–31.

Kasl, S. and S. Cobb

1966 'Health Behaviour, Illness Behavior and Sick-Role Behavior', in: *Archives of Environmental Health*, XII: 246–266

Kasteler, J. R. L., Kane D. M., Olsen and C. Thetford

1976 'Issues Underlying Prevalence of "Doctor-shopping" Behavior', in: *Journal of Health and Social Behavior*, 17: 328–339.

Kegeles, S. S.

1967 'Attitudes and Behaviour of the Public Regarding Cervical Cytology: Current Findings and New Directions for Research,' in: *Journal of Chronic Disease*, 20 (December): 911–922.

King, Maurice (Ed.)

1966 *Medical Care in Developing Countries. A primer on the medicine of poverty and a symposium from Makerere.* Oxford University Press, Nairobi.

Kirscht, John P.

1974 'The Health Belief Model and Illness Behavior', in: M. H. Becker (Ed.), *The Health Belief Model and Personal Health.* Society for Public Health Education, Inc., San Francisco: 387–408.

Kleczkowski, B. M. and R. Pibouleau

1977–78 *Approaches to Planning and Design of Health Care Facilities in Developing Areas.* World Health Organization, Geneva, Vol. I & II.

Kleinman, Arthur

1973 'Medicine's Symbolic Reality: on a Central Problem in the Philosophy of Medicine', in: *Inquiry* 16: 209

1975 'Medical Psychiatric Anthropology and the Study of Traditional Forms of Medicine in Modern Chinese Culture', in: *Bulletin of the Institute of Ethnology and Academia Sinica* 39: 107.

1978 'Concepts and a Model for the Comparison of Medical Systems as Cultural Systems', in: *Social Science and Medicine*, Vol. 12, 2B: 85–93.

1980 Patients and Healers in the Context of Culture. University of California Press, Berkeley.

Kleinman, A., P Kundstadter, E. R. Alexander and J. L. Gate (Eds.)

1978 *Culture and Healing in Asian Societies.* Schenkman, Cambridge, Mass.

Kleinpenning, J. M. G.

1980 *Drie Maal Derde Wereld. Een inleiding tot de verschiedenheid van de ontwikkelingslanden.* Van Gorcum, Assen.

Kloos, H.

1974 'The Geography of Pharmacies, Druggist Shops and Rural Medicine Vendors and the Origin of Customers of such facilities in Addis Ababa', in: S. Chojnacki and R. Pankhurst (Eds.), *Journal of Ethiopian Studies*, Vol XII, 2: 77–94. Addis Ababa, Ethiopia.

Kohn, Robert and Kerr L. White (Eds.)

1976 *Health Care. An international study.* Oxford University Press, London.

Koos, E. L.

1954 *The Health of Regionville.* Columbia University Press, New York.

Kosa, John and Irving Kenneth Zola (Eds.)

1976 *Poverty and Health.* Harvard University Press, Cambridge, Mass.

Koumaré, M.

1983 'Traditional Medicine and Psychiatry in Africa', in: R. H. Bannerman, J. Burton and Ch'en Wen-Chieh (Eds.) *Traditional Medicine and Health Care Coverage; a reader for health administrators and practitioners.* World Health Organization, Geneva: 25–33.

Krause, E. A.

1977 *Power & Illness, The Political Sociology of Health and Medical Care.* Elsevier, New York.

Kroeger, Axel

1983 'Anthropological and Sociomedical Health Care Research in Developing Countries', in: *Social Science and Medicine*, 17, 3: 147–161.

1985 'Response errors and other problems of health interview surveys in developing countries', in: *World Health Statistics Quarterly*, Vol, 38, No. 1: 15–37.

Kuls, W.

1958 'Beiträge zur Kulturgeographie der Südäthiopischen Seenregion', in: *Frankfurter Geogr. Hefte*, 32.

Kuper, Leo

1975 *Race, Class, and Power. Ideology and revolutionary change in plural societies.* Aldine Publishing Company, Chicago.

Kurian, G. T.

1979 *Encyclopedia of the Third World*. Vol. I & II. London.

Lambo, T. A.

1978 'Psychotherapy in Africa', in: *Human Nature* 1: 32–39.

Landy, D. (Ed.)

1977 *Culture, Disease and Healing: Studies in Medical Anthropology.* Macmillan, New York.

Lave, Charles A. and James G. March

1975 *An Introduction to Models in the Social Sciences.* Harper & Row, New York.

O'Leary, D. D. de Lacy

1964 *How Greek Science passed to the Arabs.* Routledge & Kegan Paul Ltd., London.

Leavitt, Frank

1979 'The Health Belief Model and Utilization of Ambulatory Care Services', in: *Social Science and Medicine*, 13A: 105–112.

Leeuw, J. de

1973 *Canonical Analysis of Categorical Data.* Doctoral dissertation, University of Leiden.

Leeuw, J. de and I. Stoop

1979 'Secundaire Analyse "Van Jaar tot Jaar" met Behulp van Niet-Lineaire Multivariate Technieken,' in: J. Peschar (Ed.) *Van Achteren Naar Voren. Achterstandssituaties in het onderwijs.* Staatsuitgeverij, 's-Gravenhage: 118–158.

Lefley, H. P.

1979 'Prevalence of potential falling-out cases among the Black, Latin and non-Latin white populations of the city of Miami', in: *Social Science and Medicine* Special Issue on The Transcultural Perspective in Health and Illness, Vol. 13B: 113–115.

Lefton, M. and W. R. Rosengren

1966 'Organizations and Clients: Lateral and Longitudinal Dimensions', in: *American Sociological Review,* 31 (December): 802–810.

Leininger, M. (Ed.)
1976 *Transcultural Health Care Issues and Conditions (Health Care Dimensions)* F. A. Davis Company, Philadelphia.
1978 *Transcultural Nursing: Concepts, Theories, and Practices.* John Wiley & Sons, New York.
Lerner, M.
1968 *Data on Social Background, Medical Care Utilization and Attitudes of Outpatients by Hospital, New York City Municipal General Hospital Outpatient Study.* Columbia University.
Leslau, W.
1963 *Etymological Dictionary of Harari.* Berkeley.
1976 *Concise Amharic Dictionary.* Wiesbaden.
Leslie, Charles (Ed.)
1977 *Asian Medical Systems. A Comparative Study.* University of California Press, Berkeley.
1978 'Theoretical Foundations for the Comparative Study of Medical Systems'. Special Issue in: *Social Science and Medicine,* Vol. 12, 2B.
1980 'Medical Pluralism'. Special Issue in: *Social Science and Medicine,* Vol. 14B, 4.
Levine, Donald N.
1974 *Greater Ethiopia. The evolution of a multiethnic society.* The University of Chicago Press, Chicago.
Lewis, Herbert S.
1962 'Historical Problems in Ethiopia and the Horn of Africa', in: *Annals of the New York Academy of Sciences* 6, 2: 510–511
1965 *A Galla Monarchy, Jimma Abba Jifar, Ethiopia.* Madison University of Wisconsin Press.
1966 'The Origin of the Galla and Somalia', in: *Journal of African History,* Vol. VII, 1: 27–46.
1970 'Occupational Caste in Ethiopia', in: A. Tuden and L. Plotnicov (Eds.) *Social Stratification in Africa.* Free Press, New York: 182–185
Lewis, I. M.
1960 'The Somali Conquest of the Horn of Africa', in: *Journal of African History,* Vol I, 2:213–229.
Lewis, O.
1955 'Medicine and Politics in a Mexican Village', in: E. Paul (Ed.), *Health, Culture and the Community.* Russel Saga Foundation, New York: 403–434.
Lieban, Richard W.
1967 *Cebuano Sorcery: Malign Magic in the Philippines.* University of California Press, Berkeley.

1973 'Medical Anthropology', in: J. G. Honigmann (Ed.), *Handbook of Social and Cultural Anthropology.* Rand McNally, Chicago.
1977 'The Field of Medical Anthropology', in: D. Landy (Ed.) *Culture, Disease and Healing.* Macmillan Publishing Company, New York.

Lieberson, Stanley
1963 *Ethnic Patterns in American Cities.* The Free Press, Glencoe, Illinois.

Lier, R. A. J. van
1949 *Samenleving in een Grensgebied. Een sociaal-historische studie van de maatschappij in Suriname.* Martinus Nijhoff, 's-Gravenhage.
1968 *Report to the F.A.O. on Social Problems Connected with the Planning of the Development of the Awash Valley in Ethiopia.* Addis Ababa.
1971 *Frontier Society. A social analysis of the history of Surinam.* Martinus Nijhoff, 's-Gravenhage.
1977 *Samenleving in een Grensgebied. Een sociaal-historische studie van Suriname.* S. Emmering, Amsterdam.

Lipsky, George A.
1967 *Ethiopia. Its people, its society, its culture.* HRAF Press, New Haven.

Logan, M. H.
1977 'Anthropological Research on the Hot-Cold Theory of Disease: Some Methodological Suggestions', in: *Medical Anthropology,* 1:4.

Logan, M. and E. Hunt
1978 *Health and the Human Condition: Perspectives on Medical Anthropology.* Duxbury Press, North Scituate.

Ludwig, Edward G. and Geoffrey Gibson
1969 'Self Perception of Sickness and the Seeking of Medical Care', in: *Journal of Health and Social Behavior,* 10 (June).

Luijk, J. N. van
1979 'Profile, Expectation and Satisfaction of Outpatients (1970–72). Health Services Research in Kenya, in: *Tropical and Geographical Medicine*, 31: 33–59.

Mannheim, Karl
1940 *Man and Society in an Age of Reconstruction: Studies in Modern Social Structure.* Harcourt, New York.

Marcus, Harold G.
1975 *The Life and Times of Menelik II, Ethiopia 1844–1913.* Clarendon Press, Oxford.

Mark, D. F. W. van der (Ed.)
1971 *Ethiopië.* Landendocumentatie Koninklijk Instituut voor de Tropen Nr. 140, Staatsuitgeverij, 's-Gravenhage.

Markakis, John
1975 *Ethiopia. Anatomy of a traditional polity.* Oxford University Press, Addis Ababa.
1987 *National and Class Conflict in the Horn of Africa.* Cambridge University Press, Cambridge.
Mbithi, P. and Rasmusson, R.
1977 *Self Reliance in Kenya: a case of Harambee.* Scandinavian Institute of African Studies, Uppsala.
McGavran
1979 In: Barton, W. L., World Health, *WHO Monthly Magazine,* Geneva.
McEwan, Peter J. M. (Ed.)
1982 *Utilization of Indigenous Healers in National Health Systems.* Special Issue in: *Social Science and Medicine,* Vol 16, 21.
McKinlay, J. B.
1970 *Some Aspects of Lower Working Class Utilization Behavior.* Unpublished doctoral dissertation. Aberdeen University, Scotland.
1972 'Some Approaches and Problems in the Study of the Use of Services – an overview', in: *Journal of Health and Social Behavior* 13, 2: 115–152
1981 'Social Network Influences on Morbid Episodes and the Career of Help Seeking', in: L. Eisenberg and A. Kleinman (Eds.) *The Relevance of Social Science for Medicine.* Reidel Publishing Company, Dordrecht.
McKinlay, J. B. and S. M. McKinlay
1972 'Some Social Characteristics of Lower Working Class Utilizers and Underutilizers of Maternity Care Services', in: *Journal of Health & Social Behavior*, 13 (December): 369–381.
Mead, Margaret (Ed.)
1953 *Cultural Patterns and Technical Change.* World Federation for Mental Health, UNESCO, New York.
Mechanic, David
1972 *Public Expectations and Health Care.* Wiley-Interscience, New York.
1978 *Medical Sociology.* The Free Press, New York.
Messing, Simon D.
1970 'Social Problems Related to the Development of Health in Ethiopia', in: *Social Science and Medicine,* Vol. 3: 331–337.
1972 *The Target of Health in Ethiopia, a Holistic Reader in Applied Anthropology.* Southern Connecticut State College.
Milkias, P.
1980 *Zemecha* – an Assessment of the Political and Social Foundations of Mass Education in Ethiopia, in: *Northeast African Studies,* 2, 1: 19–30.

Minocha, Anneeta A.
1980 'Medical Pluralism and Health Services in India', in: *Social Science and Medicine,* Vol. 14B, 4: 217–223.
Mohseni, M.
1979 'Attitudes towards Modern and Traditional Medicine in an Iranian Community', in: *Social Science and Medicine,* 13A: 499–500.
Molnos, A.
1973 *Cultural Source Material for Population Planning in East Africa,* Vol. I. East African Publishing House, Nairobi.
Monteiro, Lois
1973 'Expense is No Object . . .: Income and Physician Visits Reconsidered', in: *Journal of Health and Social Behavior*, 14 (June): 99–115
Morley, David
1976 *Paediatric Priorities in the Developing World.* Butterworths, London.
Morris, J. N.
1967 *Uses of Epidemiology*. Livingstone, Edinburgh.
Moser, C. A. and G. Kalton
1979 *Survey Methods in Social Investigation.* Heinemann, London.
Muhammad Hassan
1973 *The Relation Between Harar and the Surrounding Oromo Between 1800–1887.* Unpublished thesis in partial fulfilment of the requirement for the Degree of the Bachelor of Arts in Education. Haile Selassie I University, Addis Ababa.
Murphy, M. and T. M. Baba
1981 'Rural Dwellers and Health Care in Northern Nigeria', in: *Social Science and Medicine*, 15A: 265–271.
Myrdal, Gunnar
1968 *Asian Drama: an Inquiry into the Poverty of Nations*, Vintage Books, New York.
Nas, P. J. M., Van Renen, Darmayanti and Sjamsir
1981 'Indonesian Cities, a Typology of Kotamadya's', *ICA Working Paper* Nr. 3, University of Leiden.
Navarro, V.
1974 'A Critique of the Present and Proposed Strategies for Redistribution Resources in the Health Sector and a Discussion of Alternatives', in: *Medical Care* 12, 1: 721–742.
Nelson, H. D. and I. Kaplan
1980 *Ethiopia, a country study.* The American University, Washington, D.C.
Newell, K. W. (Ed.)
1975 *Health by the People.* World Health Organization, Geneva.

Noel Buxton
1932 *Slavery in Abyssinia*. London.
Nuyens, Yvo
1980 *De Eerste Lijn is Krom. Gezondheidszorg tussen onderzoek en beleid.* Van Loghum Slaterus, Deventer.
Nuyens, Y., R. Creyf, A. M. Ampe and M. Defever
1973 *Medisch Sociologische Verkenningen.* Universitaire Pers Leuven, Leuven.
Nuyens, Y. (*et al*)
1978 *Eerste lijnsgezondheidszorg.* Nationaal Programma Sociale Wetenschappen. Deel IA tot IH. Programmatie van het Wetenschapsbeleid. Brussel.
Ortiz, Fernando
1970 *Cuban Counterpoint. Tobacco and sugar.* Random House, New York.
Osofsky, J. H.
1968 'The Walls are within: An Examination of Barriers between Middle-class Physicians and Poor Patients', in: I. Deutscher and E. J. Thompson (Eds.), *Among the People.* Basic Books, London: 239–257.
Pankhurst, Richard
1965 'The Beginnings of Modern Medicine in Ethiopia', in: *Ethiopia Observer*, Vol. IX, no 1.
1968 *Economic History of Ethiopia, 1800–1935.* Haile Selassie I University Press, Addis Ababa.
1973 'The Medical History of Ethiopia During the Italian Fascist Invasion and Occupation (1935–1941')', in: *Ethiopian Observer,* Vol. XVI, 2.
Paul, Benjamin D. (Ed.)
1955 *Health, Culture and Community. Case studies of public reactions to health programs.* Russel Sage Foundation, New York.
Paulitschke, Philipp
1888 *Harar, Forschungsreise nach den Somâl – und Galla – Ländern Ost-Afrikas.* F. A. Brockhaus, Leipzig.
1893 *Ethnographie Nord-Ost Afrika.* Berlin.
Pearce, Ivy
1972 *Letters of Health.* Oxford University Press, Addis Ababa.
Penchansky, Roy and J. William Thomas
1981 The Concept of Access. Definition and relationship to consumer satisfaction, *Medical Care,* Vol XIX, 2: 127–140.
Peng, J. Y. (*et al.*)
1974 *Role of Traditional Birth Attendants in Family Planning.* International Development Research Centre, Ottawa.

Perham, Margery
1948 *The Government of Ethiopia.* Oxford University Press, New York.
Philips, J.
1955 'The Hookworm Campaign in Ceylon', in: H. M. Teaf Jr. and P. G. Franck (Eds.), *Hands across Frontiers: Case Studies in Technical Cooperation.* Cornell University Press, Ithaca: 265–305.
Piovano, Giovanni
1942 'Nomi Galla di Vegetali', in: *Rasegna di Studi Etiopici,* Vol. II.
Polderman, A. M.
1975 *The Transmission of Intestinal Schistosomiasis in Begemder Province, Ethiopia.* Doctoral dissertation, University of Leiden.
Pope, Clyde R.
1979 'Illness with a High Emotional Component and the Use of Medical Services', in: *Medical Care,* Vol. XVII, 12 (December): 1182–1195.
Press, J.
1969 'Urban Illness: Physicians, Cures, and Dual Use in Bogota', in: *Journal of Health and Social Behavior,* 10: 209–218.
1980 'Problems in the Definition and Classification of Medical Systems', in: *Social Science and Medicine,* Vol. 14B: 45–57.
Rademaker, L. (Ed.)
1978 *Sociologische Encyclopedie.* Deel 1–4. Het Spectrum. Utrecht.
Rahe, Richard H, R. J. Biersner, David H. Ryman and Ransom J. Arthur
1972 'Psychosocial Predictors of Illness Behavior and Failure in Stressful Training', in: *Journal of Health and Social Behavior,* 13 (December): 393–397.
Ram, E. R. and B. K. Datta
1976 'A Study on the Utilization of Primary Health Centre and Sub-centre Health Services by the Rural People of Miraj Taluka', Maharashtra, in: *Indian Journal of Public Health*, 20: 134–143.
Rance, P. L. L.
1981 'Chinese and Western Medical Care in China's Rural Commune: a Case Study', in: *Social Science and Medicine,* Vol. 15A: 137–148.
Read, Margaret
1966 *Culture, Health, and Disease.* Tavistock Publications, London.
Redfield, Robert
1956 *Peasant Society and Culture. An anthropological approach to civilization.* The University of Chicago Press, Chicago.

Redfield, R., R. Linton and M. J. Herskovits
1936 Memorandum on the Study of Acculturation, in: *American Anthropologist,* Vol. 38: 149–152.
Redlener, I. E. and C. S. Scott
1979 'Incompatibilities of professional and religious ideology: problems of medical management and outcome in a case of pediatric meningitis', in: *Social Science and Medicine* Special Issue on The Transcultural Perspective in Health and Illness, Vol. 13B: 89–95.
Reid, M. B.
1969 *Persistence and Change in the Health Concepts and Practices of the Sukuma of Tanzania, East Africa.* Doctoral dissertation, The Catholic University of America.
Reminick, Ronald A.
1977 'The Evil Eye Belief among the Amhara of Ethiopia', in: David Landy (Ed.), *Culture, Disease and Healing.* Macmillan, New York: 218–226.
Rifkin, Susan B.
1981 'The Role of the Public in the Planning, Management and Evaluation of Health Activities and Programmes, including Self-Care, in: *Social Science and Medicine,* Vol. 15A: 377–386.
Rifkin, Susan B. and Raphael Kaplinsky
1973 'Health Strategy and Development Planning: Lessons from the People's Republic of China', in: *The Journal of Development Studies,* Vol. 9, 2: 213–232.
Robinson D. and S. Henry
1977 *Self-Help and Health.* Martin Robertson, London.
Rodenson, M.
1967 *Magie, Médicine et Possession à Gondar.* Paris
Rosengren, William R.
1980 *Sociology of Medicine: Diversity, Conflict, and Change.* Harper & Row, New York.
Rosenstock, I.M.
1969 'Prevention of Illness and Maintenance of Health,' in: J. Kosa, A. Antonovsky and I.K. Zola (Eds.), *Poverty and Health.* Harvard University Press, Massachusetts: 168–190.
Roth, J.
1969 'The Treatment of the Sick', in: J. Kosa *et al.* (Eds.), *Poverty and Health*, Havard University Press, Massachusetts: 214–243.
Rubel, A.J., C.W.O'Neill and R. Collado-Ardón
1986 *Susto, a Folk Illness.* University of California Press, Berkeley.
Russel, H.B.L.
1958 *Final Report, the Pilot Mobile Health Team, Ethiopia.* World Health Organisation, WM/PHA/62. Geneva

Sarder, A.M. and L.C. Chen
1981 'Distribution and Characteristics of Non-Government Health Practitioners in a Rural Area of Bangladesh', in: *Social Science and Medicine*. Vol. 15A: 543–550.
Schaffer, B.
1975 'Editorial', in: *Development and Change*, Vol. 6, 2: 3–12.
Schaffer, B.
1975 'Distribution and the Theory of Access', in: *Development and Change*, Vol, 6, 2: 13–26.
Schaller, K.F. and W. Kuls
1972 *Ethiopia, a Geomedical Monograph*. Springer, Heidelberg.
Schneider, Harm
1975 *Leprosy and other Health Problems in Hararghe, Ethiopia*. Doctoral dissertation, University of Groningen.
Schulpen, T.W.J.
1975 *Integration of Church and Government Medical Services in Tanzania: effects at district level*. African Medical Research Foundation, Nairobi.
Scott, C.S.
1975 'Competing Health Care Systems in an Inner City Area', in: *Human Organization*, 34: 108–110.
Segall, M.
1972 'The Politics of Health in Tanzania', in: Uchumi Editorial Board (Ed.) *Towards Socialist Planning*. Tanzania Publishing House, Dar es Salaam.
Segers, J.H.G.
1975 *Sociologische Onderzoeksmethoden. Inleiding tot de structuur van het onderzoeksproces en tot de methoden van dataverzameling*. Van Gorcum, Assen.
Seo, K.
1976 'Some Determinants of the Health Service Utilization and Health Care Expenditure in Rural Families'. Department of Public Health, Yonsei University, Korea (mimeo).
Sheldon, A.
1970 'Toward a General Theory of Disease and Medical Care', in: A. Sheldon, F. Baker and C.P. McLaughlin (Eds.), *Systems and Medical Care*. MIT Press, Cambridge, Mass.: 84–125.
Shortell, Stephen M., William C. Richardson, James P. Logerfo, Paulo Diehr, Barbara Weaver and Kathy E. Green
1977 'The Relationships among Dimensions of Health Services in Two Provider Systems: a Causal Model Approach', in: *Journal of Health and Social Behavior*, 18 (June): 139–159.

Sidel, Victor W. and Ruth Sidel
1975 'The Health Care Delivery System of the People's Republic of China', in: Kenneth W. Newell (Ed.), *Health by the People*. World Health Organization, Geneva: 1–12.

Sigerist, Henry E.
1951 *A History of Medicine. (Vol. I: Primitive and Archaic Medicine; Vol. II: Early Greek, Hindu, and Persian Medicine).* Oxford University Press, New York.

Simmons. O.G.
1958 'Implications of Social Class for Public Health', in: *Human Organization*, 16: 7–10.

Slikkerveer, L.J.
1982 'Rural Health Development in Ethiopia. Problems of utilization of traditional healers', in: *Social Science and Medicine*, Vol. 16, 21: 1859–1872.
1985 '"Urban Bias" en Ontwikkeling van Gezondheidszorg: een case-study over "Cultural Revivalism" in Zuid-Sulawesi, Indonesië'. *ICA Working Paper* No. 74, University of Leiden.
1986 *Ethiopië*. Landendocumentatie Koninklijk Instituut voor de Tropen Nr. 3, Staatsuitgeverij, 's-Gravenhage.
1987 'Neo-ethnogeneeskunde, een transcultureel perspectief op het proces van nationale gezondheidsontwikkeling in de Derde Wereld'. *ICA Working Paper* No. 85, University of Leiden.

Smith, M.G.
1965 *The Plural Society in the British West Indies*. University of California Press, Berkeley and Los Angeles.

Sparer, Gerald and Louise M. Okada
1974 'Chronic Conditions and Physician Use Patterns in Ten Urban Poverty Areas', in: *Medical Care*, 12 (July): 549–560.

Speckmann, J.D.
1966 'De Plurale Surinaamse Samenleving', in: A.N.J. den Hollander (*et al.*), *De Plurale Samenleving. Begrip zonder toekomst*? J.A. Boom en Zonen, Meppel.

Spicer, Edward H. (Ed.)
1977 *Ethnic Medicine in the Southwest*. University of Arizona Press, Tucson.

*Statistical Abstract of Ethiopia.*
1981 Central Statistical Office, Addis Ababa

Stiehler, W.
1943 *Beiträge zur Wirtschafts- und Siedlungsgeographie der Äthiopischen Hochländer vor ihrer Besetzung durch die Italien.* Doctoral dissertation, Bonn.

Stoeckle, J.
1969 'The Future of Health Care', in: J. Kosa; A. Antonovsky and I.K. Zola (Eds.), *Poverty and Health*. Harvard University Press, Massachusetts (Chapter 10).

Stoop, Ineke
1980 *Sekundaire Analyse van de 'Van Jaar Tot Jaar' Data met Behulp van Niet-Lineaire Multivariate Technieken: Verschillen in de Schoolloopbaan van Meisjes en Jongens*. Doktoraal Skriptie. Vakgroep Methoden en Technieken in de Psychologie. University of Leiden.

Straus, R.
1957 'The Nature and Status of Medical Sociology', in: *American Sociological Review*, 22: 200–204.

Suchman, E.A.
1964 'Sociomedical Variations among Ethnic Groups', in: *American Journal of Sociology*, 70 (November): 319–331.
1965 'Social Patterns of Illness and Medical Care', in: *Journal of Health and Human Behavior*, 6: 2–16.
1966 'Health Orientation and Medical Care', in: *American Journal of Public Health*, 56 (January): 97–105.

Susser, M.W. and W. Watson
1971 *Sociology in Medicine*. Oxford University Press, London

Taylor, Carl E.
1977 'The Place of Indigenous Medical Practitioners in the Modernization of Health Services', in: Charles Leslie (Ed.), *Asian Medical Systems: a Comparative Study*. University of California Press, Berkeley: 285–299.

Taylor Carl E., Rahmi Dirican and Kurt W. Deuschle
1968 *Health Manpower Planning in Turkey. An international research case study*. The Johns Hopkins Press, Baltimore.

Taylor, D. Garth, Lu Ann Aday and Ronald Andersen
1975 'A Social Indicator of Access to Medical Care', in: *Journal of Health and Social Behavior*, 16 (March): 38–49.

Teller, Charles H.
1973 'Access to Medical Care of Migrants in a Honduran City', in: *Journal of Health and Social Behavior*, 14 (September), no. 3: 214–266.

Teshai Berhane Selassie
1971 'An Ethiopian Medical Text-Book written by Gerazmac Gäbräwäld Arägahäñ Däga Damot', in: S. Chojnacki, R. Pankhurst and H. Relton (Eds.), *Journal of Ethiopian Studies*, Vol. IX, 1: 95–180. Addis Ababa, Ethiopia.

Theodore, C.
1968 'The Demand for Health Services', in: R. Andersen (Ed.), *A Behavioral Model of Families' Use of Health Services*. Center for Health Administration Studies, Research Series, no. 25.
Toynbee, Arnold J.
1936 *Survey of International Affairs 1935, I & II*. Oxford University Press, London.
Trimingham, J. Spencer
1976 *Islam in Ethiopia*. Frank Cass, London.
Turner, V.
1964 *Lunda Medicine and the Treatment of Disease*. Occasional Paper No. 15 of the Rhodes-Livingstone Museum, Livingstone Institute.
Twaddle, A.C.
1981 'Sickness and the Sickness Career: Some Implications', in L. Eisenberg and A. Kleinman (Eds.) *The Relevance of Social Science for Medicine*. Reidel Publishing Company, Dordrecht.
Twaddle, A.C. and R.M. Hessler
1977 *A Sociology of Health*. The C.V. Mosby Company, St. Louis.
Udupa, K.N.
1975 'The Ayurvedic System of Medicine in India', in: Kenneth W. Newell (Ed.), *Health by the People*. World Health Organization, Geneva: 53–69.
Ullendorff, Edward
1973 *The Ethiopians. An Introduction to country and people*. Oxford University Press, London.
Ullmann, Manfred
1970 *Die Medizin im Islam*. E.J. Brill, Leiden.
United Nations
1975 *United Nations Development Programme*. UNDP/PROG/FIELD/53;UNDP/PROG/HQTRS/70. United Nations, New York.
Unschuld, Paul U.
1975 'Medico-Cultural Conflicts in Asian Settings: an Explanatory Theory', in: *Social Science and Medicine*, 9: 303–312.
1977 'The Social Organization and Ecology of Medical Practice in Taiwan', in: Charles Leslie (Ed.), *Asian Medical Systems. A comparative study*. University of California Press, Berkeley: 300–316.
Uyanga, J.
1979 'The Characteristics of Patients of Spiritual Healing Homes and Traditional Doctors in Southeastern Nigeria', in: *Social Science and Medicine*, 13A: 323–329.

Vervoorn, J.D.
1974 *Tropische Gezondheidszorg in Ontwikkeling: van isolatie tot integratie*. Van Gorcum, Assen.

Vogel, L.C. (*et al*)
1974 *Health and Disease in Kenya*. East African Literature Bureau, Nairobi.

Voorhoeve, H.W.A.
1983 *Paediatrics and Primary Health Care in Zambia*. Van der Linden, Alphen aan den Rijn.
1985 *Paediatrics and Primary Health Care in Kenya*. Van der Linden, Alphen aan den Rijn.

Walsh, J.L. and R.H. Elling
1968 'Professionalism and the Poor: Structural Effects and Professional behavior', in: *Journal of Health and Social Behavior*, 9 (March): 16–28.

Walt, K.M. de
1977 'The Illness no longer Understood: Changing Concepts of Health and Curing in a Rural Mexican Community', in: *Medical Anthropology Newsletter* 8:5–11.

Wan, Thomas T.H. and Scott J. Soifer
1974 'Determinants of Physician Utilization: a Causal Analysis', in: *Journal of Health and Social Behavior*, 15 (June): 100–108.

Warren, Dennis M.
1974 *Disease, Medicine, and Religion Among the Techiman Bono of Ghana*. Doctoral Dissertation, Indiana University.

Warren, D.M., and M.A. Tregoning
1979 'Indigenous Healers and Primary Health Care in Ghana', in: *Medical Anthropology Newsletter* 11 (2): 11–13.
1982 'The Techiman-Bono Ethnomedical System', in: Stanley P. Yoder (Ed.), *African Health and Healing Systems: Proceedings of a Symposium*. Crossroads Press, University of California, Los Angeles: 85–107.

Warren, D.M., G. Steven Bova, Mary Ann Tregoning and Mark Kliewer
1982 'Ghanaian National Policy toward Indigenous Healers. The case of the primary health training for indigenous healers (PRHETIH) program', in: *Social Science and Medicine*, Vol. 16, 21: 1873–1881

Wehr, H.
1971 *A Dictionary of Modern Written Arabic*, edited by J. Hilton Cowan, Wiesbaden.

Weidman, Hazel H.
1977 'On Mitchell's Changing Others', in: *Medical Anthropology Newsletter*, 8, (14), 25.

1978 *Miami Health Ecology Project Report: a Statement on Ethnicity and Health I*. University of Miami (mimeo).

1979 'Falling-out: a diagnostic and treatment problem viewed from a trans-cultural perspective', in: *Social Science and Medicine* Special Issue on The Transcultural Perspective in Health and Illness, Vol. 13B: 85–87.

Were, Miriam

1978 *Organization and Management of Community-Based Health Care*. National Pilot Project of Kenya Ministry of Health and UNICEF.

WHO

1977 *International Classification of Diseases*. Geneva, Vol. I &II.

1978 'Formulating Strategies for Health for All by the Year 2000'. *"Health for All" Series* No. 2, World Health Organization, Geneva.

1983 'Research for the Reorientation of National Health Systems', *Technical Report Series*, No. 694, World Health Organization, Geneva.

1984 'Glossary of Terms', in *"Health for All" Series* No. 9, World Health Organization, Geneva.

WHO/UNICEF

1978 *Primary Health Care: a Joint Report by the Director General of the WHO and the Executive Director of UNICEF on the International Conference on Primary Health Care, Alma Ata, USSR 1978*. WHO/UNICEF Geneva/New York.

Wilcox, L.D.

1972 *Social Indicators and Monitoring; an Annotated Bibliography*. Jossey Bass Co., San Francisco.

Williams, Stephen J., Stephen M. Shortell, James P. Lagerfo and William C. Richardson

1978 'A Causal Model of Health Services for Diabetic Patients', in: *Medical Care*, Vol. XVI, 4 (April): 313–326.

Winick, Charles

1958 *Dictionary of Anthropology*, Littlefield, Adams & Co, Ames, Iowa.

Woods, C.M. and T.D. Graves

1976 'The Process of Medical Change in a Highland Guatemalan Town', in: *Medical Anthropology*, by F.X. Grollig and H.B. Haley (Eds.), Mouton, Paris: 331–382.

Worth, R.M. and N.K. Shah

1969 *Nepal Health Survey*. University of Hawaii Press, Honolulu.

Wurtz, R.

1898 Hygiène Publique et Priveé en Abyssinie, in: *La Semaine Médicale*, 7 (December).

Yemane Tekle Marian

1981 *Ethiopia 1974–1980: A Critical Assessment of its Rural Development Programmes*. M.A. Thesis, Institute for Social Studies, The Hague.

Yoder, P. Stanley

1982 'Biomedical and Ethnomedical Practice in Rural Zaire. Contrasts and complements', in: *Social Science and Medicine*, Vol. 16, 21: 1851–1857.

1982 *African Health and Healing Systems: Proceedings of a Symposium*. Crossroads Press, University of California, Los Angeles.

Young, Allan

1975 'The Practical Logic of Amhara Traditional Medicine', in: *Rural Africana. Current Research in the Social Sciences*, No 26: 79–89. The African Studies Centre of Michigan State University, East Lansing, Michigan.

1976 'Internalizing and Externalizing Medical Belief Systems; an Ethiopian Medical Example', in: *Social Science and Medicine* 10: 147–156.

1977 'Order, Analogy, and Eddicacy in Ethiopian Divination', in: *Culture, Medicine and Psychiatry* 1: 183–199.

1982 'The Amhara Medical System', in: Stanley P. Yoder (Ed.), *African Health and Healing Systems: Proceedings of a Symposium*. Crossroads Press, University of California, Los Angeles: 21–41.

Young, J.C.

1981 'Non-Use of Physicians: Methodological Approaches, Policy Implications, and the Utility of Decision Models', in: *Social Science and Medicine*, 15B: 499–507.

Young, James Harvey

1961 *The Toadstool Millionaires: a Social History of Patent Medicines in America Before Federal Regulation*. Princeton University Press, Princeton.

Zimmerman, M.

1980 *Foundation of Medical Anthropology*. Holt, Rinehart and Winston, New York.

Zola, I.K.

1964 'Illness Behavior of the Working: Implications and Recommendations', in: A.B. Shostak and W. Gomberg (Eds.), *Blue Collar World*. Prentice-Hall, Englewood Cliffs, New Jersey: 350–361.

1972 'Studying the Decision to See a Doctor', in: Z.J. Lipowski (Ed.), *Advances in Psychosomatic Medicine*, 8: 216.

# Index